DOCTORS REVEAL THE MISSING LINK IN NUTRITION

The Healing **Power** *of* 8 SugarS®

An Amazing Breakthrough in
Nutrition, Science and Medicine

What Doctors want *YOU* to know about
Glyconutrients ...
The 8 Sugars Vital to Your Health

D0958440

Compiled and Edited by
Allan C. Somersall, Ph.D., M.D.

Foreword by H. Reg McDaniel, M.D.

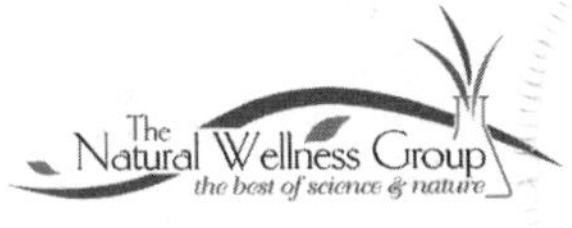

The Healing **Power** *of* ^{8}**SugarS**®,
Compiled & Edited by Allan C. Somersall, Ph.D., MD

Published by The Natural Wellness Group
A Division of GE Publishers, Inc.
2-3415 Dixie Road, Suite: 538
Mississauga, Ontario L4Y 2B1
1-905-507-6121

www.thenaturalwellnessgroup.com

All rights reserved. No part of this publication may be reproduced or transmitted in any form or by any means electronic or mechanical, including photocopying, recording or any other information storage and retrieval system, without the written permission of the publisher.

Copyright © 2005 by The Natural Wellness Group, LLC
All rights reserved
ISBN 0-9737317-0-2
Library and Archives Canada Cataloguing in Publication

Somersall, Allan C.,

The Healing **Power** *of* ^{8}**SugarS**®: An amazing breakthrough in *science*, *nutrition* and *medicine*! /Allan C. Somersall
Includes Bibliographical references and index.
ISBN 0-9737317-0-2

1. Monosaccharides-Therapeutic use. 2. Nutrition.
3. Glycoconjugates. I. Natural Wellness Group II. Title

RA784.S645 2005 613.2'83 C2005-900269-7

Manufactured and Printed in Canada

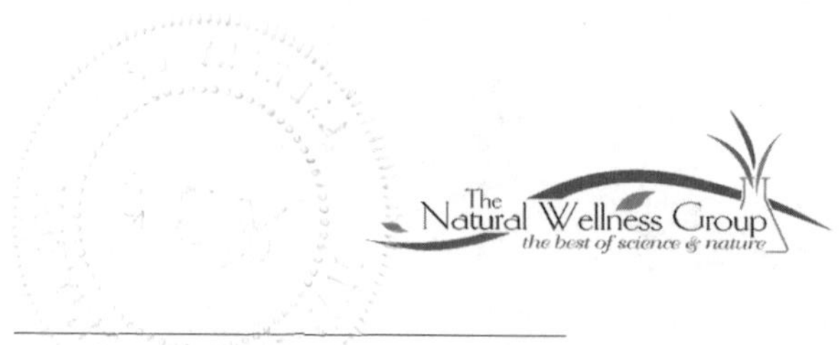

DEDICATION

to

"All the Doctors of the Future
who will give no medicine, but will interest their Patients
in the care of the human frame, in diet, and in the cause
and prevention of diseases."

-Thomas Edison

Other Books by Allan C. Somersall, PhD., MD

Your Very Good Health: 101 Healthy Lifestyle Choices

A Passion For Living: The *Art* of Real Success

Your Evolution to YES!

Understanding The Evolution of YES!

Evolutionary Tales by Dr. YES!

Breakthrough in Cell-Defense

Nature's Goldmine

The Enzyme Diet™

DISCLAIMER

This book discusses the nature, role and effects of *Glyconutrients* in the human body. This is an emerging science just entering the mainstream of clinical medicine. Several strategies are proposed throughout the book that according to early, limited scientific research, may benefit the human body in times of sickness and health. The knowledge of Glyconutrients/Glycobiology is evolving by leaps and bounds as new preventative and therapeutic possibilities become apparent. However, readers with existing medical conditions, including anyone on medication and those undergoing medical treatment of any sort, are strongly encouraged to **seek the advice of their own qualified medical professionals before making use of any of the recommendations in this book.**

The author(s), editor and publisher expressly disclaim responsibility from the use or application of any information presented in this book. It is intended and designed *for educational purposes only* but with the promising results to date, we hope that this book will prompt further personal inquiry and more professional investigation.

ACKNOWLEDGEMENTS

The Healing **Power** *of* ^{8}**SugarS®** has been a joyous - though often challenging task, and we wish to thank the following people whose contributions have made it possible:

Dr. Allan Somersall - prolific author and senior editor. He worked closely with us and brought this book to its final stages of completeness. He was instrumental at every stage along the way, keeping the whole process on track. The quality of this book reflects his significant editing, professional guidance and invaluable wisdom.

Dr. Gary Anderson - one of the coordinators on this project from its inception. He believed in the value of this project, saw the possibilities and gave us great connections. He moved the project forward at some critical points.

Dr. H. Reg McDaniel for graciously writing the Foreword. His example is an inspiration for all who have compassion and would follow the truth even when it leads down unconventional pathways.

Dr. Vicky Arcadi - a valued source of inspiration and an important center of influence.

All the doctors who contributed their knowledge and experience to this task. Their cooperation and patience under pressure were very much appreciated. The synergy was tremendous.

Virginia Somersall who first introduced us to glyconutrients and persisted to convey the message, until we saw the light. She also did a remarkable job of proof-reading and made many valuable corrections to the text.

Waplington McGall Design Group for their original cover art design.

We are truly grateful for the many other hands and hearts that made this book possible.

Publisher

From the Publishers Desk

In 1887 Paracelsus, the Father of Pharmacology said,
"Everything man needs to sustain health can be found in nature.
It is the job of science to find them."

Maybe once in a lifetime, along comes a book that makes a real difference in the life of an individual - *in your life*. **The Healing Power** *of* **^{8}SugarS®** is that book. This is a health discovery that could change your life.

When the concept of Glyconutrients was introduced to us, we were at first very skeptical. But we did our due diligence and researched the subject thoroughly. We observed one interesting factor and that was, the number of traditional doctors who were involved with glyconutrients, and in addition, recommending them to their patients.

As publishers, we aim to uncover the most up-to-date health discoveries, and reveal what they mean to you, your health and your future! Thus, the idea of bringing all of these doctors together into one book - a Co-Authored Book - was starting to take shape. We were convinced that these doctors needed to get the secret out to the world. The stories had to be told. After discussions with our team and our lead author, Dr. Somersall, we decided to bring to market the book you now hold in your hands.

Today we are discovering more about health than ever before. Nutritional science is showing that by being proactive and properly nurturing the body, it will respond.

This book has been a labor of love. We are honored to have the privilege of offering you this information, for you, your family and for all who are interested in better health. We hope you enjoy reading it as much as we have enjoyed preparing and presenting it.

Pursue health with passion!

Carolina Loren
Publisher
www.thehealingpowerofsugars.com
glycobooks@aol.com

Table of Contents

Table of Contents

Foreword©

Dr. H. Reg McDaniel

Many times in the past twenty years, I have recalled a brief excerpt from a book I had in college for a philosophy course entitled, *Philosophies Men Live By*. There was a story taken from Plato's Republic, written about 200 to 150 B.C. in ancient Greece. In the allegory, mankind is described as being inside a dark cave, strapped to a rigid chair or bench, and lined up with some means to limit one's ability to look only straight ahead at the distant wall of the cave in front of them. On this wall, the group representing society sees dark moving shapes as shadows that are their reality of life. What humanity can see and experience is limited to the appearances on the cave wall.

On occasion, by chance or struggle, one person is freed of the restraining bonds and *once free*, they are then able to look behind the group. This individual will see that on the opposite side of the cave is a fire that generates a true light of reality. Placed between the fire and the backs of the bound group is a stage on which actual shapes and characters are moved by forces unseen and unknown to the seated observers of the human drama that is projected as shadows on the wall. Seeing this, the free person will attempt to inform their peers that they cannot see reality. They see only the *shadows* of ultimate truth and therefore they must act to release themselves so that they can know and take action based on the real truth of their existence.

The reader of Plato's allegory is informed that the response of the peer group will be to reject and condemn the now free man. He will be banned from association with the majority group that is content and comfortable with their view of life and the world.

I started off my medical career as a classic, orthodox physician. However, over the years, I became increasingly aware of a 'new reality' that will be shared in this book. It reflects the central role of nutrition, and glyconutrients in particular, in health and disease. Based on my direct observation and extensive experimentation, I have had many opportunities since to recall the allegory of the cave. What I read around 1957 in college was lived out in the modern era in critical and condemning relationships with my medical peers.

There were surprising responses of patients with advanced AIDS, terminal cancer and refractory ulcerative colitis who came from different areas of the nation. These were uniformly managed patients who were locked into receiving only the same professional standards of medical practice that had failed to help other dying victims of these diseases. In particular, they were bound by a professional mind-set in that none responded well to the weak *shadows* of prescription medications which were FDA-approved and professionally sanctioned. What was audacious on my part, and what brought investigations and sanctions upon my head, was my reporting that condemned patients like these had informed me that they had found something that was not a physician-prescribed substance. It was a natural plant extract that was claimed to improve and in some cases, restore their health. I actually tested it personally on other similar hopeless patients, and to my amazement, they also improved in their health.

Contrary to my own expectations, I had stumbled upon what is described in this book as **The Healing Power** *of* **[8]SugarS**. The active ingredient of the natural plant extract claimed by the AIDS patients to be effective came from Aloe vera leaf gel. A team of analytical chemists determined that the bioactive molecule is a key monosaccharide/sugar used in cellular synthesis for innate antiviral and general defense compounds. The ingredient was mannose, a vital member of a class of necessary sugars, glyconutrients, that cells combine with proteins to form vitally important glycoproteins. We later understood that these were critical to all cellular biochemistry and physiology for defense, repair, healing and homeostasis (balance) within and between cells.

This was a new and different *fire of reality* that I, in my excitement, joy, and personal and professional sense of fulfillment, sought to share with my medical peers. I offered it to other suffering patients that had been put in hospice to die, or who were deteriorating outside any formal system. It would in time prove intolerable and unacceptable for such patients to return to their physicians who had given up trying to care for the individual. Whenever the patient returned with a restored health status and quality of life never attained in such conditions of advanced disease, their doctor who had abandoned them, suffered loss of patient and family esteem Some professionals were not amused at such maverick activity. It challenged their abilities and the established order of approved "treatment" and medical management.

In 1988 I found myself summoned to appear before the Texas State Board of Medical Examiners, accused of charges in a letter signed by no less than the dean of my own medical school. The charges made were for the "unscientific, unprofessional and unethical practice of medicine." This was for administering the active ingredient from the leaf gel of Aloe vera to dying AIDS and cancer patients, and to ulcerative colitis/Crohn's disease victims facing the surgical removal of their intestine to control relentless bleeding and pain. Apparently the worst aspect of my activity to my peers was that the unsanctioned, natural, and now recognized nutritional approach, was working repeatedly, where approved modalities sanctioned by the medical profession had failed. Such heretical and uncontrolled activity, such a trend and empowerment of the lay public, had to be stopped. A board of inquiry was conducted to evaluate the evidence and look into my fitness for being placed on probation or even keeping my medical license. It was a truly remarkable event.

In 1994, through a contrived charade, I was dismissed from the same hospital I had helped found. I had written a petition and gathered signatures from the city physicians that were presented to the City Council in 1972 for establishing the institution. In all honesty, I could have most likely avoided this early retirement by ceasing to be a persistent, unconventional thorn, if not a threat for potential embarrassment to the board, administration and other physician staff.

A very difficult and stressful event that had the entire hospital on edge, transpired in a large hospital conference room one day. An attorney flew into Dallas from the Securities Exchange Commission (SEC) that oversees publicly traded stocks. I spent a day under oath, with a court recorder, responding to charges made to the SEC that all the research I had conducted at the Fisher Institute for Medical Research was fraudulent. The allegation that was picked up and published in two business publications, all claimed that I had not seen and had no records for treatment of any patients with AIDS, cancer, and other diseases. I was described as a part of a scam designed to defraud the public into buying worthless stock in a company that pioneered development of the initial extract from the Aloe vera leaf gel.

I presented much of the same material presented in the state capital to the State Board of Medical Examiners, along with stacks of patient charts, to provide evidence that the charges were without merit. **The evidence provided spoke for itself and the charges were dropped.** But it turned out that this event did not strengthen my ability to continue my position as Chief of Pathology. One of the board members informed me that outside sources had informed the Board that I "beat the rap", but I was involved with shady characters who skirted the edge of legal activity by making claims for Aloe vera that no one in science and medicine agreed with and that they deemed absurd.

I was relieved of my duties.

However, all these events opened the door to be available in

February 1994 to start a new saga in life as Medical Director for what eventually became my mission in life: to take this micronutrient technology directly to the American public and the world.

Many hard working lay persons have since absorbed inordinate criticism, in their own efforts to share the micronutrient dietary supplement technology with their relatives and friends. In the past decade, the glyconutrient revolution has been spreading like wild fire. The reason is that micronutrients provide necessary molecules, or nutritional components, required by the trillions of cells that synthesize all the compounds for molecular structure and function of a human body. When improved nutrition is supplied to metabolizing cells, a status of better health is attainable in most people with chronic disease. Even acute disease, like infections of all types, can be prevented.

Recently I was given a copy of *Plato's Republic*, translated into English. Instead of a short summary, I read the entire allegory for the first time. The full account goes on further than what was in my text nearly 50 years ago. It describes what happens if by chance an individual is able to become totally free from the bindings of convention and finds that everyone is under the earth in a cave. That individual discovers a totally *new world* outside the cave where there is a distant horizon, a sky, sunshine by day and stars by night and life in many forms. Our now free man, with an unfettered mind and new knowledge, returns to those tethered in the cave. In good conscience and with the best of intent, the explorer seeks to inform all that will listen that there is a world out there beyond the confines of the false images that are but *shadows* of truth seen in a subterranean cave. In response, the herd rises up and kills the messenger that challenges their reality, dares to question their truths and rejects their accepted conventions.

Note that this allegory was written in ancient Greece over two thousand years ago by a philosopher, seeking to describe a means to establish an ideal, peaceful and productive society.

It has been a courageous family of messengers who have since 1994 confronted the highly educated and credentialed orthodox medicine and science establishment, bound by its own conventions of bias and self-interest. But when you reflect on it, nutrition is the original paradigm for maintaining good health and preventing disease. It has the capacity to support the instructions coded in the genes, that when optimally supported, can often correct abnormal biochemistry and physiology to restore health for many that are ill and afflicted.

I am more than delighted at the growing legion of medical and scientific professionals who now understand and choose to investigate and use micronutrients for restoring and improving life. I am pleased that a group of professionals has combined their experiences to document the facts in this book, **The Healing Power** *of* [8]**SugarS**. From different fields, they speak with a common voice about their various experiences and their appreciation for glyconutrients in health and disease. What is it that brings them together in harmony? It is the realization that drugs generally suppress symptoms by interfering with biochemistry and physiology, and thus create an illusion or a shadow of improvement. The fact is that the restoration of health is occurring at the unseen level of the cells, as the body itself attempts to correct and heal the basic problem. Improved nutrition supports the engineering and design present in cells as coded instructions located in the genes. The results shout volumes in restored lives that any and all can see and celebrate - in the newly discovered world beyond the shadows on the wall in the cave that long constituted a temporary and false illusion of better health.

The wonder of the technology of using nutrition to restore health is that in the design of human life endowed in the genome, we are surrounded in nature by the elements and nutrients required to support the cellular synthesis of life. Inorganic, lifeless ingredients like glyconutrients create organic life. Bioactive compounds are made in cells and organize the community of cells to form organs, that together form more complex systems which we know as independent living creatures - healthy *homo sapiens*.

How sweet the new reality is! The words of a new truth founded on ancient fundamentals that produce benefits beyond all dreams is now spreading like a tsunami that crushes obstructive skepticism and resistance like tiny boulders destined to be unseen tomorrow. The wonders of restored health continue to spread across a growing number of nations to form a newly discovered world of improved health for all humanity. It is a brighter, happier world far from the old planet of the painful, dismal, hope-drained cave of prior limited potential for those with chronic illnesses.

This new understanding has grown to become a beacon of knowledge that leads humanity to a new day, a better portal for lives supported by a wide array of dietary sugars. This nutritional technology now commands many millions in federal research grants and is known as Glycomics. I believe that this new science encompasses all **The Healing Power** *of* [8]**SugarS** and gives hope for better health to every citizen of our shared planet.

HRMcD

Glyco - Terminology

Glyco -	means 'sweet' (in Greek) and therefore, it is used as a prefix when describing a molecule or term that includes a sugar or carbohydrate. 'Sugar', 'carbohydrate' and 'saccharide' are all used interchangeably.
Glycoproteins	are molecules made of sugars and proteins. Most importantly, they are found coating the surface of every cell in the human body that contains a nucleus.
Glycolipids	are molecules made of sugars and fats. 'Lipid' and 'fat' are often used interchangeably. They are also associated with all membranes.
Glycoforms or Glycoconjugates	are more general terms for large molecules including sugars. Glycoproteins or glycolipids would be subclasses of these.
Glyconutrients	refer specifically to the eight monosaccharides (sugars) commonly found in glycoproteins and glycolipids. They are nutrients inasmuch as they can be supplied exogenously in dietary foods or food supplements. They are absorbed efficiently in the body.
Glyconutritionals	is a broader term which identifies the naturally occurring foods, extracts, derivates, complexes or any other dietary source of glyconutrients.
Glycosylation	is a metabolic process by which the saccharides are chemically attached to the various substrates such as proteins or lipids. These may be surface molecules or specific enzymes, for example.
Glycobiology and Glycoscience	both refer to the new emerging and promising science which seeks to understand the chemistry, biochemistry and physiology of all these glyconutrients and glycojugates, and their applications to health and disease.

Introduction

Why This Book?

Dr. Allan C. Somersall

Radical ideas provoke resistance or change ... sometimes both ... and usually, in that order. This book is about one such idea.

Never in a million years, would I have thought that nature might reserve such a crucial role for 'sugars' in all cellular biochemistry and physiology. That, at first glance, is the frivolous stuff of candy, soda pop and devilish desserts. But such immediate bias would miss the point entirely. The term 'Sugar' refers to far, far more. You cannot afford to miss it.

Today, a new understanding is changing the world of medical science. Not just an understanding of the word 'sugar', but an understanding of the role of sugars in the molecular world of cell biology. At that level, there is no taste, no sensual advertising and no media hype. It all comes down to unbiased molecular structure and corresponding function, as cells alone endeavor to promote life and health for all.

Within the past decade, scientists have found vital glyconutrients, or simple sugars, which partner with proteins and lipids to enable our cells to communicate. This cell-to-cell communication is at the heart of the body's ability to fight disease and maintain optimum health. Therefore, whether you believe you are in good shape and want to live longer, while enjoying a superior quality of life, or whether you are facing a medical challenge, -- the addition of necessary glyconutrients to your diet could make a major difference to your future.

So, this book is for you. Its message is new, but its origins go back to the earliest designs of nature for structural diversity and specificity. Such wide variety of structure that sugars make possible, enables just as wide a variability of function and with the necessary discrimination to make cellular responses unique.

'The Healing **Power** *of* **8SugarS**' removes the veil from the emerging science of glyconutrition. It introduces new concepts that are still virtually unknown to the wider medical community, much less to the general public. For some time, this exciting field was eclipsed by the promising trends of immunology in the '80s and genetics in the '90s. But now, it has emerged from the shadows with the award of three Nobel Prizes in somewhat related fields during the past decade. Glycobiology has dramatically stepped onto the front cover of *Science* magazine (2001) and *Scientific American* (2002). And consider this - it was recently heralded by the MIT *Technology Review* (2003) as 'one of the top ten emerging technologies that will change the world!'

It is no wonder then that 100+ patents have already been issued and 20,000+ papers have been published in this new field by researchers the world over.

What a way to begin this new century!

In this new book, 'The Healing **Power** *of* **8SugarS**', twenty (20) doctors from different fields combine their collective perspectives and diverse experiences to make a credible case for glyconutrients in health and disease. In easy-reading style, they reveal this new technology as an awakened giant with far-reaching potential for both prevention and treatment. Each doctor explains in a separate chapter how the new information on glyconutrients represents a major breakthrough in nutrition, science and medicine:

In **nutrition**, because carbohydrates have been taken for granted all these years as mere energy sources;
In **science**, because it relates directly to the fundamentals of cell-to-cell communication; and
In **medicine**, because there is increasing evidence of the therapeutic value of consuming these sugars as supplements to normal diets.

Of the 200+ naturally occurring sugars, surprisingly, only eight have been found to be necessary to form the important glycoproteins on cell surfaces that allow cells to interact in a specific way. Thus the concept of a 'sugar code' of biological information has arisen, with the simple sugars representing the alphabet. In other words, the different sugars combine at the molecular level to provide the 'sweet language of life' by which cells communicate.

What a way for the body to protect itself and fight back!

In 'The Healing **Power** *of* **8SugarS**', the doctors reveal the increasing weight of clinical evidence for the therapeutic benefits of glyconutrients in a wide range of medical conditions. They take a panoramic look at healthcare, from primary prevention, diet and lifestyle issues, right up to the stem cells frontier. The book is an eye-opener on complementary approaches to both health and disease. It emphasizes the surprising capacity of the body to heal itself when provided with essential nutrients, especially the eight vital sugars.

Glyconutrients is

the wellness solution

for the

21st century.

In the first chapter, the discovery of glyconutrients is described, as different scientists move across the research stage. A medical icon resolves his skepticism in Chapter Two as he faces the dramatic response of patients, up close and personal. The explanation of structure and function begins in Chapter Three but only a discussion of the immune system and the monstrous threat of infectious diseases begins to put glyconutrients in context in Chapters Four and Five. There is hope for preserving wellness in a polluted environment, with the emerging threat of 'superbugs' and the unwelcome prospect of bioterrorism.

Glyconutrients are fundamental to cell biology and therefore have implications at every age. Chapter Six focuses on improving outcomes in pregnancy and some dramatic results in young children, some with serious conditions, are reported in Chapter Seven. The unusual perspective of a doctor as Super-mom illustrates the living reality of glyconutrients in Chapter Eight.

That brings us to the three major categories of disease in affluent societies today. They all reflect degenerative conditions which to a large extent, are preventable in the ideal, and certainly manageable in the real world. Cardiovascular illness, cancer and the scores of autoimmune diseases that dominate the remaining chronic conditions, are all affected by glyconutrients. The case is clearly made in Chapters Nine through Eleven.

The evidence for glyconutrients is consistently reinforced by dozens of personal case reports that are detailed by the doctors. But the mechanism of action is at the molecular level. So further explanation is warranted and that is forthcoming. Chapter Twelve goes more fundamental and hence a little more technical, in dissecting the inflammatory process and demonstrating the essential roles of glyconutrients in the overall cascade. Fitness and sports injury is the subject of Chapter Thirteen. An unusual approach to preventive dentistry is put forward in Chapter Fourteen, while the inevitable issue of aging is addressed in Chapter Fifteen.

A Pathologist looks back in Chapter Sixteen to understand why doctors so often have unjustified bias when it comes to nutrition, while a naturopath takes the more holistic approach to disease and dispels some common myths that should turn a light on for you in Chapter Seventeen.

The goal today is optimum health and wellness. Patients want relief from pain and other symptoms but that is not enough when the resources are known in nature to get beyond the signs of dissonance and dis-ease. No wonder then that doctors are having to reassess the way they practice today in the face of both chronic illness and preventable acute conditions. One such physician bares all in Chapter Eighteen. The final chapter on clinical trials and the exciting prospect for therapeutic applications of stem cells takes us right to the medical frontiers and the increased role for glyconutrient technology in the future. After all, this is a promising hope to address the looming economic crisis of health care and the looming pandemic crisis in the developing world.

In light of all the documented evidence presented and the dozens of anecdotal but reliable reports described by the different doctors, the case for glyconutrients is so overwhelmingly credible that all health care professionals and their patients would do well to read, underline and re-read this book.

The doctors who came together to write this book have come from different healthcare fields, but we coalesce around the single idea that glyconutrients is *the wellness solution* for the 21st century. We conclude that change is on the way but first, there will be increased resistance to the widespread application of this new glyconutrient technology. However, someone else has observed, "*nothing can stop an idea whose time has come.*" This is more than an idea. It is a secret of nature now revealed and a wise, complementary choice for those who affirm that the best defense is cell-defense. And when nature speaks, we all should listen.

After all the frustrations and limitations of high tech innovation in western medicine, we forsee potential applications of simple glyconutrient technology for the complementary management of many disease states and more importantly, the required maintenance of health and wellness in the 21st century. This is clearly a revolution in nutritional therapeutics that has worldwide ramifications.

The contemporary world is in need of and waiting for such a universal panacea. Therefore, this new, safe, effective and convenient way to fortify the body has immediate implications for everyone. This book clearly illustrates that nature does not reveal her secrets easily, but when found, they appear overwhelmingly simple ... yet profound!

What a way for YOU to discover Glyconutrients and The Healing **Power** *of* **8SugarS**' - *in this new book!*

It is a must read for everyone.

Allan Somersall, PhD., MD is a physician, scientist, author and motivational speaker. He holds a first class honors degree in chemistry from London University and earned doctorates in *both* science and medicine from the University of Toronto. For over twenty years he has traveled the world promoting health responsibility and prevention through nutrition and wise supplementation. He has written eight previous books.

Chapter 1

The Discovery of Glyconutrients

Dr. George V. Dubouch

We Americans are the most overfed and undernourished people in the world. We pollute our bodies intentionally and unintentionally with unhealthy chemicals and toxins from the air we breathe, the liquid we drink and the food we eat. We are polluted to such an extent that our bodies no longer function properly. We eat too many junk foods and we fill ourselves with health-robbing poisons. We have become knotted up with emotional stress from information overload, marriage and family relationships, occupational demands, financial anxiety and a host of similar challenges.

It's no wonder then that we get sick. We come down with a cold or the flu two or three times a year. We develop headaches, indigestion, allergies, chronic joint stiffness and a long list of other nagging complaints. We are tired all the time and gain too much weight. Then, we go to the doctor, only to find that over time our body has succumbed to one or other of the endemic chronic diseases - hardening of the arteries, hypertension, diabetes, cancer, arthritis, and who knows what else. Then we are recommended perhaps to have surgery, or take drugs to block, mask or cover up our symptoms for the rest of our "natural" - or more correctly - "unnatural" lives. We do everything to alleviate our pain, regulate our natural body functions and maintain the normal activities of daily living. We aim to at least survive, at all cost.

Because so many of us are experiencing these kinds of problems, people have come to accept them as normal, unavoidable illnesses . . . but are they? Of course not! What you are about to learn could turn your health around and add years to your life.

What if you could wake up tomorrow, mentally alert and with fewer of the nagging symptoms that have become your way of life? What if you could discover a safe alternative intervention that you could apply to improve your own health now and brighten your prognosis for the future? Well, get ready for some good news! In the past twenty years, there has been a breakthrough discovery for health and wellness - perhaps even anti-aging. For the past nine years millions have been utilizing this documented scientific knowledge and the results have been absolutely amazing! And that's just the beginning.

Most doctors have not yet heard of this. You've probably never even dreamed of something like this. But as you will learn later, and just as the evidence suggests, all the world stands to benefit from it.

This discovery I'm referring to can be expressed in one single word: **GLYCONUTRIENTS!**

This discovery is not a new drug; it is not a vitamin, mineral, herb or a homeopathic remedy - In fact, it should hardly be called a discovery. It is more an awakening, a new understanding that leads to possible action. It's been there all the time. But it needed a *technology* to reduce it to common practice, to exploit it and make it happen. In that sense, it is an invention. Methods of use and different formulations are therefore patentable and to date, over 100 new patents have been issued worldwide, pertaining to the discovery of glyconutrients.

Glyconutrients are a different kind of nutrient; *glyco-* comes from a Greek word meaning sweetness; so, *glyconutrient* means sugar nutrient. This is not table sugar (sucrose). Sucrose is a disaccharide, a two-sugar molecule; it is sweet to the taste, but has limited nutritional value. Sucrose is used only as fuel for energy production and getting too much of this kind of sugar inordinately stresses the pancreas, ruins the teeth, leads to obesity and generally starves the body. Consequently, it is unequivocally unhealthy!

But do not be deceived - the exact opposite is true for glyconutrients.

The glyconutrient complex of sugars is not sweet like table sugar, but it is imperative that we get these vitally important nutrients every day. After all, they are nutrients - something we eat, or should eat - to provide the body with what it needs on a regular daily basis.

The glyconutrient complex of sugars is made up of **eight plant-based saccharides**. They are combined in the body with different substrates - especially proteins and lipids - to form some of the most important biologically active molecules. Glycoproteins, for example, are now known to be critical for all cell-to-cell communication. Furthermore, these glyconutrients are used by the body to facilitate a reversal of the underlying cause of an underactive or overactive immune system. In essence, glyconutrients work like a natural immune modulator, bringing the body into a healthy balance. In contrast to the destructive effect of too much table sugar, these sugar nutrients called monosaccharides can even help diabetics by supporting the body in its rebuilding of pancreatic function. This book will go on to tell you why and how everybody need these glyconutrients for good health, for healing and to slow down the aging process. You are indeed going to make your very own discovery of **The Healing Power *of* ^{8}SugarS**.

Serendipity

So how did this all come about? What circumstances made it happen? Was it another case of serendipity where some lucky scientist just stumbled upon something that they did not expect to find, which later turned out to be like gold? Or was it the result of blood, sweat and tears. The march of science is unpredictable, but clearly breakthroughs do come by both pathways. Which one was it here?

The story begins a long way back.

The glyconutrient complex of sugars is not sweet like table sugar, but it is imperative that we get these vitally important nutrients every day.

Dr. Bill McAnalley, a research scientist from Texas, as a little boy experienced firsthand a facial burn. In those days, for most minor complaints, the first recourse was a home-remedy. There were no superstores then, with aisle after aisle filled with a plethora of pharmaceutical synthetic preparations to relieve or cover up every conceivable complaint. Common remedies were natural remedies, and most of the time, they worked.

The gel-like fluid that was applied to young Bill's burn in this case, came directly from the inner leaf of a live Aloe plant. The benefits were readily apparent to him. The initial ordeal from his burn, the simplicity of the treatment and the positive results all impressed Bill's open mind. This unsuspecting gel turned out to be a good source of one of the first saccharides now found in the glyconutrient complex of necessary sugars. In fact, all these vital sugars turn out to be derived from natural sources. They appear to be part of the **Intelligent Design.**

The images of that experience stayed with Bill until one day many years later, as a doctor of both toxicology and pharmacology, he started to investigate polysaccharides. This opportunity came about because Clinton Howard, the founder of Carrington Laboratories (at first a manufacturer of skin care products and later, a research and development company), had earlier started the ball rolling. He had managed to raise the money to do legitimate scientific research in this field, at a time when there was very little interest in scientifically documenting even the constituents (much less the alleged benefits) of Aloe vera or any similar natural products. But why Aloe?

The Aloe Controversy

Aloe vera has been used in the healing arts for thousands of years. This medicinal plant has some recorded uses going back to the Egyptians and Mesopotamians, but it began to find much broader applications around the time of Christ. Dr. N. Moore in her short but timely book *The Miracle of Aloe Vera (1995)* quotes from Bill Coates' *The Silent Healer, A Modern Study of Aloe Vera (1984):*

> *"In 74 A.D., Dioscordes, a Roman pharmacist, in his De Materia Medica listed many medicinal cures for Aloe. Included in his list were medicinal properties such as healing wounds, repressing boils, healing bruises, eliminating skin abrasions, stopping hair loss, soothing eye sores, healing genital ulcers, ameliorating tonsillitis, healing hemorrhoids, and of course, relieving constipation or bowel problems by acting as a laxative."*

Over the centuries, the perceived benefits of the Aloe plants continued to spread across the globe. By the end of the Middle Ages it had become a common ingredient in the most widely used medicinal mixtures. By the turn of the last century, much more serious conditions were now included in the list of indications, such as irregular menstruation, diseases of the spleen, brain diseases, pneumonia, gonorrhea and rheumatism. As a topical agent, it was unsurpassed.

But despite its widespread popularity and its rampant success as a healing panacea, its mode of action remained a pure mystery. Earliest attempts to identify or isolate some active ingredient of the Aloe all proved futile. Aloin was extracted as a black and brown bitter substance in 1851, but nothing useful was forthcoming until Ikawa and Niemann determined that the Aloe gel consisted of mucopolysaccharides. That was the first clue.

But it was only a clue, for there was no understanding at all of any structure - property correlation. Speaking of properties, the results from using Aloe proved to be inconsistent and unreliable from time to time, place to place and one investigator to another. This made Aloe the subject of much controversy, which usually implies "a lot of heat, but little light." The Aloe preparations used were themselves quite varied in composition, in form and in age.

Classic insight came from some research done by the US Atomic Energy Commission at the Radiation Burn Center of Los Alamos in the 1950's. Their net conclusion was that some elusive active ingredient was present only in freshly harvested Aloe vera, but that somehow became inactive either by processing the Aloe or just storing it over time. That could explain much of the inconsistency in applied results. But it could not silence the controversy. There was still no structure - property correlation. The answer could only lie in the characterization of the 'active ingredient' and at least a rational mechanism of action.

Enter Dr. Bill McAnalley, please ...

Dr. *McAnalley graduated from San Angelo State University in 1968 with a BS in Chemistry-Math. For the next five years, he taught math and chemistry in San Angelo public schools. In 1973, he earned his MS in Natural Science from New Mexico Highlands University in Las Vegas, New Mexico. In 1978, he received his PhD in Pharmacology and Toxicology from the University of Texas Health Science Center, Dallas, Texas, where he was an adjunct faculty member from 1979-1998. Dr. McAnalley worked as a Toxicologist for the US Environmental Protection Agency (EPA) and was Director of Research at Carrington Laboratories from 1985-1995. He is the primary inventor of over 100 patents that have been issued worldwide, including use and composition of matter patents. His work has been published in over 25 peer-reviewed journals and he has written chapters in three reference books.*

The Active Ingredient

Dr.McAnalley was committed to finding this active Aloe ingredient and exploring its potential. His initial work satisfied him, if not confirmed, that the Aloe vera gel did have medicinal value as a topical application for burns and wounds at least. And he did find that the effectiveness was clearly dependent on the amount of time passed after harvesting the leaf from the plant. He also noted in the laboratory that when the Aloe plant was either cut or compressed (as was commonly done in treatment preparations), one or more enzymes were released. That enzyme he concluded would then deactivate the active ingredient.

That triggered a key idea.

Why not find a way, if possible, to deactivate the enzyme(s) to retain the effectiveness of the medicinally active ingredient(s)? That's what Dr. McAnalley managed to do, back in the late 1980's. As the director of research at Carrington Laboratories, he developed and later patented a freeze-dried dehydration process to provide a purified powdered extract from the clear gel center of the Aloe vera leaf which contains the medicinally active ingredient found only in the fresh, natural Aloe.

Dr. McAnalley turned his attention to identifying the active ingredient. By using careful chromatographic separation techniques and sophisticated analytical instrumentation, he and his colleagues were later able to characterize this elusive substance. It turned out to be a 'mucilagenous polysaccharide.' Those are rather big words that warrant further explanation.

'*Mucilagenous*' is simply an adjective pertaining to the moist, soft and viscid appearance and forms of '*mucilage*' which is a general term for various sticky preparations of gum or glue. This physical 'sticky' characteristic is a challenge to pure chemists who would usually prefer to work with nice soluble crystals, fine free-flowing powders or pure liquids. It is messy work and turns the lab bench into a messy workplace more akin to the old alchemy. But patience and diligence will usually pay off.

The stickiness is characteristic of polysaccharides. It derives from their molecular structure. Poly-saccharides actually means *many* saccharides (sugars), usually arranged in linear chains or polymers. You might think of them as the sugar equivalent of rubber or plastic but with very different physical properties.

Sugars are ring molecules, typically with 5, 6 or more carbon atoms, to which are attached hydrogen and hydroxyl (-OH) groups. The hydroxyl group is somewhat bipolar, with a negative oxygen and a positive hydrogen, and these act like tiny electrical magnets which attract each other to create the 'sticky' properties.

Polysaccharides then, consist of long chains (polymers) of sugars, linked together in different ways to form a starch-like fiber. The active ingredient that Dr. McAnalley found in the Aloe vera was a polymannose. Mannose is a simple sugar. Alexis Berendu, PhD, has been credited with developing some critical methods to isolate and characterize the molecular structure of the more complex polymannose. In polymannose, the mannose molecules are linked in a special way and designated as a B-(1,4) - linked mannan.

Just a word of explanation about commercial names for these

Aloe derivatives. The polymannans (or just mannans) derived from Aloe vera, were given the trade name *acemannan* by the US Adopted Names Council of the AMA. This name is now associated with an 'unapproved drug' by the FDA regulations. The term *Manapol*™ refers to a proprietary nutritional supplement, containing at least 56 percent polymannans.

The Mechanism Of Action

Now that Dr. McAnalley had identified and characterized the active ingredient of Aloe vera, the big remaining question was. How does it work in any of its medicinal applications? What is its 'mechanism of action'?

Enter Dr. H. Reginald. McDaniel, please ...

Dr. Reg McDaniel graduated from the University of Texas Southwestern Medical School and spent 30 years practicing anatomical and clinical pathology, including positions as the Director of Pathology & Laboratories and Director of Medical Education at Dallas-Ft Worth Medical Center.

In 1981 he began research at Fisher Institute for Medical Research using a bean extract to stimulate the immune system. He conducted the first government-monitored studies in humans using aloe polymannose (manapol®) with unprecedented results. He devoted his attention to the potential of glyconutrients and other plant micronutrients to restore health by nutritionally supporting normal biochemistry under gene control. In 1996, the American Naturopathic Medical Association recognized Drs. McAnalley and McDaniel for their work regarding glyconutrients with their "Discovery of the Year Award". For nine years Dr. McDaniel was a consultant to Carrington Laboratories and Medical Director for a company established to take this nutrient research and technology to the mass market. He has published numerous papers on glyconutritionals' effects on various disease conditions.

Now the story continues. When Dr. McAnalley developed and patented his novel method of processing Aloe vera gel to protect the polymannose, the new stabilized extract was made available in the form of a juice which could be taken orally. It was soon made commercially available and as its use became more widespread, anecdotal reports of a wide range of 'medicinal' benefits began to circulate. People with all kinds of health problems began attributing their noted improvements to this Aloe juice.

Dr. McDaniel was recruited by both Clinton Howard and Dr. McAnalley to work with the expanded research team at Carrington Labs. He consulted on a series of pilot studies with AIDS patients, using the patented Aloe extract. Those results proved remarkable and led to a number of other clinical investigations of the benefits of the active Aloe extract. They examined the effects of acemannan on over 100 different disease conditions. All the research data showed very positive results and pointed in the same direction.

By the mid '90s, it had occurred to Drs. McDaniel and McAnalley that the sugar molecule in Aloe vera might not be unique. It could just possibly be one of many "biologically active" sugars that have some important role in the body, over and above their use for energy. Remember that it was still popular throughout the western world's nutrition and medical establishment to think of all carbohydrates as essentially energy sources and at best, a source of bulky indigestible fiber in the diet. But both doctors envisaged various sugars being assembled and utilized in the cell. Could that be real?

At a conference in Virginia in 1996, Drs McDaniel and McAnalley were fortuitously introduced to two research papers on the work of a German scientist using Arabinogalactan, a freeze-dried powder from the sap of the larch tree that is rich in other 'sugars'. In fact, this product is approved by the FDA as a non-toxic food and cosmetic additive. Some mushrooms are also known to be rich in vital sugars and have been used extensively, especially in Asia, for all types of alleged medicinal benefits. Second generation sources of the necessary 'sugars' include other natural products like chitin and chitosan, as well as maitake-D fraction and polysaccharide K and P.

Now, enter Dr. Robert K. Murray, please ...

Dr. Murray received his medical degree from the University of Glasgow, Scotland and his PhD in Biochemistry at the University of Toronto, Canada, where he later became a Professor of Biochemistry. Professor Murray had a distinguished teaching and research career at the University during which he published over fifty scientific peer-reviewed papers, authored multiple textbook articles, and was one of the authors of the last five editions of '<u>Harper's Biochemistry</u>.' Since 1998, Dr. Murray has served as a consultant in carbohydrate biology and biochemistry to the nutritional supplement industry.

While Drs. McDaniel and McAnalley were musing about the possibility of other sugars being biologically active, the most formal scientific statement of the biological role of sugars first appeared in a classic article in Harper's Biochemistry, 24th Edit (1996). There Professor Murray reviewed the subject of 'Glycoproteins', making emphatic reference to the significance of the 'sugar' chains attached to proteins. He underlined their central biomedical importance and noted specifically, that of the 200+ simple sugars already known in nature, only eight are commonly found in the sugar chains of glycoproteins.

These eight known necessary monosaccharides (sugars) are:

Glucose	**Xylose**
Galactose	**N-acetylglucosamine**
Fucose	**N-acetylgalactosamine**
Mannose	**N-acetylneuraminic acid**

Further details on these sugars and their biological activity is given as **Appendix 'A'** at the back of the book.

No wonder then that Drs. McDaniel and McAnalley were the first to independently propose a novel *nutritional* supplement including all the known necessary or vital sugars in a single complex. They filed for worldwide "composition of matter" patents. The result was a formulation that outperformed all previous Aloe vera extracts in all their applications and resulting benefits.

A hypothesis for the "mechanism of action" now fell naturally into place.

First, consider **the crucial role of glycoproteins in biology**. Almost all plasma proteins in humans - except albumin - contain sugars. All cellular membranes have proteins containing sugars. A number of blood group markers are proteins with sugars. Some hormones (such as that used for confirming pregnancy tests) are proteins with sugars. The sugar chains contain many different linkage possibilities giving rise to a code of biologic information. How much more important could any class of molecules get? And that's not the whole story. But it's more than enough.

Then, if the addition of **the vitally necessary sugars makes these precursors more readily available** to the cells for inclusion in glycoprotein synthesis - that could readily explain why 'sugars' as nutrients (glyco-nutrients) could be so effective when used in supplement form. All the evidence to date seems to concur.

Applause

Now, enter the entire cast, please ...

The first **International Conference** in the new science of Glycobiology convened in 1989 at UCLA, California, sponsored by Smith Kline and French Laboratories. It brought together 180 scientists to review and explore one of the most rapidly growing fields in cell biology at that time - a field that was projected to have "a major impact on medical research and practice in the future."

The composition, structure and function of glycoproteins had been reviewed earlier in a textbook edited by Dr. Gottschalk and published by Elsevier back in 1972. But the science had become the playground of the pharmaceutical drug researchers only, exploring new concepts of drug design.

At a more fundamental level, **Nobel Prizes** in Physiology and Medicine had been awarded during the 1990s in three areas, all somewhat related to the emerging field of Glycobiology:

1991 To Erwin Neher and Bert Sakmann for their discoveries concerning the function of single ion channels in cells.
1994 To Alfred Gilman and Martin Rodbell for their discoveryof G-proteins and the role of these proteins in signal transduction of cells.
1999 To Gunter Blobel for the discovery that proteins have intrinsic signals that govern their transport and localization in the cell.

What a way to dramatize the biological 'bridge to the 21st century?' In each of these areas of cell-biology, glycoproteins were the important supporting cast. They provided the structures that determined biochemical properties of the molecules responsible key physiological functions in the cell.

As the curtain was raised on the new millennium, it was now time for real applause. And it was forthcoming.

2001 ***Science Magazine*** - Science magazine, the official journal of the American Association for the Advancement of Science and the premier journal for researchers and scientists as a whole - dedicated 12 articles in the *March issue* to educating the scientific and medical communities about glyconutrients. In that 42-page **Special Report** it emphasized that carbohydrate compounds currently in clinical trials were aimed at fighting everything from inflammation and tissue rejection to hepatitis and cancer. An article in that report, entitled "Glycosylation and the Immune System," cited rheumatoid arthritis as one example of the connection of the need for monosaccharides in various disease conditions, and the new hope for many other disease states such as cancer, diabetes and Alzheimer's.[1]

2002 ***Scientific American*** featured a **Cover Story** in July on "Sweet Medicine - Building Better Drugs from Sugars". It underscored the fact that sugars modify many proteins and fats on cell surfaces and participate in such biological processes as immunity and cell-to-cell communication. They also stated that sugars play a part in a range of diseases, from viral infections to cancer.

That same year, ***The Scientist*** carried a story entitled 'Glycobiology Goes to the Ball" The profile written by Jeffrey Perkel suggested that "new federal funding, new technologies, and a better understanding of carbohydrates' roles in biology had scientists pondering the feasibility of a Human *Glycome* Project."

Later that year, biochemist Gerald Hart of Johns Hopkins University declared "This is going to be the future. We won't understand immunology, neurology, developmental biology or disease until we get a handle on Glycobiology."

2003 The Massachusetts Institute of Technology published in its ***Technology Review*** a feature on the "**Ten Emerging Technologies That Will Change the World**." Among them was the field of Glycomics, reviewed by James Paulson. There was good reason for this excitement because 'sugars' play such a critical role in stablilizing and determining the fuction of proteins through the glycosylation process. No glycosylation, no life. The prospects of getting a handle on this could really have far-reaching implications.

Clearly, the science of Glycobiology had arrived and taken over center stage in physiology and medical science. While the drug manufacturers saw opportunities for designing new classes of drugs to exploit this emerging field, a more subtle but no less significant change was taking place. Naturally occurring 'sugars' that had been taken for granted all this time had zoomed into prominence as vitally necessary food nutrients. These glyconutrients could no longer be neglected.The spotlight in nutrition turned in that direction and the intensity and concentration have been increasing ever since.

Encore

The discovery of these unique saccharides in combination and their importance for supporting overall good health is still surprising medical science. Millions of satisfied consumers, thousands of impressive testimonials, hundreds of documented papers and abstracts, as well as a limited number of double-blind, placebo-controlled studies,[2,3] all together confirm the efficacy and effectiveness of these wonderful, non-toxic, all-natural nutritional substrates that rarely, if ever, have negative side effects.

There is now a dedicated web site containing over 40,000 references all devoted solely to providing research information on nutritional products containing monosaccharides (glyconutrition)[4]. This information provides scientific underpinnings for the use of glyconutrients and informs health professionals who are interested in learning more about the safety and effectiveness of glyconutritional supplementation for their patients. Sections are also included for the lay person who wants to know more about personal choices that they can make to affect their health and the health of their families. Finally, for the research scientist, the site assembles in one place, much of the published research concerning the role of nutritional monosaccharides in health. This growing body of knowledge comes from all over the world and spans many scientific disciplines. The site is educational in nature but is in no way intended to substitute for any doctor's care or for proven therapy.

The medical journal, *Acta Anatomica*, observed in 1998: "Many of the secrets of glycoscience are only accessible to a closed circle of aficionados, who appear to be the only ones to understand the meaningful words of a sweet language of life . . . its biological significance has long been underestimated. The last decade has witnessed the rapid emergence of the concept of the sugar code of biological information: Indeed, monosaccharides (sugars) represent an alphabet of biological information...but, with unsurpassed coding capacity."[5]

Supplementation

The fact is, all mammals need at least these eight known monosaccharides for necessary cell-to-cell communication and proper function. Humans normally get only two of the necessary saccharides from food - glucose and galactose, which are the only ones common in our modern diets. Moreover, people who are dairy intolerant may only be getting primarily one monosaccharide (glucose), since galactose is primarily in dairy products. (For *Sources of Glyconutrients, see* **Appendix 'B'**). If all the essential factors are present within the body, our systems can manufacture the other six or seven monosaccharides needed through inter-conversions of sugars. But the process is time- and energy-consuming as well as very error-prone due to the large number of enzymatic steps involved. Add to that, our nutritional deficiencies and possible cellular contamination and it is most reasonable to assert that almost everyone should supplement with glyconutrients.

The eight necessary sugars are precursors that are converted by the body into glycoforms (glycoproteins and glycolipids)[6,7] on cell surfaces, through the sensitive process of glycosylation, as mentioned earlier. When the glycoforms are present and functioning effectively, it is like turning the lights on inside your body, so to speak, so your defense mechanisms that make up the immune system can see who is friend and who is foe - which cells need help and which need to be eliminated.

Glyconutrients are the raw materials the body uses to create the glycoforms. Molecules such as proteins or lipids that have carbohydrates attached to the outer surface of cells become antenna-like glycoforms. Cells communicate one to another through the sense of touch, correct cell-to-cell docking takes place and chemical and electrical messages flow back and forth. Important coded information and translated commands from one cell to the next cell must be unimpaired, quick and clear. This communication linkage is a significant part of the body's natural recognition and defense system for maintaining good health and long life.

The breakdown of the life force and functioning character of the cell is the basis of disease. A major contributing factor is the lack of proper cellular communication. The living cell is in constant motion, undulating and absorbing as well as ejecting. It has a delicate balance. When this cellular balance is upset, interrupted or damaged, a response is eventually experienced. This response is what we call a *symptom* (subjective) or a *sign* (objective). For example, when you cut your finger, one symptom would be pain, another bleeding. But how does your healing mechanism know what happened? Who tells what systems to take action to heal the injury? How does one cell communicate to another to bring about the platelets to mesh and mend, stop the bleeding, reduce inflammation and heal the tissues? Another question to ponder: When eating a meal, how does your digestive system know what gastric juices are needed for protein, fat or carbohydrate digestion? Is it guesswork by the body, or is there a higher intelligence at work on our behalf?

The intelligence that develops a full-grown individual from a fertilized ovum is also the intelligence that heals, defends, repairs and regulates. This innate intelligence is fully self-sufficient in every living cell when its environment and constitution is healthy. **The cell is the fundamental unit of all living things**. The human body is made up entirely of trillions of cells organized into tissues, glands, organs and systems. Cell-to-cell communication is imperative! Even if you think your cells are healthy because you eat right and get plenty of exercise - guess again! If your body does not get enough of these glyconutrients from your diet because of the poor quality of available foods, it is just a matter of time before your immune system function will be compromised.

By making sure that your body gets these glyconutrients and other essentials that have been missing from the commercial food chain and normal diets - nutrients your body needs for health and healing - you can optimize your body's potential to heal itself. Hence, you can experience for yourself **The Healing Power** ***of*** **8SugarS**.

It is important to understand that the immune system is one of the most vital systems of the body for maintaining a homeostatic (balanced) condition. Without all the necessary glycoproteins on the cell surface, it is like trying to write a letter to someone without using vowels - no one would be able to read it. Or, it is like trying to talk to someone without verbs - the other words you speak will be unintelligible.

The eight vital saccharides balance and strengthen the immune system like no other natural product or combination of products found anywhere in the world. It can up-regulate or down-regulate an immune system, depending upon whether the system is underactive or overactive, bringing it into a state of balance and optimum health.[8,9,10] With proper cell-to-cell communication, the immune system can be vigilant in its surveillance and elimination of viruses, fungi, destructive bacteria, carcinogens and then defend against infections and even toxic chemicals.

Conclusion

Over 100 years ago the creative genius, Thomas A. Edison, the inventor of the electric light bulb, shed another kind of light on the doctors of the future. He said, "The doctor of the future will give no medicine, but will interest his patients in the care of the human frame, in diet and in the cause and prevention of disease." He was prophetic and right on. I put it this way: If the doctor of today doesn't become the nutritionist of tomorrow, then the nutritionist of today will become the doctor of tomorrow. Hippocrates, the father of modern medicine, told all of us 2,500 years ago: "Let your food be your medicine and your medicine be your food."

Glyconutrients are essentials in food. They represent nutrients that are limited in our normal food supply. They provide the missing link in nutrition - a health-building, non-toxic nutritional complement for all mankind. Their discovery and widespread use as supplements will alter the health and wellbeing of generations to come. However, I also believe that one day, in the not-too-distant future, metabolic therapy using glyconutrients will become the professional standard-of-care. Today, at age 65, I expect to be alive to welcome that historic day.

If the doctor of today does not become the nutritionist of tomorrow, then the nutritionist of today will become the doctor of tomorrow.

About the Author
George V. Dubouch, Ph.D.

Dr. George Dubouch holds a Bachelor's degree in Community Health and a Master's in Nutritional Science. He earned his Doctorate degree in Communications from Columbia Pacific University in 1983. He is the author of the book Science or Miracle? *The Metabolic Glyconutritional Discovery.* He has traveled the world exploring diet, nutrition and optimum health. He runs a nutrition clinic out of Talent, Oregon.

Editors note:

You will now go on to learn more about this new discovery from a medical icon - a practicing physician for many years - who refused to concede to this new technology, until he could do no less ...

Chapter 2

Confessions of a Medical Skeptic

Dr. Rayburne W. Goen

I have been a medical doctor for over 60 years. When I first heard about glyconutrients six years ago, my reply was simply: "*Hogwash*". I declared that anyone who claimed that oral administration of supplements was of striking benefit to people suffering from *a long list of unrelated diseases* or ailments, had to be a quack. They would be in the same class as all the others making such claims - whatever the modality. Nothing could be effective for the relief of a multitude of ailments, even though so many products are blatantly proclaimed and touted to be so in the many brochures and catalogs arriving in the daily mail.

To my mind, I was already well versed in that kind of hype! After all, I had previously tried a number of them myself, for my own ailments, thinking I had nothing to lose. So, why not? Enthusiastically at first, I used the highly acclaimed glucosamine, chondroitin sulfate, cetyl myristoleate, MSM, SAM-e, blue green algae, alfalfa tea, olive leaf extract, colloidal silver and other natural remedies. I consumed each one as my eyes toiled over lots of "ink," but they did not seem to help me in any significant way.

With that track record of disappointing claims, I became close-minded. You could call me skeptical, dubious or cynical - as you may be now and as the vast majority in my profession would have been, and probably still are. I was, however, receptive enough to read some pertinent articles from prestigious medical journals which were offered to me. To put it mildly, I must admit that I was a little jarred by the implications of what I read. I began to look into what turned out to be, an overwhelming amount of related literature. I soon found out that carbohydrate (*glyco-*) metabolism had suddenly become a hot subject. Over **20,000 papers** had been published on Medline in three short years, 1996-1998, and a greater number since. Most of them are in what could be classified as *specialty research journals*. These are journals that most of us, as practicing physicians, do not subscribe to or read. To be honest, in most cases, neither do we easily understand. The *clinical* articles published thus far have been mainly *retrospective* or *prospective*. That means that they are essentially *case reports* of different series of patients with different disease conditions, and with suspiciously high percentages of positive results. I read many of these articles. I could not believe that doctors were frivolously documenting something if it were so fundamentally powerful.

But it was hard to accept that a mere food supplement ('sugars' at that!) could correct an unknown deficiency in our diet, so vitally important as to control the mechanism of all **cellular communication** in our body. This was the *glyco-* ("sweet") part of glycoproteins which enable so many metabolic and biologic functions that occur in the marvel of all creation ... the human body. I speculated that if this were true, it would become the most momentous discovery in medicine during the past 100 years. It would rank up there with the discovery of essential amino acids, fatty acids, vitamins and minerals. But it could have even more far-reaching implications than the few known conditions which ensue from deficiencies of those initial four classes of essential nutrients.

Physician Heal Thyself

I therefore proposed to *try* glyconutrient supplements for a list of 21 ailments I could identify in myself. Even to the doctor, most of these could be attributable simply to "old age," since I was 85 years old at the time. But, 'what the heck,' I had nothing to lose either. I could be my own guinea pig and with absolute informed consent. I was being neither neurotic nor masochistic - just trying to be somewhat scientific. I had identifiable problems. I now had a prospective treatment option and the opportunity for first hand 24/7 clinical observations. I could be both doctor and patient,all at the same time. So, why not?

None of my ailments completely disabled me, except for the arthritis of my knees, which required aspiration of fluid and instillation of cortisone more and more frequently. Eventually, I had to have injections every three months first for one knee, and then the other. Only after those treatments, would I again be functional. I also had a peripheral neuropathy (nerve disorder), which impaired my balance and walking, and greatly disturbed my sleep because of my restless legs. Then there was a right shoulder rotator cuff tear; low back pain; degenerative cervical disc disease, which affected the nerves radiating out from the spine. I also had an inflammatory osteoarthritis of my hands. I could not shake hands properly without hurting for the next three days. Add to these, high blood pressure (190/105); elevated cholesterol (320mg) for many years; nocturia (with four to six trips to the bathroom during the night); urinary urgency and incontinence; prostate cancer; cataracts in both eyes, etc. I was a 'mess' - an 'old mess'. Other than all that, I was a perfect specimen, in fine shape. Yes, right! But my mind was still alert and I was thoughtful enough to put what I had read in the journals to my personal test.

So, I added glyconutrients to my daily diet!

Within four months, I became virtually symptom-free of most of these 21 complaints. I was subsequently able to discontinue all the eight prescribed drugs I was taking. I also stopped all over-the-counter medications, except for a baby aspirin every other day which I took since I had a coronary back in 1990. This too was discontinued in 2003 when I started taking fish oil and flaxseed oil, since they also have an antiplatelet effect. Over the years, drugs had been effective to a degree, but all had side effects that were either disagreeable or even intolerable, at least in my case.

There are ***BAD sugars*** *and* *there are* ***GOOD sugars!***

I was delighted. Now I had experienced it for myself. I could not negate the effective value of glyconutrients for dealing with my own variety of chronic disorders. But that result was still not enough to convince me. This had to be some sort of "fluke'. It was not mind over matter for sure. But maybe just coincidence. Placebo? Not for a skeptic like me and not with such memorable experiential benefits.

Just maybe I had latched on to something beyond my wildest dreams.

One Patient At A Time

I resolved to still disprove this "stuff" by persuading a "know-it-all" former patient who scoffed at the idea of taking supplements like these for his refractory Raynaud's Syndrome. He experienced cold-sensitive fingers that turned purple and agonizingly painful upon exposure. He also had uncontrolled Type 2 Diabetes with serious adverse effects from insulin and his oral anti-diabetes drugs. He also had elevated cholesterol and developed diabetic nerve complications, worsened by all the "statin" drugs he used for cholesterol reduction. He was scheduled for replacement surgery on both knees, each of which had been operated on twice before for old injuries and loss of cartilage. His knees had shown poor response to NSAID drugs, which also had intolerable side effects. Unfortunately, he was in a bit of a mess.

He had sworn he was going to discontinue all the drugs he was taking. He would rather die than live this miserably. I reminded him that dying is an easy out. Furthermore, he might not soon die, but he could be disabled by heart attack, stroke, amputations, blindness, or renal failure and dialysis. I managed to induce him to try glyconutritionals for four months, with the assurance that they absolutely could not harm him.

He reluctantly agreed.

Three weeks later, he reported that he was free of knee pain and all those tingling sensations in his limbs (paresthesias). He was having normalized blood sugars even though he was down to taking just the one oral anti-diabetes drug he had tolerated. That drug had not previously controlled the high blood sugar. Now on glyconutrients, his vision and mental clarity were improved. He neglected however, to reorder the supplements, and the symptoms all recurred within two weeks. Upon resumption of the supplements, the symptoms again abated.

I was still not convinced!

I did cautiously offer glyconutrients to several other former patients, including two diabetics with complications who did not respond to my usual management. I observed similar salutary effects. They showed not only arrest of their downhill course, but actual improvement to the point where they could return to useful function! From all my medical experience, this was impossible! All previous management modalities were able to slow deterioration, but nothing my patients had done had ever reversed any of their symptoms significantly. After taking glyconutrients for almost a year, they experienced results that I could only describe as incredible.

I was nearly convinced, but not quite yet.

The Case That Did It

I gave glycosupplements to Z., a patient whom I had "doctored" for almost 50 years with muscular dystrophy of the spinal atrophy type. Her brother had died at age 13 with similar disease of the Duchenne type. She was in total care since the age of three, unable to do anything for herself. She had impairment of swallowing and was on oxygen 24 hours a day. She was able to do some ceramic painting, with her right arm supported on a table. But she could only manage that for two hours, at most twice a week. I offered to supply the supplements and she readily agreed.

Four months after starting glyconutrients, she could, for the first time in almost 50 years, now feed herself. She swallowed easily. Yes, she could brush her own teeth, and was now off oxygen for 3-4 hours daily. She could now paint 6-8 hours per day, and up to 6 days a week! She stated "I have so much energy, I could do more. But I know I should rest some, whether I feel the need or not!" She has sustained this improvement, and for the first time ever, she has not been treated or hospitalized for respiratory failure or infection in over a year, despite a flu outbreak disabling two of her own nurses and her roommate!

This was indeed enough to convince me that this stuff was for real! When the clinical consequences of a genetic defect of this magnitude and duration were favorably modified to this extent, all my doubts were gone.

I was no longer a skeptic. I became committed!

The Ecstasy & the Agony

B., a former surgical technician in the military, developed Type 2 Diabetes after returning from overseas in the 1980's. When originally diagnosed, his blood sugars were in the 900's. It remained uncontrollably high (above 500) for many years, despite multiple injections of Regular Insulin up to 200 units daily, plus Ultra-Lente (long acting) Insulin 120 units daily. He developed retinopathy (eye damage), requiring Laser cautery every 3 months for years. He also experienced peripheral neuropathy of both legs and arms and complications of diabetic ulcers on his legs and feet. Amputation was advised. But this he refused. He also noted muscle deterioration, with leg cramps (claudication) and chest pain (angina) on attempting to walk just half a block. He gained weight up to 330 lbs, with the resultant inactivity. Despite being on multiple antihypertensive medications, his blood pressure averaged 200/115 for years. That was dangerously high. He developed arthritis, especially in his hands.

After 4 years, he acquired an electrified "scooter" that enabled him to get around. In the early 1990's, over a 3-4 month period, he had a series of strokes with some permanent left-sided weakness, migraine headaches and double vision. Sleep apnea and shortness of breath at rest, necessitated six inhalers, including nasal and tracheo-bronchial steroids. He experienced heart failure with edema of the lower limbs. For years he had been on a multiplicity of antibiotics - even a month without any was considered a "good month"! His kidneys began to excrete albumin, and his BUN and creatinine (blood test results) became elevated. Those are signs of approaching renal failure that would require dialysis.

Because of the seriousness of his combined health problems, he "realized this would prove *terminal* in a short period of time". He became severely depressed because of his condition and by what it was doing to his family. Despite the efforts of twelve doctors and specialists, nothing seemed to help. He was in really bad shape.

If effective, never discontinue the glyconutrients!

Then just as he had "given up all hope and was making arrangements for his funeral", the minister who would conduct his funeral introduced him to glyconutritionals. B. decided, as a last resort, to try some. He was not expecting anything to happen. After all, nothing else had helped.

Three months later, his vision was improving. The ulcers on his feet and legs were appreciably healed. The pain and swelling, the weakness (including the left sided stroke weakness), the shortness of breath and angina were all no longer real problems. He was off all six inhalers and his joint pains from arthritis were all but gone. He was even able to walk without depending on the scooter or a cane and he was back to driving his car. The migraines resolved, as did his chronic sinusitis, and he needed no more antibiotics. His blood pressure then averaged 130/85. Albumin was no longer found in his urine, and the creatinine levels had not increased, indicating stable renal function rather than the previously noted downhill progression. He lost weight - from 320 to 280 pounds - and continued to lose fat and regain muscle mass. The insulin was reduced to 10-50 units daily, of Regular; plus Ultra-lente, 60 units twice per day. The blood sugars were then running 105-125, and the glycohemoglobin (A1c) showed an incredibly low measurement (5.1). This last index is a measure of the biological level of glucose saturation of the red blood cells. That number (5.1) is very, very good. He could no doubt have reduced his weight and insulin further by following a low glycemic diet. He started to exercise more. His severe depression was over.

After more than four years of such dramatic improvement in his condition, B. had a most unfortunate accident. He was doing some home repairs and falling timber gashed his back. Meningitis was initially suspected and his **doctors stopped his glyconutrients** during the course of his hospitalization, workup, operations and finally rehab. He deteriorated rapidly, with diabetes uncontrolled, paralysis of bladder and stools, massive bedsores, ulcerations and bleeding. Sad to say, he died after months of suffering, *without glyconutrients*.

Too little, too short

M., is a 65 year old housewife who had breast cancer in 1984. She was treated with bilateral mastectomy (ie. both breasts were removed). The cancer recurred in the abdomen and stomach 16 years later, for which she received six chemotherapy treatments in 2000. These were poorly tolerated and did not improve her condition. She developed obstruction of her colon, necessitating a colostomy. Then a blockage in the stomach outlet resulted in abdominal swelling, with loss of appetite and rapid weight loss. She was told there was nothing more to do. Under the circumstances, hospice was utilized for pain control with injections of narcotics and expectation of death within six months. Three months passed, with a steady downhill course, despite her using herbal remedies. While in palliative care, glyconutrients were offered to her and in desperation, she began to take them. Within two weeks she was out of bed and going to church. A week later she insisted on going to a garage sale! She was then up and about doing her housework and delighting in her cooking. She again enjoyed eating. She was now in little pain and the abdominal swelling had disappeared.

Unfortunately, after eight months of such comfort and activity, glyconutrients were not available for two weeks, during which time she rapidly declined. When they became available again, she could no longer swallow or retain, and within another two weeks, she succumbed and died. Perhaps there really is a lesson here. There was for me, at least. The lesson: if effective, never discontinue the glyconutrients.

An Incredible Story

Here's another remarkable anecdote from my own experience. K. is a seven year old with severe cerebral palsy. Her hands were tightly clenched, her arms and legs were spastic and crossed. Her head and eyes turned upward and out, and she is unable to speak.

Glyconutrients were started, and within one week her hands were unclenched. Her arms and legs were uncrossed in another week, and she was picking up things. Another three weeks later, she was trying to talk. This was frustrating to her, and she became almost violent in her actions for the next six weeks. I did not hear about her for another four months.

Then I was told that her normal older brother received a new bicycle for his birthday. He was admiring and riding it. The report is that K. walked over to the bicycle, picked it up, straddled it, and began to pedal. She did not know how to guide, balance or stop, so when she precariously reached the curb at the end of the street, she stopped pedaling and fell over. She was not hurt. She got up, turned the bike around, got on, pedaled back, stopped pedaling and fell over again. A month later I watched a video of her riding the bicycle. She was guiding it, turning the handlebars and braking with coordination.

What's going on here? No one really knows. Somehow the glyconutrients are enabling her body to heal itself. But that's medically impossible. Thank God, the body can begin to reverse a lifetime defect, when given what it needs.

Dumb and dumber

I have done some dumb things in my later years. Here's a classic: I roofed a house at age 87.

Yes, the roof of our cottage on Lake Ft. Gibson was beginning to leak after 28 years. I contacted some roofers and contracted with one of them to repair the roof. He did not get around to it and after several reminders, he said he could not do it until January. I told him that was too late and the contract was cancelled. I tried several other roofers, but nobody could get to it any earlier. So I decided I would do the job myself. I had worked for my father, a home building contractor, on many weekends and during the summers, since I was thirteen years old. Therefore, I figured I could do it.

I went to my local Home Depot, looked at fiberglass composition shingles and decided on the one with the longest warranty: 40 years! At my age. I did not want to be doing this again any time soon. I made a deal with the man delivering the 60 bundles of 50 pound shingles, to hoist them up to me on the roof. But the hydraulic fluid in his machine leaked out on our first try and he was unable to perform the task. I would not be daunted. I carried each one of the bundles up a 10 foot ladder by myself and distributed them onto the lower portion of the front and back of the roof. I finished the job in three weeks. No knee or back problems. No one else would ever guess what I did.

But there was even more to come.

Six months later, my radiologist daughter in Oklahoma City called me bemoaning that her lawn was burning up with the heat. I asked her, "How could it be? Your lot borders on a lake, with a submersible pump and a circular sprinkling system." She replied that her system was like a golf course. It had sprinkler heads that needed to be pushed down and twisted, five heads at a time, which were 60 feet apart.

She would have to do this, go to the control box and turn the pump on. Then she could go to bed, setting her alarm for one hour. She had forty sprinkler stations, which meant getting up eight times during the night. She was exhausted. I asked her why she had not called a local lawn irrigation service to break up the circle into eight stations, with a line and control for each. She said she had, but nobody could get to it until the next January. I told her I could do it. In fact, I reminded her that I had installed the lawn irrigation system at our Lake Cottage, with the help of my two sons, and it worked fine. She said "Daddy, you can't do this. It has been 104-109 degrees every day, and it has not rained for three months. The clay is as hard as concrete." I insisted I could do it, that I was reared in the Altus area, the hottest, driest, windiest part of Oklahoma.

I used her shovel to try to dig the first ditch, and it literally bounced off the hard clay. I got a sharpshooter and it was not much better. I concluded that the only way I could do it was to jump high into the air, and land heavily on the sharpshooter, when it would dig about three inches. With three or four more jumps I got it to the fourteen inch freeze line. I lifted the three inch strip out, moved back three more inches and repeated. In similar fashion, I dug 600 feet of ditches in this manner. That took over 10,000 jumps and the job was finished in two weeks. I would get up, start work at 7 a.m. and labor until 7 p.m. with ten minutes rest every hour, to tank up on water, wipe off the sweat, and berate myself for having volunteered to do the job. I was, however, a man of my word and was not about to give up. The system worked admirably, and the lawn was saved.

But that's not the end of that story.

A year later she married a doctor in Okarche, OK, about 25 miles northwest of the city, and sold her home. I could have killed her. But he is an admirable man and I love them both, so all is forgiven. Again, I had no trouble with the knees or back, or heart. Should I wonder why?

Above All, Do No Harm

The only thing that convinces us doctors is *consistent, safe results*. We have all been led down the primrose path with promising new drugs. These are synthesized, tested in animals and then in humans, over a period of up to ten or more years, and with typical expenditures of millions of dollars before being approved by the FDA. Then we have seen some of them - even after widespread use - withdrawn from the market years later because of dire effects on important organs like the heart, liver, kidneys, bone marrow, GI tract, or during pregnancy, or whatever. How many do we daily prescribe which result in occasional idiosyncratic side effects, even with approved doses and within the acceptable risk-benefit ratios.

But according to a report in the *Journal of the American Medical Association* for July 26, 2000, in the year 1997 alone, over 106,000 patients died inside, and 180,000 died outside hospitals from reactions to properly prescribed and taken drugs. This is the third leading cause of death in the United States, outnumbered only by cardiovascular disease and cancer.

I have seen unwanted side effects with patients in my practice, as have most doctors who prescribe for patients. It has been devastating enough to me and to other healthcare professionals, but how much more so to the patients and their families. The debacle this past year with drugs like Vioxx, Bextra, Celebrex and others, should cause chills to the spine of every doctor prescribing and every patient using prescription medications. Now even the older, non-steroidal NSAIDS including aspirin, Aleve, Naprosen and Ibuprofen have been associated with significantly increased incidence of heart attack and stroke.

Every prescription drug has fine print attached. The Physicians' Desk Reference is packed with millions of warnings, contraindications, side effects and the like. It's the nature of pharmacology and therapeutics.

Yet doctors are constrained by their Hippocratic Oath to "above all, do no harm". That is the ideal. In the real world, prescribing synthetic drugs is usually a choice between the lesser of two evils. It is always using the presumed benefits to the patient to justify the attendant risks. It is an equation we dare not overlook, but one that is often weighted by common practice, by patient expectations and by manufacturer's propaganda.

The Missing Link

The necessary monosaccharide sugars are teamed up with other nutrients enabling body protection, regulation, repair, nourishment and elimination. Glyconutrients are fully documented to be safe, non-toxic and do not interfere with prescription drugs. We are noting across the board, on average, one-third of those taking glyco-supplements show striking improvement; one-third require longer, or larger amounts; and one-third may not respond. Such results as those I described earlier, and now many others, I have not seen before in my 65 years as a doctor!! Nothing is ever 100% - but there must be some other *unknown* essentials, as well as the known. We need oxygen, water, and food: i.e., amino acids, fatty acids, carbohydrates (as fiber and starch) vitamins, minerals, trace elements. None of those known essentials are now likely deficient within our current diet, if we include the increasingly popular and traditional supplements.

But there is something else missing from this list of necessary nutrients. This *missing link* is not really new. It has been there all the time but unfortunately, nutritionists and doctors have taken it for granted, even though it was seen almost everywhere that the cell biologists looked.

The missing link turns out to be nothing more than simple carbohydrates - vitally important 'sugars'. In our sugar-addicted culture we were blinded by the obvious, because we failed to recognize that 'all sugars are not created equal.' Despite all the time we spend advertising and consuming the empty, refined table sugar (sucrose) in all its forms and disguises, we never get beyond its sweet deception. Perhaps our minds were seduced and constrained by our taste buds. Even now, the word 'sugar' brings one thing to our minds, whereas the most important value of carbohydrates remains obscure to almost everyone.

You must now do everything to avoid that trap. You should keep in mind that **there are BAD sugars and there are GOOD sugars!** Just as we had to learn that there was good and bad cholesterol.

Carbohydrates were always acknowledged to be useful in the diet, but just for energy. Not any more. These simple sugars which we now know to be *necessary* for maintaining good health, represent a kind of molecular code. The variety of language, if you like, that allows cell-to-cell communication, derives from the many variations in structure at the molecular level of these different sugars. The term 'necessary' here means indispensable, the body cannot do without it, or else you would have dysfunction, you would be sick or dying.

How important is all this?

VERY IMPORTANT! Do you realize, for example, that human blood types differ in only one small detail: galactose is the terminal 'address' on a glycoprotein found on the surface of the type B red blood cell; then, there is instead N-acetylgalactosamine on the type A. Transfusing a Type A patient with Type B blood (or vice versa) results in a very acute immune-type reaction that can be fatal. Another example: fluid from a rheumatoid arthritis joint shows absence of one terminal glactose molecule in a mild case, and two on examination of the immunoglobulin IgG in a severe case. In principle, could this not be restored to normal and the arthritis relieved upon taking glyconutritionals? Oh, but we recall that galactose is not one of the missing monosaccharides. It's usually available in the normal diet. So what is wrong here? One of the 30+ enzymes required to properly attach galactose is called galactose isomerase, for example. Suppose that this or any of the other 30+ enzymes is inadequate or ineffective in getting the job done, then the galactose is not attached appropriately, and disease occurs anyway: rheumatoid arthritis.

Similarly, interconversion of the different sugars is possible. But the processes are complex, requiring lots of enzymes and also energy. For example, it takes some fifteen enzymatic reactions to convert galactose to fucose. What if there are inborn errors of metabolism and some enzyme is lacking? What if there is a deficiency of the specific vitamins which are 'essential' co-factors for the different enzymes to work? Where does all the energy come from to do all this, just to provide a building block? What if the 'supplier' is late getting to the assembly line? Any of these factors could make the synthesis of the vital 'building-block' glyconutrients (sugars) insufficient or ineffective. It would therefore make consummate sense to make these particular eight necessary sugars readily available in the diet, and to be sure, as regular supplements.

Glyconutrients are safe, non-toxic and do not interfere with prescription drugs.

Conclusion

I am now retired, but I can't deny my love for medicine. Neither can I ignore the recent monumental advancements in the science of nutrition, and especially the role of monosaccharides in the formation of glycoproteins, so vital in the function of the cells of the human body. At age 90+, I am enjoying a new career - to share with everyone I meet, this nutritional breakthrough, and its effect on immune function. Medicine has advanced beyond the primitive treatments of disease, to immunizations, wonder drugs, incredible surgery, organ transplants, and DNA/genomes. We have great expectations from the latter, but the promised wondrous cures are yet years away from application. Even the initial genetic modifications are fraught with the same old side-effects that other synthetics have exhibited.

Glyconutrients are already available, here and now. They are proven safe and effective, awaiting but the eventual universal recognition by all health professionals! The new nutrition: diet, supplementation and exercise, is the keystone of prevention and wellness. I can only predict that it will eventually become the new focus in the practice of medicine.

I may yet see that.

For years, I felt helpless and frustrated, when patients would come to me for advice and relief of their pain and suffering. I was unable to prescribe a safe drug that would relieve or cure them. As a doctor, I trusted in the axiom "*for every disease, a cure*." However, in my whole life as a doctor, I have never seen anything so awesome as I am now seeing: that taking these nutrients orally has enabled patients with all kinds of diseases to improve their condition, sometimes more dramatically than others. I am so excited that now, in my retirement, I have an opportunity to introduce this, to the benefit of more people than ever I did in my 60+ years of practice in the medical profession!

About the Author
Rayburne Goen, MD

Dr. Rayburne Goen earned his Bachelors and medical degrees from the University of Colorado with honors. He served during WWII and later became a Diplomate of the American Board of Internal Medicine; a Fellow of both the American College of Physicians (FACP) and the American College of Cardiology (FACC). He was a Clinical Associate Professor of Medicine, University of Oklahoma School of Medicine, and a Past Vice President and President of the Medical Staff, St. John Medical Center and of St. Francis Hospital, Tulsa, OK, respectively. Two of his four children and one grandson are now following in his medical footsteps. He is a legend in his own time.

Editors note:

The structure of these 'super sugars' you now know as glyconutrients, critically determines their function. You will learn more about this next from one whose personal story and practice reflect daily a structure and function relationship ...

Chapter 3

Structure and Function of Glyconutrients

Dr. Stephen Summey

As a doctor of Chiropractic care for over 25 years I have had keen interest in the benefits of good nutrition on overall health. I have been more impressed with the overall scope and benefit of glyconutrients than any other nutritional supplement that I've encountered in all my years of practice. To be perfectly honest, more than four years ago when I was first introduced to this field, I was very skeptical.

Like most of us, I was taught that we had too much sugar in our diet and we needed to minimize carbohydrates and sugar intake. Besides the fact that we have an overabundance of sugar in our modern over-processed and green-harvested diet, we were convinced that "sugar is a source of energy, and that is the end of the story." I soon learned how wrong this teaching was.

I began to research Glycoscience and found an overwhelming amount of information in the scientific literature that is growing by more than 50 professional papers per day world wide! Yet I learned a long time ago that "What you *know* is not as important as what you *do* with what you know." Taking *action* after reading the information in this book is the most important thing to remember. That's what I did. I used glyconutrients in my own family and soon incorporated them in my clinical practice.

My Personal Experience

As I began to understand that we don't get an adequate quantity and variety of these necessary sugars in our modern diet, I started to supplement my whole family's diet with a convenient complex of these saccharides'. There were also a few other plant based phytonutrients, phyto-sterols and anti-oxidants that I used to complete what may be called an 'optimal health system'. I noticed an increase in my energy very quickly and after six weeks of supplementation, my allergies went away, with no recurrence in over four years. My chronic back and neck pain and stiffness improved noticeably. Needless to say, I was very impressed.

As I said earlier, I was indeed quite skeptical in the beginning, because of all the anecdotal stories I was hearing. There were many dramatic anecdotes of people who were given up by the traditional medical system and who later showed incredible results with glyconutrients. The list of conditions that were helped by such supplements spanned all areas and they seemed to benefit all the body's functions and systems. This intrigued me and I was determined to get to the bottom of this and prove that it was nothing more than some kind of 'snake oil' or other fraud.

Like most medical doctors and chiropractors, I knew the big difference between simply chasing (suppressing or covering up) the symptoms, and treating the cause of patients' problems. I had studied nutrition for over 25 years and yet in so many cases, we were still trained to treat the symptoms with nutrition. After all, it was better than using toxic chemicals or pharmaceuticals - one drug for one disease or symptom - but we were nevertheless still chasing the symptoms with nutrition.

But I had a bigger problem. Many times patients would leave the office with a large quantity of nutritional supplements worth $300 to $400. These patients needed to be supplied with what I considered to be high quality, 'professional line' products. Our inventory grew to $10,000 which required constant monitoring and re-stocking. I realized my front office was becoming a small health food store. The mark up on these products had to be 50% to 100% for this to be profitable. When my patients went to the local stores or mail order sources for their supplements, I lost business. I then had to find more patients to 'unload' my inventory or the products' shelf life would expire. This was becoming more of a burden than I cared for and I decided I wanted no part of being a glorified vitamin salesman. Besides, this was taking me off purpose from my professional practice.

Perfect Timing

My background and training included many professional courses in nutrition. My orthopedic and sports medicine post-graduate certification courses taught me the important role that nutrition played in both recovery from injury and performance on the field. After a few years out of the nutritional arena, I wanted to get back to educating my patients and the public about the critical value of supplementation to health and wellness. It seemed that the timing could not have been better when a patient of mine had me watch a 12 minute video called "Winning the Battle Within".

This video was all about the importance of our immune system and how an award-winning glyconutritional supplement helps our cell-to-cell communication process. Dr. Nugent (President Emeritus of the American Naturopathic Medical Association, ANMA) said on this video "We (the ANMA) gave the glyconutritional complex the award of the year in 1996 and if we had an award of the century, we would have given it this award also!" I saw the video nearly five years ago and it was the start of my educational journey in this new science. It has added benefits to my family, my patients, their families and friends in this town and across the USA and beyond, more than anything I've ever seen!

Sports Takes a Toll

I went to Western State College in Gunnison, on the western slope of Colorado, on an athletic scholarship. I played football for seven years as a running back and line backer, through high school and college. I wrestled for nine years, and pole vaulted competitively for five years. Wrestling and football took a huge toll on my body, leading to eight dislocations of my left shoulder over a two year period. The rotator cuff was so unstable that this shoulder would dislocate at night while I slept! I had reconstructive surgery and missed my sophomore year of wrestling in college to allow the shoulder to recover. In my junior year I finished 3rd in the RMAC (Rocky Mountain Athletic Conference) and qualified for nationals. In my senior year, I experienced a season-ending injury to the left side of my rib cage while wrestling against an opponent at Air Force Academy. I played 15 years of competitive softball until I was 39 years of age. Our team won the State of Colorado A-B open, for the 35 years-and-older division.

I know it was a combination of physical conditioning, diet, and sports performance nutrition which kept me in good physical health all these years. These three things promoted recovery from injuries and allowed me to enjoy overall health and vitality for 25 years of competitive athletics. I was a Nautilus Fitness Instructor while at Logan College and I started a multidisciplinary rehabilitation facility in Longmont, Colorado. This allowed me to maintain good physical conditioning throughout these years.

Another Shoulder, Another Injury!

Four and a half years ago, however, I was rollerblading with my daughter in Boulder, Colorado and I fell twice and dislocated my right shoulder (the good one) both times. Due to its instability, it dislocated three more times that weekend! Five full dislocations

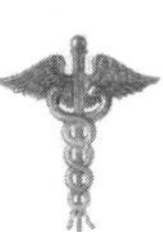

in one weekend and I was thinking "here comes another reconstructive surgery, plus six weeks of disability and six months of rehabilitation" like my other shoulder went through. Fortunately for me, that did not happen because of this new glyconutrient technology and a very special man you are about to meet.

Guidance from an Olympian

I had recently been to a seminar in Denver given by Freddie Williams, a very talented athlete and Canadian Track & Field record holder in the 800 meter event. As I recall from his seminar, he had held the record for ten years and had retired five years before at 38 years of age! He attributed much of his recovery ability, his Canadian records and his Olympic qualification to the use of the glyconutritionals. They were both legal in sport and safe. He related the story of a woman who was an ultra-marathon runner (50 mile races!) who tore her Achilles' tendon and was faced with a career-ending surgery. She used the same glyconutrients internally and topically on the tendon and she was running in two weeks! I remembered this amazing story and figured "what do I have to lose, except for the six weeks of disability and lost income, the cost of the surgery and all the risks involved?" I thank Freddie Williams for all the support, encouragement and guidance he showed and gave to us in that seminar.

I learned there is no toxicity with glyconutrients and that we can get too little of them, but not too much. The amount needed depends on the individual needs at the time. I was desperate and believed my need would be high and I didn't want to mess around with just normal amounts for normal healthy people. My shoulder was not normal and it was not healthy. Therefore, I started on an aggressive program. I used large amounts of the glyconutrients and a sport recovery product; a phytonutrient complex to support the adrenal glands; as well as a topical formula with similar ingredients and a multi-vitamin/mineral supplement with glyconutrients to promote nutrient bioavailability.

Results in Record Time!

In three days, my need for pain medication was gone. I practiced normally with a full load of patients that next week. Within two weeks the shoulder stabilized and no longer wanted to slip out of place or subluxate and I began light rehab exercises. In six weeks, my shoulder was 90% back to normal strength and range of motion, and within 12 weeks after five full dislocations, I was back to even higher levels of strength and mobility than before my injury.

I have a rehabilitation department in my office and I track my workouts daily. This is just not supposed to happen! My orthopedic and sports medicine training taught me that with three dislocations before 30 years of age, surgery is inevitable!' If it had happened to someone else and they told me this story (without an understanding of the science of glyconutrients) I would not have believed them. Yet it happened to me and I was very happy and thankful someone had shared this technology with me.

I was still wondering how the impossible happened to me. How did the shoulder heal without surgery when all my training told me, rotator cuff tears and shoulders with five dislocations don't just tighten up and heal without major surgery? More specifically, they certainly don't do this in 12 weeks! I remembered my first injury and reconstructive surgery to my left shoulder. It took six weeks of immobility in a sling, plus another six months of rehabilitation, and even then it was not more than 90% back to normal.

That was when I really got serious about finding more information regarding this science. I searched on the internet and found a peer reviewed article on inflammation by Doris Lefkowitz PhD[1], and thousands (7,600 as of this printing) of referenced books, journals and articles, about half of them linking to Medline.[2] I printed the inflammation article, read it, re-read it, highlighted it, underlined it and after about five readings, I knew this was the key to how my body healed correctly without reconstructive surgery. I began to "wake up" to the fact that inflammation and the proper functioning of our immune system is a major key to the resolution of many of the top killer diseases!

Abnormal Functioning

It is the normal functioning immune system that recognizes bacteria, viruses, fungus, cancer and *damaged tissue.* When an injury occurs (or when inflammation is present), this sets off a number of biochemical reactions. The neutrophil is one of the first immune cells to arrive at the site of injury. The macrophages, B cells and T cells are a part of this process. If there is lack of or slow healing, this results in chronic inflammation. In other words the inflammatory process does not resolve as it normally should. This is like getting a cut or external wound on your hand and not cleaning it up. This will slow or stop the healing process. Dirt, debris or inflammatory substances, when not "cleaned up" by the immune system, will lead to chronic or unresolved inflammation. This can be mildly annoying or severely disabling, depending on how widespread it is and which tissues are involved. My tissue damage had been truly widespread, clearly recurrent and potentially, severely disabling!

> ***The*** **structure** *of 'sugars' (glyconutrients) determines the* **function** *of glycoproteins which are ubiquitous in cells.*

The 7 years of football, 9 years of wrestling, 15+ years of competitive softball and a total of 13 dislocations have all taken a toll on this 51 year old body. X-rays reveal that I have two discs in my neck that are 50% degenerated (dehydrated) and one disc in my lower back that is 85% degenerated. There is a decrease in the openings for the nerves in my neck and lower back, bone spurs in both areas and I have degenerative arthritis in my spine as a result of all the physical stress and abuse I put my body through.

With this injury to my musculo-skeletal system and subsequent degeneration, I would normally expect to have constant and/or chronic pain and inflammation in my spine, shoulders and many other joints and muscles. However, again fortunately for me, *I am 98% symptom free!* Why, do you think? I believe my level of health and wellness is a combination of good nutrition and supplementation, plus keeping the spinal joints functioning well - in other words, having correct biomechanics of the spine and other joints. Regular chiropractic wellness care is a must here! Regular exercise, in proper combination, helps to stabilize the joints as well as keep them moving, which is the major factor in keeping them 'lubricated'.

A Computer Analogy

For this analogy we will compare a computer to the human body. The hard wiring of a computer must have good connections. The CPU (central processing unit) must have good connections in the back of the computer, with the keyboard, monitor, mouse, printer and other peripherals. The Central Nervous System (CNS) of a human being (brain & spinal cord) is like the CPU or computer's brain. Now in operational terms, the CNS must have good structural connections with the rest of the body (autonomic nervous system & peripheral nervous system). The connecting points are the 24 movable vertebrae of the spine. If there is excessive stress (physical, emotional or chemical) our neuro-musculo-skeletal system will reflect this as physical symptoms like muscle tension, headaches, back aches, numbness, tingling, muscle spasms and pain.

Stress in an electrical system, like a power surge, will blow a fuse or burn out a component. The spine is like a circuit breaker, various stressors will affect our nervous system, then our muscular system, which will cause our joints to malfunction or fixate (get stuck, lock up), or dysfunction. We will know if our *structure* is affected because our *function* will be affected eventually.

Structure vs Function / Hardware vs Software

This *structure vs function* analogy of glycoproteins, from a microscopic point of view, will be covered later in this chapter. What I'm referring to here is our body's structure vs function. That is the macroscopic view. Good posture and muscle tone will support good spinal structure which will lead to good function of our neuro-musculo-skeletal system. If our "hardware" has good "structural" connections it will function well.

Now, let us cover the equally important "software". On a microscopic level our nutrition or malnutrition will affect us biochemically. From the computer analogy, there is only one (software) operating system that runs (most of) our computers and it's called "Microsoft" ™. The software or communication system that "runs" our body is glyconutrients. These necessary nutrients are the communication building blocks which are involved whenever any two cells come together.

Let's ask a question? Which is most important on your computer (assuming you have one) - software or hardware? The obvious answer is that *both* are critical to the proper functioning of your computer. The same is true of our bodies. We are complex products of both structure *and* function at both the macroscopic (anatomical) level and the microscopic (physiological) level. One derives from the other, and *vice versa*. Let's put that in the form of two equations:

At the **macro** level:

BIO-MECHANICS = **ANATOMY** + **'Hardware' Conections**
(Function) **(Structure)**

At the **micro** level:

BIO-CHEMICALS + **'Software' Connections** = **PHYSIOLOGY**
(Structure) **(Functions)**

Bio-chemicals are derived from adequate nutrition (fuel) to provide the molecular structure that is critical for the proper software connections of our immune system. That keeps inflammation under control. And that's just one of the major functions of glycoproteins. We will look at several others later in this same chapter.

So, let's pose another similar question like we did before. Which is most important in our body, bio-mechanics or bio-chemicals? Again, the obvious answer is that *both* are critical for health and wellness.

Biomechanics may refer to the overall *function* of the body as a flexible mobile machine with interdependent parts. But that is clearly derived from the anatomy (structure) of all the body parts. Similarly, bio-chemicals may refer to the molecular *structure* of the cellular components, especially the glycoproteins, with interdependent communications. But that clearly leads to the momentary physiology (function) of all the body's cells. In other words, there can be no separation between structure and function at either macroscopic or microscopic levels. The *structure* of 'sugars' (glyconutrients) determines the *function* of glycoproteins which are ubiquitous in cells. They are therefore the key players!

Genomics vs Glycomics

You have already learned that only eight simple but super sugars are commonly found in the oligosaccharide (more complex sugar) chains of glycoproteins.[3] In fact, only a few decades ago we did not have the technology (such as gel permeation chromatographs and scanning electron microscopes) to know what these saccharides (sugars) were, much less their structures.

When studying the individual components of our DNA and in understanding the genetic code, scientists studied proteins and their amino acid building blocks and nucleic acids. The Genome Project set out to identify and characterize all the genes that make up human chromosomes, which obviously determine the essential variables of cell physiology and therefore all health and disease. It will continue to be important in the future, regarding our understanding and exploitation of human genetics. But the focus has remained on proteins and nucleic acids. Until recently, sugars were simply thought of as unimportant and got cleared away chemically.

Although everyone is familiar with the term 'genetics', we could use the term '*Genomics*' instead, to refer to the study of the structure and function of genes and how they determine all characteristics which manifest in health and disease. *Glycomics*, or the study of how sugars are involved in vital functions in our body, may be understood by the following simple analogy: DNA is the "blue print" of our body like the actual blue prints (or plans) of a new house being built. The general contractor must know how to read the blue prints in order for him to communicate to the subcontractors what needs to be done. For this to happen, the contractor must communicate with all the subcontractors. That's where the vital sugars come in, since they enable the cells to do just that.

Glycoscience refers to the investigation and the understanding of this communication "alphabetic language" of the cells. Glyconutrients are key building blocks of the language of this cellular communication code. Just as important as the alphabet is to the English language, so are the glycoproteins, glycolipids, and proteoglycans (the three main classes of glycoconjugates in our body), to this cellular code. These 'glycoforms' as they are sometimes referred to, surround every cell in the body and according to Professor Murray, "*Glycoproteins are Critical Molecules for Health*". In an article with this title, he talks about the significance of these "sugars attached to proteins" or glyco-proteins.

As we consider further these necessary glyconutrients (sugars) that the cells use to make the variety of *critical glycoprotein molecules,* lets look at the question of structure a little more closely. That will then lead us to their all-important function.

Structure

As previously stated, there are only eight vital sugars known to be present in human glycoproteins. They are all simple sugars or mono-saccharides. Probably the most known and widely accepted and used glycoprotein today is *glucosamine*. Did you ever think of glucosamine as a sugar? Well, glucose is the number one, most prevalent sugar in our diet. When the amine group (compare: like in amino acids, the simple building blocks for proteins) is combined with glucose we get this over-the-counter, naturally-derived product used commonly in the treatment of osteoarthritis.

Glucosamine (as a sulfate or hydrochloride) is actually derived from marine exoskeletons or produced synthetically. It is required for the synthesis of other glycoforms including mucopolysaccharides, which comprise the body's tendons, ligaments, cartilage, synovial fluid, mucous membranes, and structures in the eye, blood vessels and heart valves. Glucosamine stimulates the metabolism of chondrocytes in the articular cartilage and of synoviocytes in the synovial tissues. Of special interest, glucosamine has been demonstrated to stop and possibly even reverse degenerative joint disease. It is often used in conjunction with chondroitin (as sulfate) which belongs to a class of very large molecules called glyco-aminoglycans. They are found in cartilaginous tissues and serve as a substrate for the formation of the joint matrix structure. As such then, the *properties* and use of these saccharides seem to derive essentially from their *structure* and not as much from their unique biochemical activity per se. Clinical and research evidence from all over the world continues to validate the effectiveness of this glycoprotein in helping to support joint health in both animals and humans. And that's just the tiny tip of a huge iceberg.

> *Glycoproteins are critical molecules for health.*
>
> *-Prof. R.K. Murray*

Glycoprotein molecules are structured in so many ways that science is just beginning to understand their complexity. The significance of this has been greatly underestimated until the last few years. The diversity of the structure of glycoproteins is found in the geometric shape of these sugars. There are 5 carbon atoms in xylose, 6 carbon atoms in fucose, galactose, glucose, mannose, N-acetylGalactosamine, N-acetylGlucosamine, and 9 carbon atoms in N-acetylneuraminic acid. These typical ring structures provide several points of attachment for other sugars, fats and/or proteins. As mentioned previously, this variation gives rise to the different glycoforms: namely glycoproteins, glycolipids, and proteoglycans.

Actually, to be more precise, these 'ring' structures are not flat or circular. They are three-dimensional arrangements of the six atoms (including one oxygen) that are more adequatedly described as a 'chair' or 'boat' conformation. But that's probably a bit more chemistry than the typical reader would want or need to know.

Glycosylation

The significance of these simple sugars attaching to proteins (by a process called glycosylation) is evident throughout this whole book, but basically they allow a multitude of biologic properties which greatly affect human health as well as disease. **The great variation of biologic properties that glycoproteins offer is due to the virtually unlimited combinations in which these sugar chains can attach to protein chains and to themselves.** This process of glycosylation requires specific enzymes to attach and detach the sugars to the proteins. The deficiency of an enzyme (for example, lactase), a genetically determined deficiency, will result in lactose (milk sugar or dairy) intolerance, with the well-known accompanying symptoms of bowel gas, cramps and diarrhea. There are many congenital defects in various enzymes which can have profound effects on our health.

Coding Complexity

To give a point of reference for the complexity of sugar chains vs protein chains, we look to the bonding types and sites. For the reader who is interested in the basic science - amino acids have two characteristic groups that are attached to a single carbon atom and give them their name: an amine $-NH_2$ group and a - COOH acid group. These opposite groups combine to form the so called peptide bond.

$-NH_2$	+	$-COOH$	=	$-N(H)CO-$	+	H_2O
amine		carboxylic acid		peptide bond		

In this way, amino acids, the building blocks of proteins, bond together by these peptide bonds to form proteins. There have been 22 different amino acids identified with 10-12 known as 'essential' (must be supplied outside the body from food sources) for survival. By combining amino acids by their simple peptide bonds the most complicated combination is A + B or B + A, or A + B + C, or B + C + A, or C + A + B, etc. In effect then, 4 of these amino acid combinations will produce up to **24** possible combinations.

The critical sugars, on the other hand, are ring molecules with 5, 6 or 9 carbon atoms each of which provides a possible site of bonding with other molecules. Therefore, if we just take 4 sugars combined with their 5, 6, or 9 possible sites of attachment the result is over **124,000 possible combinations**! By combining the eight of these necessary sugars found in glycoproteins, this brings virtually unlimited coding combination possibilities, especially when you add the 20+ different amino acids in proteins and various lipids to this mix. Hence, the possibility for amazing diversity and coding with these sugar moieties attached to proteins.

So much for structure, let's move on to function and explore what these glycoproteins actually do in real life.

Function

The list of functions associated with glycoproteins is already quite extensive and growing all the time. Moreover, many of these functions are critical to cell physiology, especially in terms of cell-to-cell communication.[4]

The structural diversity of glycoproteins directly affects their functional diversity. In simple terms, **structure affects function**. When structure is abnormal, malfunction will follow. Health (and disease) can be considered from the molecular level in terms of this structure-function model. As Professor Murray observed in *Glyconutritionals: Consolidated Review of Potential Benefits,* "All diseases are manifestations of abnormalities of molecules, chemical reactions or processes." The importance of glycoproteins and their function in our body, in particular, is related to the fact that whenever cells communicate with each other, glycoproteins are involved in some way.

Glycoproteins hold cells together (cellular adhesion) to make different tissues, organs, organ systems etc. They allow our immune cells to identify bacteria, viruses, fungus, cancer, foreign material or debris from damaged tissue, and to destroy these invaders and clean up the mess left over from infection or injury.

Glycoproteins are involved in cell signaling - a fact that was not even understood by Southerland and associates, who in 1971 won the Nobel Prize in Physiology or Medicine for discovering the mechanism by which hormones interact with the cell. They thought there was some sort of lock and key mechanism involved. It is now known that glycoproteins form the communicating links that interact with the cell surface membrane, and that hormones don't have to enter the cell to "turn on" various functions of the cell. This is how many hormones work and it explains why such a small amount of any hormone can have such profound effects.

> *Glycoprotein molecules are structured in so many ways that science is just beginning to understand their complexity.*

Glycoproteins are involved in the normal development of the nervous system. There are several congenital disorders of glycosylation (CDG) identified at this early stage in this emerging science, many of which will have mental retardation as a major characteristic sign.

The liquid medium of our blood, the so-called plasma, is mostly glycosylated. So are the clotting factors and the HDL and LDL group of lipoproteins (or the so-called "good and bad cholesterol"). [3]

Communication

All molecular and cell biologists agree that the human cell membrane is composed of a bi-lipid layer, which keeps the extracellular fluids separate from the fluids and structures found inside the cell. There are many different glycoproteins which are an integral part of this membrane.

The structures of molecules on the surface of any given cell are characteristic of that cell and give them virtual ID-tags. Wherever that cell goes, it is assessed as 'friend or foe' and treated with the specificity determined by its ID-Tags. This can have life and death implications. Let's take the most obvious illustration.

Blood transfusion is practiced in almost every hospital in the world everyday. The key to its application is to do a compatibility match between donor and receiver by the characteristic blood groups. The most important (most widely used) system is that of the ABO typing. Now, here's the surprise! The only difference between Type O blood and Types A and B blood is that the glycoproteins on the cell surface of the red blood cells of the Types A and B blood contain one additional sugar molecule. Further, the difference between Type A and Type B blood is only the difference between the sugar on the end of the extensive molecular complex. The Type A blood has an additional acetyl group that Type B does not. The wrong match could be fatal! That's the living difference - all determined by a sugar! And that's only one of them.

That's the living reality of glycoproteins!

Cell to cell "communication" is done by chemical interaction with the cell surface to enable our immune system to properly identify self vs non-self, cancer vs healthy cells, damaged tissue or inflamed tissue which needs to be cleaned up before the body can rebuild and fully heal. This area of cell signaling is a major area of research going on at this time in both the biomedical and pharmaceutical arenas.

To underline its importance, several Nobel Prizes have already been awarded. There are several "sugar" drugs already on the market which have synthetic glycoproteins connected with the bioactive ingredient to provide us with so-called "smart" drugs. Antibacterial classes of drugs, for example, can be made more effective by targeting more specific tissues with glycoprotein technology. This could have major implications for the individual patient. This 'smart' drug technology could spare the healthy microorganisms when fighting bacterial infection. For the world at large, this could reduce the growing threat of 'super bugs' developing because of the overuse and abuse of antibiotics. Some serious biologists have warned that this potential threat exceeds that of nuclear annihilation over time.

Then there is cancer treatment. Everyone knows that one in three persons in industrialized societies is likely to develop some form of cancer. The management options today are classically - chemotherapy, radiation or surgery. Chemotherapy is a feared monster. The side effects are often horrendous with nausea, headaches, weakness, hair loss, weight loss, tissue and sometimes organ damage, etc. That is because anti-cancer drugs are indiscriminate. They affect all cells - both healthy and cancerous. But with glycoprotein technology, as adjuvant therapy, the benefits could in principle be targeted to the specific cancer receptor sites of the diseased tissues. There's hope!

Finally, we should refer to glycoproteins as gatekeepers. Glycoproteins have a regulating effect on ions allowing sodium, potassium, calcium and chloride into and out of the cells. This can have a profound effect on many conditions. One such condition for example, is cystic fibrosis (CF). There is a transmembrane regulator which has glycoprotein to regulate these ions. These ions are responsible for the viscosity of the mucus in the lungs and digestive organs such as the pancreas. Clinical observations have been remarkable regarding the improved digestion, respiratory function and immune regulating effects of glycoproteins on many CF cases. An old name for the condition was 'mucoviscidosis' as mucus plays an extremely important role in this disease. Mucins are also heavily glycosylated, by the way. A more thorough explanation of this process has again been given by Dr. Murray and Jane Ramburg.[5]

Inflammation in Health and Wellness

Inflammation is a normal process which affects all living organisms. It is a response to tissue injury and is a beneficial response if the correct components (nutrients) are found in adequate quantity in these living organisms. If there are missing nutrients or deficiency in certain key glyconutrients, in particular, inflammation can become a major problem. This has only recently been given adequate attention and is being documented by a rapidly growing mountain of scientific research articles and many books on this subject.

One such book is Dr. Fleming's "*Stop Inflammation Now*!" He has over 400 references in his book and speaks of the science of cell-to-cell communication indirectly when he states on page 11, "whenever the cells of your immune system spring into action, they have to communicate with each other in order to coordinate their attack on a disease-causing agent or cancer cell."[6]

One would imagine that this is an intuitive observation. The immune response can be compared to going to war! And you really don't have to go through military college or officers training to realize that a key strategy in any war is to knock-out and dismantle the enemy's communication lines as quickly as possible, while doing everything to protect and preserve your own. Effective communication is indispensable in war! And therefore, for any effective immune response, cell-to-cell communication is paramount. It is a coordinated response with extreme specificity. Each cell must be fulfilling its own role, but must also be in concert with all the other cells. They must all know **when to act** and certainly **when to stop acting**.

Dr. Fleming has pointed out 12 factors that link in a chain reaction which perpetuates or normalizes the critical process of inflammation. Many of these links are directly affected by glycoproteins. We also know now that factors like serum cholesterol, triglycerides, excess body weight, antioxidants, the immune system and other important physiological processes, are positively influenced by a proper combination of supplemental levels of glyconutrients. A balanced and adequate diet is of course the most important factor and by consuming 6 to 9 servings of fresh vegetables and tree-ripened fruits, we dramatically reduce undesirable inflammatory components (like free radicals) in our blood. Moderate regular exercise can also go a long way to bring other factors mentioned under control.

To sum it up Doris Lefkowitz, PhD stated in a previously mentioned article "*Glyconutritionals: Implications in Inflammation*" that "Inflammation is a condition to which we all can relate ... good nutrition enables the body to deal more effectively with many pathologic conditions, including inflammation." [1]

Conclusion

Physiologically, *structure* and *function* are interrelated at both the macroscopic and microscopic levels.

The unique molecular structure of monosaccharides is exploited in nature to maximum advantage. The eight necessary and vital sugars combine with proteins (and peptides) to provide a wide diversity of

structures that allow the 'language' for cell-to-cell communication to coordinate and control many important physiological ***functions*** - that is indeed the '*sweet language of life.*'

About the Author:
Stephen R. Summey, DC., FACO., CCSP

Dr. Stephen Summey obtained his Bachelor's in Biology, Psychology and Health Education, from Western State College of Colorado and his Doctor of Chiropractic from Logan College, St. Louis. He is also certified in Chiropractic Orthopedics and Sports Injuries. He runs an active, reputable chiropractic practice and has also been a contributor and proctor for the Colorado State Board of Chiropractic Examiners.

Editors note:

By now you must be getting the idea that glycoproteins have a major impact on the body's immune (defense) system. You're certainly right. An expert, previously employed by the US Patent Office, will spell it out more clearly in the next chapter ...

Chapter 4

Glyconutrients and the Immune System

Dr. John Rollins

I came to know about glyconutrients some twenty years ago in connection with my employment at that time. In 1982 I went to work as a Chemical Patent Examiner at the United States Patent and Trademark Office (USPTO) in Washington, DC. My docket consisted primarily of patent applications which disclosed compositions comprising Bio-Affecting Plant extracts and carbohydrates. Prior to my tenure at the USPTO I was a member of the faculty of the College of Medicine in the Department of Microbiology at Howard University in Washington, DC. My examining and management experiences at the USPTO exposed me to many of the leading pharmaceutical and nutritional discoveries of the last two decades. The invention that most captured my interest and imagination during that time was the discovery of the important role that certain dietary sugars played in human health. These sugars are being studied vigorously and the impact of their role in cell communication and adhesion, fertilization, inflammation, differentiation, immune system function and human disease is now coming to light.

Some Watershed Patents

During the mid 1980s, I began examining a series of patent applications submitted by a Dr. Bill McAnalley and some other colleagues. Dr. McAnalley is a research pharmacologist and toxicologist from Dallas, TX. He and his research team had been studying the gel of the Aloe vera plant with the hope of discovering the active healing agent present within the gel. Derivatives of Aloe vera had been used for centuries, both topically and internally, and a wide variety of health benefits had been widely attributed to their use. This research team made the discovery of the principal healing component and a means of stabilizing this component. Also, included in these applications, were formulations of compositions comprising the newly found active component, methods for using the composition and processes for preparing and stabilizing the active component. Dr. McAnalley's breakthrough discovery was identified as a long-chain carbohydrate molecule consisting primarily of a sugar called mannose. For this new discovery, and those that followed, more than 50 patents, both U.S and international, were awarded to Dr. McAnalley and his group.

This discovery was revolutionary because it was completely contrary to what scientists believed at that time. Most bio-medical researchers and educators had their focus on nucleic acids and peptides as the major active biological molecules. In fact, molecular biology had essentially become the study of genes, nucleic acids in DNA, and the synthesis and deployment of the proteins that they directed. "Sugars" on the other hand, were the stepchild of science. The primary and most important role of sugars was to provide energy for the cell. It was believed that all sugars in the body are converted to glucose and then, glucose is converted into all other biological sugars, sometimes called the **'glucose only' theory**. That was standard dogma.

This discovery was derived from an edible food product - not a synthetic drug - and so it laid the foundation for an entirely new class of necessary nutrients to be later called glyconutrients. By the mid 1990's, Professor Robert Murray observed that of the 200 monosaccharides that occur in nature, no more than 10 different ones are commonly found associated with proteins and lipids within the cells of the body, as well as on their important surfaces, and in the extra cellular fluid.[1] These sugars are identified throughout this book and by now you are becoming acquainted with them.

Dr. Murray also reasoned that these sugars might somehow play a key role in cellular communication. These observations and those of other scientists confirmed the speculations of Dr. McAnalley, Dr. H. Reg McDaniel and others, who had begun studies on the possibility that other sugars in addition to mannose might be beneficial for human supplemental consumption and that they might also support the immune system. These studies led to the formulation and patenting of the only complete dietary supplement composition comprising all eight of the known necessary sugars identified above.

Coming Home

This brings me back to a more personal note. During the time that I was examining patent applications for the first generation of glyconutrients, my wife was diagnosed with having systemic lupus erythematosus. This is the disease condition commonly known as lupus. It is a systemic illness whereby the immune system malfunctions in such a way that the body treats many of its own cells as though they were 'foreign'. It mounts an inflammatory immune response to fight back against itself, as it were. As such, it can affect almost any organ at any time. It takes different forms but generally, the patient with lupus tends to have periods of exacerbation and remission. Good medical management is essential, but unfortunately, sometimes even with the best of care, the disease is aggressive and the patient's condition can deteriorate irreversibly.

My wife's condition was such that her immune system was destroying her own red blood cells. In other words, her immune system did not recognize her red blood cells as her own. In the 1980s as well as now, the major course of treatment has been the administration of potent immunosuppresive drugs, particularly prednisone. Her future health did not look promising. That was so until she began a regimen of the same patented glyconutrient composition. After having been on prednisone for eleven and a half years with all its side effects, then with only two months of consumption of glyconutrients and phytonutrients, her rheumatologist began to wean her off prednisone. This process took a year. During this time she did not experience any drug withdrawal symptoms or any signs of lupus.

Today, my wife has been off prednisone and remains lupus free for more than seven years. You can therefore appreciate why I hold some convictions about the value and efficacy of supplementing one's diet with glyconutrients. You might also appreciate why I chose to contribute a chapter on this particular title for this composite book.

Components

A thorough treatment and consideration of the workings of the human immune system, one of the most complex and complicated systems in the body, is virtually impossible in the limited space of one chapter. Therefore, I will limit the discussion here to the general issues, with a few specific examples of the role that glyconutrients play in the structure and functioning of the immune system.

The immune system is comprised of both specialized cells (in the *cellular* response) and specialized cellular secretions (in the *humoral* response). The cellular components consist of several types of white blood cells known as neutrophils, macrophages, natural killer cells, and T- and B- cells. The humoral components comprise cytokines and other glycoforms. (Note the *glyco-* prefix immediately here, it implies 'sugars' are involved.)

Neutrophils are small white cells that are part of our first line of defense. They are small but numerous and are the first to arrive at an injury site. There they engulf the invading microbes via phagocytic action. Neutrophils also produce enzymes that digest surrounding damaged tissue. These cells sacrifice themselves to protect the injured or infected tissue.[2]

Macrophages, sometimes called the 'big eaters', are the largest of the white blood cells. The main function of the macrophage is to evaluate and destroy pathogenic invaders by engulfing them. Macrophages are found in all our organs and tissue systems and after a while they become specialists in protecting "their" organs. When macrophages are activated they move into action. Macrophages are constantly on patrol, looking for damaged cells, aging cells, foreign invaders, etc. They do this by touching their surfaces with the surfaces of the cell they are assigned to protect. It is like reading or feeling the "Braille" of the cells' surface.[3] During this process of touching, they are actually comparing the information found on their surface glycoproteins with the glycoproteins of their host cells! (Note the *glyco-* again. It implies 'sugar'.) An amazing amount of information is obtained by the macrophages during this constant touching. They can determine if the cells are healthy, damaged, infected or cancerous. These macrophages are more tenacious than their little brothers, the neutrophils. They can live a long time and can engulf larger pathogens and larger amounts of cellular debris.

You may be itching to find out more already, but I will address the role of glyconutrients in more detail, later in this chapter.

The next groups of cells that are found in our immune system are the so-called "*Natural Killer Cells*" or NK cells. These cells do not destroy by engulfing, but by chemical means. They are able to use enzymes and other chemical weapons to destroy the enemy. However, NK cells can misfire. They have been known to destroy host tissue as they fight their battles. As we grow older, their numbers decrease and they can be overcome by conditions such as AIDS and cancer.[4,5] However, glyconutrients have been shown to increase the numbers and the activity of NK cells.[6] There we go again with glyco-nutrients.

Now it's time to introduce the generals among the immune cells. If neutrophils, macrophages and natural killer cells are the soldiers of the force, B- and T-lymphocytes are the generals. They are the most elite specialists of our immune system. *B-cells* produce the target specific antibodies of the immune system. Antibodies are part of the humoral immune response and are found in the blood and other body fluids. *T-cells* are in charge of the cellular immune response. They have the knack of personally taking charge of neutralizing and destroying invaders such as bacteria, viruses, fungi and unwanted particles.

There are other highly specialized T-cells such as *helper* T-cells and *suppressor* T-cells. Helper T-cells stimulate an immune response and suppressor T-cells suppress or stop a response. Space does not allow us to elaborate further, but if either of these groups of cells is out of balance or malfunctions, autoimmune disorders or immunodeficiencies can develop. Lupus, cancer and AIDs are just three examples, but there are literally hundreds of known diseases attributable to a dysfunctional immune system. Many chronic diseases in particular, like rheumatoid arthritis, MS, diabetes, thyroditis, etc. are believed to have autoimmune causes.

Lastly we have a group of specialized chemical components known as *cytokines*. This group includes interleukins, tumor necrosis factors, lymphokines and interferons. The various cytokines assist B- and T- cells in identifying their targets. Glyconutrients make it possible for our cells to increase the supply of cytokines.[7] By now, that must be no surprise. Macrophage activity is stimulated by glyconutrients. Mannose, galactose and polysaccharides containing these sugars have been shown to activate macrophages.[8,9,10] Activation means that these cells are primed to go into action and perform their functions. These activated macrophages set a series of immune functions in motion by the production and release of cytokines. These cytokines carry and convey specific messages that direct, for example, T- and B- cells to specific sites so that they can attack foreign invaders and particles.[11,12,13] In cancers, for example, activated macrophages can produce tissue necrosis factor that specifically targets the cancer at hand.[14]

Challenges

Our world today confronts us with many challenges. Many of these environmental and pathogenic challenges did not exist during our grandparents' and great-grandparents' generations. We are faced with high levels of stress, toxins, pollutants, poor nutrition and increases in metabolic diseases and disorders. These conditions are thought by some to be, to some significant extent, the result of today's nutritional deficiencies!

Most of us today know that we need nutrients such as amino acids for proteins, fatty acids to build lipids and fats, plus vitamins and minerals for enzymes and much more, all in our diets. We have known that these nutrients are 'essential' to our health and well-being. The majority of the population even uses some form of supplementation to ensure adequate supplies of these essential nutrients in a convenient form.

Yet, our overall health is nowhere near optimal. Chronic diseases are on the rise and medical science is not providing viable or cost-effective solutions. Something, is generally "missing" in our diets. More and more research findings are linking disease states with weak and imbalanced immune systems. At the same time, other scientists are finding that properly glycosylated proteins and lipids are 'essential' for the proper operation of our cells and especially our immune systems. In other words, the more we learn about health and disease states, the more we become aware of the importance of having a strong and healthy immune system. In addition, we are learning that a special class of carbohydrates, necessary sugars or glyconutrients, may be the other missing and even 'essential' nutrients in our diets.

Technically, the term '**essential**' may have a double meaning in this context. First, these nutrients are essential in that human life as we know it could not exist without them. But further, the term also implies that the body can do nothing to substitute for these nutrients if they are not consumed. In other words, the body cannot make them. Therefore, in the true sense, all 22 amino acids for example, are essential in the first sense but only a limited number, perhaps 10 or 12, are essential in the second sense, since inter-conversion is possible. In the case of sugars, we know that they are essential, in the first sense at least, although perhaps 'indispensable' would be a better term, but again inter-conversion by enzyme reactions is possible. However, this inter-conversion process is rather complex, enzyme dependent, energy consuming and prone to error. At least we can underline their importance if we emphasize that the glyconutrients are necessary and indeed, vital to human health.

Research is linking many modern diseases with poor or malfunctioning immune systems and clinical research is also finding that the addition of glyconutrients to the diet can correct many of these conditions. The following is a list of some of the conditions that are responding positively to improving the health of the immune system with dietary glyconutrients:

- cold viruses, flu viruses, herpes viruses;
- bacterial, fungal and parasitic infections;
- allergies, asthma, burns, topical wounds,
- fibromyalgia and chronic fatigue syndrome,
- arthritis, diabetes, lupus, multiple sclerosis and other autoimmune diseases,
- cancer, hepatitis, HIV, premature aging,
- sexual dysfunctions, Alzheimer's, ADHD, depression,

- hypertension, heart disease, etc. ..

This is by no means a complete list. When we look for the underlying link, we find insufficient amounts of glyconutrients/or glycosylation problems and malfunctioning immune system components could very well be at fault.

Researchers have shown that administering a proprietary complex of glyconutritionals can enhance the immune system of rodents. Their findings show that glyconutritional-treated animals exhibited tumor regression and an increased number of animals recovered completely. Animals that recovered from tumor transplants rejected subsequent tumor transplants.[15] In his later chapter on glyconutrients and cancer, Dr. Emil Mondoa presents an extensive review of the role of glyconutrients in the course of many cancerous conditions. Dr. Mondoa shows that not only do glyconutrients enhance the immune response to tumors but also improve the body's tolerance of chemotherapy and radiation.

Virus infections are very common in our modern world. Viruses are very small biological entities that are comprised of nucleic acid (DNA or RNA chains) and protein, while some have lipid or fatty coats. Viruses cannot reproduce or live outside a living cellular host. Therefore, they depend on a host cell to reproduce themselves and to exert their biological effects. Viruses can be specific in their preferred host animal and even for particular cells within the host. Cold viruses (rhinoviruses), for example, prefer the respiratory tract cells. Other viruses prefer other tissues and organs.

The more we learn about health and disease, the more we become aware of the importance of a strong and healthy immune system.

Viral infections are very difficult to treat; they are not sensitive to antibiotics. Medical science has developed only a few antiviral agents. However, they are not always effective and their use in treatment is very expensive. That leaves us with dependence on our immune systems. Fortunately many viral infections are self-limiting and do not kill their host. Many viruses have the uncanny ability to undergo subtle genetic changes that make mounting an effective defense rather difficult. Minor changes or variations in the antigens of viruses demand adjustments in the agents and/or antibodies needed from immune cells for the effective removal of the invaders. If outside intervention is difficult or nonexistent, that leaves us with the need to strengthen our immune systems.

Let's take a look at our old friend, the cold virus, again. This virus is known to gain entry into our bodies by attaching to specific receptors on the surface of mucosal cells, like those lining the nasal passages, the mouth and the eyes. Researchers have known for many years that if these cold virus receptors could be blocked, the viruses would not be able to attach and enter the cells. If they cannot enter the cells they cannot infect the cells and cause colds.[16]

Two studies at Johns Hopkins have confirmed the ability of saccharides to prevent colds in children.[17,18] Oligofructose compounds were used in studies to determine their effect on the occurrence of gastrointestinal problems in children. The investigators were observing the increase or decrease of stomach and intestinal problems with oligofructose supplementation. To their surprise, they noticed that children who received the oligofructose supplements had fewer colds than those in the placebo-controlled group. Those in the treatment group who did get colds, had fewer colds and milder symptoms, and the duration of those symptoms was shorter than in the control group. Similar studies with the influenza virus have been performed in mice. These studies showed that glyconutrients could protect animals against the flu or help later to fight it off.[19,20]

Dr. McAnalley, and his group, in their Australian patent showed that **glyconutrients can have a positive health promoting effect in patients with a wide variety of disease conditions.**[21] When we consider that all disease states begin at the cellular level, it is not difficult to see how glyconutrients could play such an important role in our health and well-being. Our bodies are comprised of cells that must work together, as each carries out its individual function. These individual functions are not carried out in isolation but in harmonious cooperation. Cellular interaction and communication require a system that is precise, specific and fast. Each cell must have all the communication tools available to it, at all times, on demand.

Imagine that you have just scratched yourself. Within a few seconds the wound begins to sting and in a few more seconds, it becomes red and begins to pull the edges together before your very eyes. This event begins the influx, or as some call it, the cascade of immune cells and cytokine reactions. Now, what if your immune system was impaired, or your cells in the wounded area were not able to communicate their needs? What would be the consequence? The consequence of course, would be infection and/or disease.

Imagine this same sequence happening in one or more of your joints. Somehow there has been a change in the antibodies that are near your knee cartilage and they think that your knee belongs to someone else. Remember their job is to protect you from foreign invaders. Now your knee joint is thought to be the foreign invader and the antibodies attack your cartilage. What could cause this? Some researchers think that rheumatoid arthritis (RA) results from a bacterial infection and your immune system mistakes your cartilage for the bacterium.

Dr. John Axford at the Royal Academy of Medicine in Great Britain has found malformed antibodies in patients with RA. His studies grew out of observations of pregnant women who have arthritis. Surprisingly, during their pregnancies and during breast-feeding, they had no RA symptoms. We now know that the arthritic diseases are a group of inflammatory disorders in which improper *glycosylation* seems to be at the core. Also, decreases in galactose residues are seen in the related IgG immunoglobulins. The mechanisms of improper glycosylation are beyond the scope of this chapter. However, just a little of the science is important to note. Dr. Axford's work is leading to techniques that can distinguish between various rheumatoid diseases. Results suggest that each disease is associated with a specific mechanism that gives rise to alterations in the normal glycosylation pattern of IgG. 'Sugar printing' of IgG is therefore a potential means for the differentiation of rheumatic diseases and may provide insight into their origins."[22] In other studies, Dr. Axford has observed that when galactose is added to the diet of patients with aberrant IgG molecules, the RA symptoms are abated.

Author Rita Elkins, in her booklet Miracle Sugars, states that "*correct immune system response is complicated even further by the fact that many infectious agents routinely mutate, confusing the immune system. This explains why we can catch multiple colds and flu over the course of time. Each time there is a mutation, a new antigen needs to be developed. This requires a complex communication cycle between T-and B- immune cells. The faster this occurs, the faster the immune system can prevent and heal damage from mutated infectious agents. Once the new antibody signature is learned by the immune system, it stays in the memory forever. Having a ready supply of glyconutrients may also help the body speed up this process.*"[23]

Many researchers around the world are doing extensive studies on determining the structure and content of glycoproteins and glycolipids found on the surface of cells. Some studies involve the study of the association between glycosylation and immune complex formation in various disease groups. They isolate immune complexes and IgG from serum and evaluate the carbohydrate content using very sophisticated methods. Researchers are finding more of the N-acetylglucosamine sugar in complexes from patients with rheumatoid arthritis than in those from patients with systemic lupus erythematosus, Crohn's disease, or infectious endocarditis, or from normal controls. Much of this kind of research is leading to the conclusion that immune complexes from various disease conditions are distinct from each other. This kind of information, referred to by Dr. Axford as sugar printing, may yet lead to the development of various new diagnostic tools.

Also, as we and others have stated, glycosylation has a very important effect on the activity of immunoglobulin molecules. One of the earliest observations of these differences was that of Bond and coworkers.[24] They also noted that the carbohydrate composition of immunoglobulins associated with RA lacked terminal galactose sugar residues. This terminal absence of galactose residues may be responsible for inducing rheumatoid factor production and immune complex formation. Axford's work has led to an understanding that when galactose (a glyconutrient) is added to the diet of many of these rheumatoid patients, this malformation can be repaired and immune complex formation does not occur.

Glycosylation Is Key

Many proteins critical to normal cell physiology are glycosylated (have sugars attached), and variations in their glycosylation pattern often lead to changes in their function. Most major diseases are associated with a change in the glycosylation pattern of a critical protein structure. Researchers are exploring these changes both in health and disease. They are developing new methods and techniques so that they can be investigated more efficiently. They are trying to find out what the implications are to further understanding disease mechanisms and treatment. These studies are very important to gain better knowledge of how glyconutrients work in our cells. However, we already know enough to realize that these nutrients are very important to our health and well being. Of that, there should be no longer any doubt.

As this new century begins, many discoveries will be made that will increase lifespan and improve the quality of life. However, there are many diseases such as cancer, autoimmune conditions, immunodeficiency disorders and congenital conditions that continue to be a scourge on mankind. Medicine as we know it today, may not have sufficient answers. Several new emerging therapies and "tools such as immunotherapy or immunoceuticals, can now be included in the general category of nutraceuticals, or dietary supplements."[25]

There have been many new discoveries made and those found in naturally occurring substances are proving to be keys in this new disruptive approach to wellness. At the center of these discoveries is and will be, dietary or necessary carbohydrates. For example, more than 50 mushroom species have yielded potent immunoceuticals, particularly as anticancer agents. Kidd and his research team have proposed a mechanism of action for mushroom glucans.[25] Many of the details of the actions of glyconutrients are still unclear, but the ongoing research will provide more precise information in the future. However, based upon what we know today the following is a simplified sketch of a possible glyconutrient/immune system interaction.

In this scheme, a foreign invader or toxin comes in contact with the skin. Keep in mind that there are many pathways that may exist in the immune system. Dendritic or Langerhans cells residing in the skin, for example, are capable of detecting a foreign threatening assault and mobilizing an appropriate immune response. According to Kidd and others, due to their widespread localization throughout tissues, dendritic cells are the first cellular line of defense of the immune system. They are likely to be the first host cells to contact incoming glycoform material. As these sugar components enter the mouth, for example, they can be sampled by the Langerhans cells present in the oral mucosa, and then by dendritic cells in the stomach and intestines. Following absorption and circulation to the liver, glyco-materials are sampled by the dendritic-like Kupffer cells. These glycoforms assist the different cell types in carrying out their protective functions. Carbon-14 studies have shown that large oligosaccharide molecules (containing a few sugars connected together) can be absorbed directly from the small intestines into the blood stream.

So much for detection and protection. Now, here's a brief, simplified outline of how the immune response cascade might work.

Glyconutrients stimulate neutrophils and macrophages into action to put them on alert. This activation results in heightened immune response. Once the glyconutrients are picked up by dendritic cells and other antigen-sorting cells, they are primed to go into action. Then, after the macrophages and other cells are activated, they may also encounter other stimulants such as specific antigens from the invader or from tumors. Some macrophages may go on to attack the invader or tumor cells directly while others may present samples of the foreign antigens to T-lymphocytes (helpers). These helper cells can now go on to stimulate cytotoxic T-lymphocytes while other helper cells stimulate B-lymphocytes to make specific antibodies. Others stimulate Natural

Killer cells. All these activated cells may go on to attack the invader or tumor cells. The stimulated T-cells have long-term memory and will know which antibodies to produce when they encounter the specific antigens again. When the response and attack is complete, a healthy immune system produces suppressor T-cells to stop the response. This last step is crucial, because any kind of 'overkill' or overactive immune response would be seriously self-defeating in the end.

When All Else Fails

No review of the immune system in this generation would be complete without discussion of the modern pandemic we know as Acquired Immuno Deficiency Syndrome (AIDS)

Over the past twenty years, we have witnessed the spread of this pandemic, now known to be caused by the human immunodeficiency virus (HIV). The retrovirus gets into cells of the immune system and destroys them with devastating consequences. Patients suffer from fatigue, intermittent fever, weight loss, opportunistic infections and more. Management protocols have been devised after aggressive research in this area and today, a triple cocktail of anti-retroviral drugs has proved lifesaving for many who can afford them. But we are a long way from conquering this disease.

Most major diseases are associated with a change in the glycosylation pattern of a critical protein structure.

Early in this new pandemic, some anecdotal reports from AIDS patients who had consumed a stabilized Aloe vera beverage, indicated that they had experienced significant clinical benefits. Dr. Reg McDaniel led a team of researchers to explore this possibility further. Aloe extract was given to 41 patients who improved their Walter Reed Staging for AIDS by 71% in three months and those who stayed on the program showed consistent improvements for up to 6 years.

McDaniel and his group verified that the same active ingredient, now known to be polymannose (PM) was involved. They used sophisticated methods to demonstrate a dose-response (ie. more PM, more results) for PM induction of interleukins 1, 2 and 6, gamma interferon, tumor necrosis factor, along with granulocyte/macrophage growth factor in mixed leukocyte cultures in the laboratory. They also showed that AIDS patients who were deteriorating despite being on the triple-cocktail, when given polymannose and micronutrients that support cytokine synthesis, showed significant reduction in their clinical symptoms. Viral loads also declined.

The next investigative step in examining the potential for a non-toxic complex saccharide to improve the quality of life and prognosis for AIDS patients was carried out in Belgium. In a small, double-blind pilot study, minimally symptomatic HIV-positive patients were given the drug AZT, oral aloe polymannose, each alone and in combination. The nausea and vomiting of AZT administered patients were reduced and evidence of bone marrow toxicity was also reduced. In this case, however, clinical improvements were not statistically significant. At least, this was suggestive of the value of polymannose as possible adjuvant therapy in AIDS patients.

The Canadian HIV Trials Network conducted a randomized, placebo-controlled pilot study in approximately 100 advanced AIDS patients with CD4s of less than 200, suffering chronic progressive deterioration from both HIV-1 and drug toxicity. The rate of deterioration of the patients was noticeably reduced by the rate of decline in CD4 helper lymphocytes and there were noted improvements in their quality of life.

Further investigations for using aloe polymannose in AIDS patients was abandoned due to the lack of dramatic benefits in independent pilot studies, lack of research funds, and a predictive pilot study which indicated that patients with a CD4 helper lymphocyte count of less than 200 and a highly elevated viral load would not respond to the polymannose glyconutrient. Some AIDS patients were clearly more responsive than others.

When one considers the nature of this AIDS pandemic, the exorbitant costs of standard antiretroviral drug therapy; the comparatively low cost of glyconutrient preparations; the virtual absence of toxicity (and especially compared to the drug cocktails); the magnitude of need in economically depressed populations around the world and the immeasurable cost in human suffering and potential life lost - there is an urgent cry for further research in this area. Could glyconutrients offer at least some hope in this bleak and desperate situation? That question demands attention, funding, research and hopeful application. That is a critical challenge in our generation.

Conclusion

Glyconutritional supplements support normal healthy structure and function of the body. They support cell-to-cell communication and modulate the immune system. Much more research is needed to uncover how glyconutrients work in our cells. This is the focus of the emerging science of Glycomics. The immunologists, cell biologists, developmental biologists and others will one day be able to understand far more than they can today about Glycomics and Glycobiology. Also, the pharmaceutical industry will have developed more targeted glycoform drugs as the complex sugar codes are decoded.

However - and here's the important bottom line for you - you don't have to wait! There are effective glyconutrient foods and supplements already available. Remember the data now shows that the eight necessary sugars and derived glycoforms are involved in almost every process that takes place in your cells and your immune system depends on them, not only for its proper structure but also, for its critical functioning. As such, these necessary sugars could not be any more vital to your health. That's news! Great news!

About the Author

John W. Rollins, Ph.D.

Dr. Rollins received his BS degree from Norfolk State University, Norfolk, VA in Biology; his MS degree from Tuskegee University, Tuskegee Institute, AL, and his MA and PhD degrees from the State University of New York at Buffalo in Developmental Biology. He did two years of Postdoctoral studies in Chemical Carcinogenesis at the New York University College of Medicine, Dept of Pathology. He has held positions as a research Assistant Professor, Dept of Pathology, NYU College of Medicine; Assistant Professor, Dept. of Microbiology, Howard University College of Medicine; Chemical Patent Examiner , Patentability Review Examiner and Quality Assurance Specialist at the U.S. Patent and Trademark Office. His specialty was Bio-affecting plant extracts and carbohydrate compositions. Dr. Rollins is married with three adult children and two grandchildren.

Editors Note:

The biggest threat to the immune system on a constant basis is that of infection by unhealthy microorganisms. As you are about to learn next, that threat is much bigger than you might think ...

Chapter 5

Glyconutrients and Infectious Diseases

Dr. Daniel Fouts

In the beginning -

1929	Penicillin is discovered.
1946	Penicillin becomes available commercially and miraculous recoveries from bacterial infections begin.
1948	Penicillin resistant bacterial strains have already appeared.
1960's	Over 25,000 antibiotics are available for doctors' use.
1970's	Rapid emergence of methicillin resistant *staphylococcus aureus* (MRSA).
1980's	Predictions made that infectious diseases will be conquered by the end of the century.
1990's	Superbugs are now defeating the most powerful antibiotics we have.
2002	"VRSA: The Worst Has Finally Happened" the development of vancomycin resistant *staphylococcus aureus*.
2004	Washington News Conference: "Bad Bugs, No Drugs: As Antibiotic Discovery Stagnates - A Public Health Crisis Brews." Of 506 new drugs in Development, only five are new antibiotics.
2005	'Super MRSA' is now community acquired.

The Saga continues....

July 23,2002 - Chicago Tribune headline: "Unhealthy Hospitals - 103,000 Preventable Deaths in the year 2000", with the following observations:

- 50-60% of the more than 2 million nosocomial infections each year are caused by antibiotic-resistant infections. Nosocomial - means 'originating or taking place in a hospital' - in this case, nosocomial infection (that is, you got it after you went to the hospital).

- Results in 103,000 deaths from infections that could not be treated and also a health care system cost of $5 - 30 billion.

Here come the Viruses ...

- Few effective antiviral medications exist.
- Rapid viral mutations constantly render medications ineffective.
- Viral released enzymes alter our tissue cell surfaces making us more susceptible to opportunistic bacterial infections as well.
- AIDS virus kills 1.2 million in sub-Saharan Africa alone.
- Hepatitis C poses a bigger potential threat worldwide than AIDS.

November 25, 2004 - WHO Warns of Dire Flu Pandemic

- The World Health Organization has issued a dramatic warning that the bird flu virus will trigger an overdue international pandemic that could kill up to 7 million people. Between 25-35% of the world population would likely fall ill.

- Three pandemics occurred in the 20th century-
    - 1918-19 Spanish Flu - as many as 50 million people died worldwide - some developed symptoms in the morning and were dead by nightfall.
    - 1957 - Asian Flu - nearly 700,000 in US and 1 million worldwide died.
    - 1968 - Hong Kong Flu pandemic - nearly 1 million died worldwide.

Of course there are still the yeasts, parasites and other pathogenic organisms waiting their turn to wreak havoc on our bodies - and we haven't even mentioned the genetically-altered potential bioterrorism bugs yet!

The above could easily provide plenty of script ideas for a host of Hollywood horror movies. Unfortunately for many people, it is more like participating daily in an infectious disease episode of 'Reality TV.'

To say that we desperately need more options for controlling and managing today's infectious diseases would be a major understatement.

New Options

Fortunately, recent discoveries relating to how our bodies prevent and fight infections give us at least some new options. We've gained a lot of knowledge about the immune system that protects us naturally. However, the old adage that "Knowledge is Power" is actually not true. It's the ability to *apply* that knowledge that gives one the power. It's important that you learn about those options but far more important that you take the next step and apply the knowledge.

When you say 'carbohydrate' or 'sugar' today - most people immediately start thinking about junk food, or the Atkin's Diet, or diabetes and sugar avoidance, or other negative thoughts. However, just as there is good cholesterol and bad cholesterol, it turns out that **there are good sugars (bioactive, structural, building blocks) and bad sugars (empty calories, devoid of vital nutrients).** The pharmaceutical industry recognized this principle in the past few decades, as you will notice from the following quotes from medical and scientific journals.

• "New carbohydrate technology will provide novel products for treating a broad range of diseases, including immune disorders, cancer, infectious diseases and cardiovascular conditions." ***Biotechnology***, Vol 9, July 1991.

We desperately need more options for controlling and managing today's infectious diseases.

• "The day may not be far off when antiadhesive drugs, possibly in the form of pills that are both sugar-coated and sugar-loaded will be used to prevent and treat infections, inflammations, the consequences of heart attacks and perhaps even cancer." ***Scientific American***, Jan 1993, p89

• **Glycocompounds '98**, Intertech's Business Development Forum on Bioactive Carbohydrates brought together in Vancouver, Canada, 22 of the top pharmaceutical, biotechnology and multi-national chemical companies worldwide. Their purpose was to map out a path for glyco-drug development of the anti-cancer, anti-infective, anti-inflammatory, anti-biotic and anti-viral potential of glyconutrients.

• "Recognizing the importance of sugars in health and disease, increasing numbers of researchers in academia and the biotechnology industry have recently stepped up efforts to learn the details of their structures and activities and translate those findings into new therapeutic agents." ***Scientific American*** July, 2002 p42.

While all nutrients are important - and obviously, the body

requires many different nutrients - recent studies suggest that glyconutrients are by far the single most important class of nutrients in both preventing and overcoming infections. As you saw in the last chapter, glyconutrients are involved in almost every aspect of the body's defense strategies.[1] In fact, glyconutrients were busy protecting us as infants even before our body's immune system had had time to develop its own defenses.[2]

How We Get Infected

First, we'll look at the initial mechanism of infection. It's a common expression to hear someone say that I "caught" a cold or I "caught" the flu. That's commonly stated, but it's wrong nonetheless. Important pioneering research in Israel during the mid 1970's by Ofek and Sharon actually demonstrated that quite the reverse is true.[3] The bacteria, viruses, yeast, toxins, parasites etc., quite literally "catch" us. The principle of how that works is seen in the diagram that follows.

All our cells have antennae-like structures sticking out from them called cell surface receptors. These antennae are constructed from the special bioactive sugars that are attached to a protein backbone in

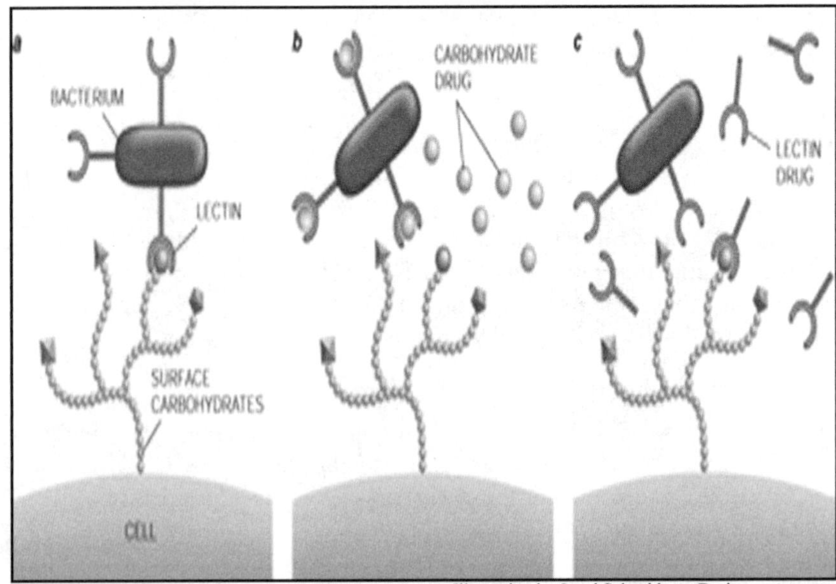

Illustration by Jared Schneidman Design - by permission

literally millions of potential combinations. In effect, the bioactive sugars have a puzzle-piece-like attachment site on them. Those puzzle-piece attachment sites are used for many different functions like holding cells together; recognizing sites for proper identification by our immune defense cells, and as docking sites for hormones and other signaling molecules to send their instructions into the individual cells - just to name a few. Unfortunately for us, the infectious organisms and toxins have a matching protein puzzle piece, called a lectin, which they use to "catch" the cell surface antennae (bioactive sugar) puzzle piece. If the organism "catches" (adheres to) you, an infection can occur. If it doesn't catch you, then there is no infection. This concept is the driving force behind the investment of many millions of dollars in ongoing research and development of a new class of pharmaceuticals called anti-adhesion carbohydrate drugs that will someday be used to both prevent and treat infections.

Sugars to the Rescue

The operative word here is someday. Even though the research has been going on since the mid 1970's, the drugs still don't exist. However, the entire principle of anti-adhesion drug development is based on the fact that competitive or decoy soluble bioactive sugars can mechanically block the organism from catching you.[4-12] Incredibly, research also demonstrated in both animal cell culture and human models that the soluble bioactive sugars could even "kick off" or dislodge the infectious organisms after they had attached to the cell surface receptors. Thus, the glyconutrients have the ability to not only prevent infections but to also treat infections. [4,10,13]

In various animal model studies, researchers found that if they pretreated the animals with a bioactive sugar specific for the adhesion mechanism of the infectious organism involved, they could literally prevent infections from occurring in animals given lethal doses of certain bacteria. In other animal studies, the animals were given the bioactive sugar after they were infected and were able to quickly recover without the spread of the infectious organisms into critical organ systems.

Because the decoy bioactive sugars only mechanically block attachment - and do not interfere directly with the life cycle of the infectious agent - it is unlikely that resistance by the infectious agent could develop. Another beneficial aspect that the pharmaceutical companies are pursuing is the fact that a non-attached bacterium is easier to kill with an antibiotic. Combination therapy using an anti-adhesion drug with an antibiotic may allow for smaller doses of antibiotics over shorter periods of time and hopefully, that should result in the development of lower levels of antibiotic resistance by the bacteria.

Unfortunately, after almost 30 years, anti-adhesion drugs are still only in the research and development stages. That's the bad news. Now, here's the good news - **the glyconutrients on which all these drug developments are based, are available now!**

Interestingly, while carbohydrate biochemistry research seems to be daily bringing about a greater understanding of the human body and consequently, more therapeutic options, the body itself has always utilized the naturally-occurring, bioactive sugars to prevent and fight infections. Consider the following examples of this.

- The first line of defense against many infectious diseases consist of decoy oligosaccharides (bioactive sugar groups) in saliva, tears, urine, sweat, breast milk and in the mucous layers that line all of the exposed epithelial cells in the digestive, respiratory and genitourinary tracts. The organism attaches harmlessly to the decoy sugar, thus preventing attachment to a cell that could lead to a consequent infection.

- Bioactive, sugar-bound pathogens are cleared by the physiological mechanism of the tissue in question - e.g., mucociliary action in the airway or bulk fluid movement in the GI tract.

A Breast Milk Secret

Human breast milk is interesting in that five of the eight bioactive sugars are present in it in significant quantities. All infants are born with an immune system that is immature since it has not yet been exposed to various pathogens and thus, has not yet developed specific antibodies that will later protect them as they get older and their immune system matures. The bioactive sugars in human breast milk provide protection against infections, especially in the respiratory and digestive tracts of the infant, while at the same time, they help to enhance immune system development to resist possible future infections. A mixture of approximately 130 unique oligosaccharide combinations from those bioactive sugars makes human breast milk totally unique in the mammalian kingdom. No other formula or mammal's milk can give the human infant the same kind of protection that human breast milk can. In addition, the bioactive sugars help stimulate the growth of friendly probiotic bacteria in the infant digestive tract.[15] These probiotic bacteria, predominantly *bifido* bacteria and *lactobacillis*, then help provide defense against various pathogenic organisms. They also release substances that stimulate the baby's immune defense cell production and development.

In babies who cannot breastfed for various reasons, adding a complete glyconutrient supplement to their formula can help supply the infant with the necessary bioactive sugars required by their immature immune system. An additional major benefit is that those same bioactive sugars are also required for ongoing brain development in the infant. Because the bioactive sugar content of human breast milk can vary 2-4 fold due to the genetic makeup of the mother, additional supplementation with a complete glyconutrient complex might also have some clinical benefit to the breastfed infant. Several studies have demonstrated distinct differences in brain development and learning ability in breastfed versus formula fed infants.

'Sugar' Supplements

Multiple studies in the 1980's and 1990's proved the effectiveness of administering the bioactive sugars either in an oral supplement form or even used in inhalation therapy for respiratory infections. For example, a 1997 study suggested the possible use of specific bioactive sugars that could be used in inhalers to assist in the management of *pseudomonas* infections in cystic fibrosis and critical care patients. In 2001, inhalation therapy with two bioactive sugars was used to totally eliminate an antibiotic resistant *pseudomonas* infection in a German infant who was also undergoing chemotherapy for a brain tumor.

A July, 1991 medical article by Karlsson proposed that the receptor binding sites on the influenza virus and other viruses are retracted and narrow, thereby avoiding the recognition by antibodies. This may explain why many viruses, and possibly several bacteria and parasites escape immune surveillance. Vaccinations are not likely to succeed, so the use of soluble low molecular weight substances that block the binding site may be an alternate approach. The soluble glyconutrients have already been shown to do exactly that.

The ability of the sugars to mechanically bind up toxins released by bacteria and viruses as well as displace them from where they attach to cell surface receptors is well documented. This is critical from a recovery standpoint, since in many infections, it is the toxins released by the pathogen that cause all the damage. *While we have many antibiotics, we don't have effective bacterial and viral "antitoxins"*.

Remember that with eight bioactive sugars there are eight possible puzzle-piece adhesion or target sites for infectious organisms to "catch" us. Often these organisms have the ability to attach to more than one sugar-puzzle-piece. The pharmaceutical companies recognized early on that with multiple possible target sites, an anti-adhesion drug would need to provide a "cocktail" of inhibitors to be effective.[16] The same is true for a glyconutrient supplement. It is important to provide the body with a supplement containing ALL the eight potential bioactive sugars it requires to help block attachment (adhesion) by the various human pathogens and toxins. A prime example is Echinacea which only contains a few of the glyconutrients. It may work great one time, but the next time does not seem to help at all. Echinacea can only be effective against a pathogen that targets and attaches to two particular sugar-puzzle-pieces. Other infectious organisms that target other sugars cannot be blocked by Echinacea. The same holds true for other natural products like Shiitake and Maitake mushrooms and some of the tropical fruits.

Your body knows all there is to know about health, even if your mind is limited in understanding how and why it works.

Glyconutrients are also involved in another role to block adhesion by infectious organisms. The bioactive, structural, building-block sugars are used to assemble many different cellular components - one group in particular is called glycoproteins. A 1989 study demonstrated that normal human serum possesses natural anti-adhesins which are represented by the glycan parts of the serum-glycoproteins.[6] No surprise by now that it is the sugars that play the critical role there. It is now an apparent pattern in cell physiology and biochemistry.

Glyconutrients are absolutely necessary for building immune system cells, for carrying out immune surveillance, and then activating and regulating the defense against infectious diseases. Dr. Rollins explained in the last chapter that the immune system is incredibly complex in both structure and function, and bioactive sugars are involved in every aspect of its execution.

Sorry, we cannot avoid the slightly more technical part here - but since your body already knows how to do this - you can ignore this next section if you wish. It is very important and worthy of repetition here.

Glycoproteins in Defense

Glycosylation is the process in which the bioactive sugars are attached to proteins in the manufacturing facilities inside our cells to make glycoproteins and other glycoforms. Consider the following.

- Almost all the key molecules involved in the innate and adaptive immune response are glycoproteins.
- In the cellular immune system, specific glycoforms are involved in the folding, quality control, and assembly of peptide-loaded major histo-compatibility complex (MHC) antigens and the T- cell receptor complex.
- In the humoral immune system, all of the immunoglobulins and most of the complement components are glycosylated.

The bottom line is that the bioactive sugars are critical to build glycoproteins and other glycoforms which are used to:

- Build the immune system defense cells.
- Build the cell surface receptors on the defense cells involved in immune surveillance (recognizing good guys vs. bad guys).
- Begin and regulate the inflammatory cascade which is the initial immune system response to an infection.
- Build the chemical signals that both activate and regulate the immune system (cytokines, lymphokines, interleukins, interferon, etc.).

The marketing / advertising for other types of supplements, herbal and otherwise, may claim to enhance immune system function. However, it is important to put the suspected mechanism of action pertaining to any such claims into the overall context of immune response. Remember, from a pure biochemistry standpoint, *your body requires glyconutrients to first properly build defense cells that have immune surveillance capability.* This must happen before another supplement / nutrient can start to enhance their function. Also, activation of the immune system by other supplements usually requires communication through a cell surface receptor that is constructed inside the cells with glyconutrient building blocks. In this context, glyconutrients obviously play the pivotal role.

Your Body Knows All

Additional uses of glyconutrients by the immune system are

many and varied but realistically, they are beyond the scope of this chapter. As we noted above, the good news for us is that the body already knows how all that complex immune system structure and function work. The bad news is that critical glyconutrients necessary to both build and regulate defense cells are now generally missing from our diets. An important concept is that the body does not get 'stupid' and forget how to get the job done. Your body knows all there is to know about health, even if your mind is limited in understanding how and why it works.

Our cells are pre-programmed to do what they do. The major limiting factor for cells to be built and work properly is simply that they get the necessary raw material nutrient tools from the diet to do exactly that! Since most of our defense cells live only thirty days or less, many billions of them are being replaced on a daily basis by newly built cells. The challenge for the body is to find the necessary glyconutrients to constantly and properly build new defense cells. Therefore a glyconutrient supplement which provides all the necessary glyconutrients that are missing from our diets, helps to maximize the body's potential to constantly build, maintain and regulate its immune system defenses.

In the daily war against infections and other health challenges, I certainly advocate using as many nutritional weapons as you can afford. However, no other nutritional component can substitute for or replace glyconutrients. Because glyconutrients are missing and will continue to be missing from our modern diets, the only practical solution is to use a supplement that provides all the bioactive sugars.

Glyconutrients clearly represent the missing link in nutrition today! Remember, the concept that we are talking about is *not* the ability of a glyconutrient supplement to cure, treat or mitigate a disease / infection *but* to supply the body with the appropriate raw material (nutrients) to perform a number of critical defense functions:

- Act as decoys.
- Displace already attached infectious organisms.
- Build defense cells.
- Enhance immune surveillance capabilities.
- Initiate inflammatory cascade response to infection.
- Build the chemical signals that activate and regulate the immune system.
- Build cell surface receptors on the defense cells to which chemical signals communicate their instructions.

Real People, Real Results

As with any technology, research articles and various studies can be impressive, but even more remarkable are real results in real people. I have had the opportunity for a number of years to travel and lecture about glyconutrient technology in particular, and nutraceuticals in general, all over the US, Canada and overseas. I am constantly amazed at the body's ability to overcome various health challenges, including infectious diseases, when properly supported with glyconutrients. Significant improvement in many different infectious diseases following glyconutrient supplementation have already occurred. Listed below are some areas where improvements in health have been noted:

- Infection prone children, including those with recurring otitis media (middle ear infections).
- Recurrent Pseudomonas infections in cystic fibrosis children and adults.
- Chronic Lyme's disease.
- Strep-induced toxic shock syndrome.
- Recurrent urinary tract infections.
- Bronchiolitis Obliterans Organizing Pneumonia (BOOP).
- Infections in Down's Syndrome patients.
- Lung infections in patients with COPD.
- AIDs patients and children in AIDs orphanages in Africa and Malaysia.
- Chronic sinus infections.
- Significant decrease in malaria exacerbations in African orphanages using glyconutrient supplements.
- Frequency and duration of colds and flu.
- Candida infections.
- E. coli O157:H7 food poisoning.
- West Nile virus

And many more...

Conclusion

This book is full of *personal experiences* from credible professionals. First hand detailed *anecdotes* are presented to illustrate the benefits of these vital sugars. More formal *case reports* are also referred to, where the clinical data was followed responsibly and reliably. A few *clinical trials*, done by the most rigorous of methods, also confirm what the preliminary results have suggested. Put it all together, and the evidence all seems to point in the same direction. We are just beginning to appreciate the true value and benefit of these vital sugars that together we call glyconutrients.

Again, knowledge is only power when it is applied. A complete glyconutrient supplement providing all the missing bioactive sugars is the single most important additional option available to help you in your war against infectious diseases. As the threat of epidemics and super-infection continues to grow, the wisdom of applying this glyconutrient option for your increased protection makes more and more sense!

About the Author
Daniel Fouts, DC

Dr Dan Fouts received his undergraduate training at Kent State University in Ohio followed by professional training at National College of Chiropractic where he graduated in 1973 with a BS in Human Biology and a Doctor of Chiropractic degree. In addition to his many years of clinical practice, Dr. Fouts served as Team Physician for the Palm Beach County (Florida) Youth Football League and was an Examining Doctor for the Florida Board of Chiropractic Examiners. In 1991 Dr Fouts participated in a Pilot Research Study on sEMG - Videofluroscopy in conjunction with the Radiology Department of Memorial Medical Center / Cancer Treatment Center of Tulsa. This was followed up in 1992 with Dr Fouts participating as a lecturer at the Second Multi-disciplinary Symposium on Cervical Soft Tissue Injury - Identification and Documentation, Tulsa,OK. Dr Fouts has lectured on glyconutrient, antioxidant and nutraceutical technology all over the United States and Canada, as well as Puerto Rico, St Thomas, Australia, New Zealand and the UK.

Editors Note:

Clearly, the earlier we start to protect ourselves, the better. In fact, true fortification of our bodies begins in the womb, as all our essential elements are formed in pregnancy. You will be treated next to a novel approach for increasing outcomes in pregnancy ...

Chapter 6

Improving Outcomes in Pregnancy

Dr. Vicky Arcadi

The definition of pregnancy, according to *Dorland's Medical Dictionary*, is "the condition of having a developing embryo or fetus in the body, after union of an ovum and spermatozoon." Trite as it may be, that definition is an appropriate starting point in this chapter because it underlines the three key elements in a healthy pregnancy. First, the host's body is the environment or stage where secondly, the sperm and egg unite and produce finally, the embryonic fetus which establishes its home there - at least for several months.

To improve the outcomes of pregnancy, the first important step in the planning of a pregnancy is therefore preconception health. Not only do we need to consider achieving and maintaining optimal health *during* pregnancy, but we also must strive for health *before* the sperm meets the egg. This would only make sense. Preconception health is something that must be discussed as it is important for a healthy pregnancy *and* a healthy outcome for both mother and baby.

Before Conception

If both prospective parents have not practiced good health through their lifetimes, then it is time, before conception, to take a serious look at their health. If this period has already passed, then perhaps it can be addressed for the next baby. Why is this so important? The nutritional diet and health of the individual at the time of fertilization will have a direct effect on the vitality of the sperm and the egg. The healthier the parents are at the time of conception, the healthier the sperm and the egg, the healthier the fetus, the healthier the baby, the healthier the child, and, ultimately, the healthier the adult.

One's diet needs to be abundant with adequate amounts of the essential nutrients for the sperm and egg to directly benefit and favor fertility.[1] Actually, normal physiology demonstrates that the preconception nutrition is more important than most people realize. Pre-pregnancy nutrition can determine if the fertilized egg "sticks" or not. That's a crude way of describing how the embryo implants inside the uterine wall and continues to develop. If and only if that process is effective, then we will have a real pregnancy. Otherwise, there will be a very early miscarriage. The reason is, upon union of the sperm and the egg, the embryo depends almost exclusively on the *preconception nutrition* and the nutritional quality of the lining of the uterus (called the decidua) for its ability to be nourished *after* implantation in the *uterine lining*. According to *Guyton's* Medical Textbook of Physiology, "During the first week after implantation, this is the only means by which the embryo can obtain any nutrients whatsoever, and the embryo continues to obtain a large measure of its total nutrition in this way for eight to twelve weeks, though the placenta also begins to provide slight amounts of nutrition after approximately the sixteenth day beyond fertilization (a little over a week after implantation)."[2] This is called *Trophoblastic* nutrition. Then, between weeks twelve and sixteen, the placenta is formed and begins to take over the function of supplying *all* the nutritional needs for the developing fetus, based on what the mother-to-be is eating. This is termed *placental* nutrition.

Placental Nutrition

So, when a woman experiences a miscarriage during the first four months, which is not uncommon, it could just be that her nutritional intake, prior to conception, was not adequate to support the needs of the embryo. The trick is to get the embryo implanted in a uterine lining that is rich with nutrients and then build a big, healthy placenta from what is already there. The placenta can then support the needs of the fetus for the duration of the pregnancy. Later on in the pregnancy there could, of course, be other complications that may contribute to a miscarriage or premature labor. We are not going to get into those problems in this chapter. Nevertheless, a woman must take her nutrition very seriously as she is building a baby. The placenta must be sustained with good nutrition so that the baby will have his or her reserves during labor and delivery as well.

The placenta is the only known organ with an abbreviated lifespan. It must be nourished to become as healthy as possible. A midwife's goal in the prenatal care process is to get the placenta to be as big and beefy as possible. Why? The placenta must be able to function at optimal levels during labor and delivery. Not only must the baby grow and be nourished and oxygenated by this incredible organ, but also, when the time arrives for labor and delivery to take place, it is the placenta that must maintain reserves to nourish the baby.

The medical approach, unfortunately, often does not emphasize the nutrition of the pregnant woman quite as much in prenatal care. The drug companies simply provide a pre-natal, synthetic vitamin preparation and that's it. How unfortunate! The medical approach has too often been reactive, assuming that if anything goes wrong with the baby, then the consequences can be dealt with in the hospital. Perinatal care and neonatal intensive care, in particular, have come a long way. Technology is now sophisticated to the point that in tertiary care hospitals, even premature babies who are delivered at 24-26 weeks and fit in the palm of the hand, can now be successfully managed, with good survival rates.

But that misses the point entirely. Pregnancy is a natural event and not a medical condition! An intense focus on supplying the needs of the pregnant woman to prepare for the labor and birth seems to make more sense.

Using nutrition as the main concern in prenatal care, over the last twenty-one years of our practice, has yeilded very favorable results. The mother and baby definitely benefit from proper nutrition. Some cases have been more difficult than others. Sometimes, one kind of commercial food supplement would work for one woman and yet would not work the same, or as well, for another. However, over the last nine years, while utilizing glyconutrients with pregnant women, the results we have seen have been very different. These nutrients resulted in improvement with every case - *without exception*. With every pregnancy, there was a consistent result. This was not expected. The outcomes were so much better than we had ever seen. Women responded and their babies responded. Based on these results, clinically, it made sense to assume and it emboldens us to assert, that every pregnant woman would benefit from adding these nutrients to her diet.

Non-Toxic Sugars

It would now be appropriate to briefly comment on these nutrients specifically. A more thorough discussion of glyconutrients was given in earlier chapters. Glyconutrients have proven themselves to be a necessity in every aspect of pregnancy. This includes *preconception nutrition*, for all the reasons stated earlier, as well as *prenatal nutrition*. What must be emphasized here, however, is that we are dealing with supplementary nutrition that is non-toxic at any level and at any stage. We know that at least five of the eight vital glyconutrients are found in mother's breast milk.[3] In a longitudinal study, Hanson found that breastfeeding not only provides good nutrition and protection against infections during lactation, but it "actively stimulates the immune system of the child to provide better host defense, including improved protection against various infections and enhanced vaccine responses, after the termination of breastfeeding."[4]

Now if these nutrients are found in human breast milk, then wouldn't a pregnant woman *also benefit* from these nutrients? The answer is, of course, yes. The truth is that *any one of us would benefit* from the nutrients found in breast milk. Years of clinical applications have shown, most importantly, that these glyconutrients are safe for pregnant women and safe for babies.

'The Birds And The Bees'

Glyconutrients, or monosaccharides, are the building blocks of carbohydrates. They are also known as sugars, or healthy sugars. *Mono-* means single and *-saccharide* means sugar. The essential elements of carbohydrates are found most abundantly in plants. They are not the same as table sugar per se, but are sugars that make up the nutrient-rich carbohydrates from foods. We should get at least eight, but unfortunately, due to urbanization and industrialization, we only get generally an adequate supply of two of the eight in our diets.

The main function of these glyconutrients is to be the front line of communication between cells. Without these nutrients, there can be no communication. Needless to say, sperm and egg need to communicate. They need *detection, recognition, attraction, association, consummation* and finally *fertilization.* Each step is critical and cannot be taken for granted. These are coded molecules interacting in a charged medium in three-dimensional space. This is reproductive life expressed. There is no room for error or falsehood. The sperm cannot find the egg, and certainly cannot fertilize the egg, without adequate amounts of these nutrients being present.

Pregnancy is a natural event and not a medical condition.

Once the sperm finds the egg, a lot of molecular activity must take place. Cell surface interaction gives rise to stimulation and molecular synthesis. This is more than 'the birds and the bees.' It is a complex biochemical interplay that produces a new combined entity with amazing specificity. We can then have *conception* which will lead to early *multiplication*, then *implantation* and a growing *embryo*.

Pregnancy, for most women, is an incredible experience. After all, it is a miraculous process. Most women love being pregnant, but because the woman's body is dynamic and constantly changing to accommodate her baby, she might experience discomforts that are common in pregnancy. Because she is "with child," a pregnant woman cannot take most toxic medications or drugs. She ought not to be radiographed or x-rayed and, for the most part, she would very seldom have surgery. She is, therefore, in a very precarious position. She is like an island, alone and having to fend for herself. And it seems that everyone is afraid for her. Not to worry, however, because the most effective approach for a healthy pregnancy, proven over and over again, relates simply to proper nutrition. It's the least an expectant mother can do.

Nutrition is a natural requirement, just like breathing, rest, exercise and all other aspects of personal body-care. It is dangerous to neglect any of these during pregnancy.

Discomforts In Pregnancy

With pregnancy, as we know, there are many discomforts associated with the continuous changes that a woman's body must endure. If we look at pregnancy by trimesters, we can see what is happening and why these discomforts are present.

First Trimester

In the first trimester (weeks 1-12), as we noted, the placenta is being formed. With the production of hormones skyrocketing to keep the lining of the uterus intact, this is a time when mother might experience morning sickness. If morning sickness is severe, we call it *hyperemesis gravidarum*. This is the extreme case and is somewhat rare. These women could be so sick that they are unable to keep anything down and usually end up hospitalized for dehydration and weight loss. The vast majority of women, when mildly afflicted, usually have nausea and vomiting mostly in the mornings, hence the term "**morning sickness**." Based on clinical cases, several postulates have been made for why morning sickness occurs at all. Within the last eight years, there has been more reason to believe that we are dealing with hormonal issues and, consequently, possible blood sugar-handling problems.

If and when they have morning sickness, pregnant women only seem to want to nibble on crackers - white, nutritionally-poor soda crackers. That's not a great source, even in desperation. Neither is sipping on ginger ale - flat or not. Nutritionally, the one food group that helps to build a big, healthy placenta is carbohydrates. Glyconutrients, when taken at baseline levels, seem to dramatically reduce the symptoms of morning sickness. Why? Studies have shown that glyconutrients do have an effect on hormonal issues in women as well as on their blood sugar levels. [5,6,7] The best combination would be adding glyconutrients along with an electrolyte drink that the mother can sip. This combination has anecdotally shown great success with curbing the symptoms of morning sickness. In athletes, this combination has also been known to affect blood sugar and hormone levels.

Another discomfort of pregnancy that will come and go is **fatigue**. With fatigue, generally, we are dealing with a deficiency. Initially, in the first trimester, fatigue could be due to all the dramatic changes that are occurring in the body all at once. In addition, dietary needs become more evident. In normal physiology, a rise in progesterone levels in the body diminishes the digestive enzymes and hydrochloric acid output. This reduction in enzyme secretion can contribute to dietary deficiencies, such as anemias. If food cannot be broken down, then the mother will not absorb her food. Iron and protein absorption is essential to prevent anemia, especially at a time of increasing blood volume. Fatigue is a great sign that this is not happening. Confirmation of anemia is accomplished by taking a blood test, which the doctor or midwife does frequently during the pregnancy. Anemia is a very common occurrence in pregnancy and is readily handled, in the majority of cases, by dietary changes. Glyconutrients simply help the body do the job it was meant to do by giving it the tools. The doctor or midwife may recommend iron tablets or specific foods to add to the diet. In any case, *glyconutrients will enhance the desired result.*

The glyconutrient complex is necessary in the diet to form enzymes in the body.[8] Proteins, calcium and iron must be broken down or assisted by enzymes to become bioavailable in the body. It is not hard to see, then, how important glyconutrient supplementation is to the mother and her growing fetus.

Another clue that enzyme production is not optimal, besides fatigue, would be **cramping** in the calves when resting and cramping of the feet while in the shower. Cramping can occur throughout the pregnancy. When this happens, the calcium is not being absorbed and assimilated into the tissues. Blood circulation may also not be as efficient. Hence, the muscles can cramp, especially the muscles carrying the largest weight which are most frequently found in the calves and feet.

We have found that when we supplement with the complex of monosaccharides necessary for cellular communication, the mother experiences relief and a return to more normal energy levels. This has been shown clinically in hundreds of pregnant women. Since the half-life of the glyconutrient complex is 72 hours, improvement is usually seen within days.

Another recurrent discomfort beginning in the first trimester of pregnancy is **lower back pain**. This is quite common as the pregnant woman is secreting a hormone called relaxin intermittently throughout the pregnancy and up to six months postpartum, depending on whether she is breast-feeding or not. Women also secrete this hormone during their menstrual periods and often experience back pain at that time. Did you ever wonder how a woman's pelvis expands to accommodate an eight-pound baby? The hormone relaxin, as it is secreted, acts on the ligaments in the pregnant woman, to allow the joints to be malleable and the ligaments to soften. Her pelvis will be forever changing during these forty weeks of gestation and back pain will come and go, as there are growth spurts in the developing fetus. Glyconutrient supplementation promotes the cell-to-cell communication in the body and has been shown, clinically, to help reduce the pain and inflammation. Chiropractic care has demonstrated effectiveness in the elimination of back pain.[9,10] However, we have also found that adding glyconutrients has clinically provided a much better and more rapid result.[9,10] A more optimally nourished body will be better able to handle the discomforts of pregnancy.

One of the most important concerns with pregnant women, regardless of gestation time, is their **immune system**. Infections, influenza and other illnesses, can pose a risk to a pregnant woman, and her baby. There are limitations on what can be recommended to a pregnant woman for treatment. Only a limited number of antibiotics are relatively safe in pregnancy and most medications are not advisable for pregnant women in any case, as they can be harmful to the baby. Therefore, the best scenario is to prevent her from initially getting sick. One of the best ways demonstrated to enhance and modulate the immune system is through the addition of glyconutrients to the diet. These nutrients help the body to work at the cellular level including the recognition and elimination of viruses and bacteria.[11] After following hundreds of pregnant women taking these nutrients, what has been noted is that they usually don't get sick. This is truly remarkable because pregnant women are commonly stressed and it is not uncommon for them to get frequent colds, sore throats and respiratory infections. For the immune system alone, glyconutritionals are extremely beneficial and help allow for an uneventful pregnancy.[12,13,14]

Second Trimester

As a woman enters her second trimester (weeks 12-24) things begin to get exciting. At this point, she starts to feel life. The placenta is most likely formed by now and the mother is supplying the nutrition to the baby. She will probably feel hungrier and she might also feel more tired. The baby will wake up and become very active when it is hungry. Mom will begin to have her "cravings" in this trimester. Any stress she has will be felt dramatically. She might fatigue easily as she is now feeding two. This is when diet plays a huge role in how she herself will progress.

Glyconutrients need to be looked at like a staple of the mother's diet during this trimester. Centuries ago, glyconutrients from foods was the staple in our diets. These glyconutrients are foods we no longer get through our diets in our industrialized world. Their benefits are so numerous that there could come a day when it might be a requirement for all physicians and midwives to recommend every pregnant woman take them, along with other supplements. To put this in context, just imagine introducing the suggestion in the last century, that all doctors should prescribe prenatal vitamins when hardly anyone was routinely prescribing them.

Glyconutrients should be taken 2-3 times a day, just as other food would be taken. Because they are food, in carbohydrate molecular form, they burn off, just as pasta or bread would. This is like any other food that must be taken every day. There is no difference, except that these nutrients help all our cells in the body to communicate. Without them, we cannot function optimally.

Who would have thought that foods put on this planet would play such a role in our health? We were meant to eat these foods. Since they are not readily available in our stores and food chains, we must supplement. This could not be more important for the pregnant woman. She is eating for two. This is the reason why, perhaps someday in the future, these nutrients will be on the list of necessary supplements, along with the prenatal vitamins that every practitioner routinely prescribes now for pregnant women.

In this second trimester, there are a few discomforts that must get mentioned. These discomforts, if not handled and managed, can lead a woman into the next and final trimester with a struggle. It is worth mentioning here that all the prenatal appointments must be kept. Prenatal care is critical for the success of the pregnancy. These visits will help the practitioner keep a careful watch on the progress and health of both mother and baby. Good, regular and consistent prenatal care is the best safeguard for a healthy, happy pregnancy.

One of the discomforts commonly seen in the second trimester is the early onset of **edema**. Edema can be caused for many reasons. **Hypertension** is another condition we might see surface during this time. If a pregnant woman has these two conditions, along with protein in the urine, then we have a possible clinical condition called preeclampsia. This is an early form of toxemia in pregnancy that, if seen during the last part of pregnancy, the physician will elect to do a caesarean-section on the mother. There is no discussion in these circumstances, as the risk of vaginal birth would be too high. If the mother is already adding glyconutrients to her diet, it is more than likely that the symptoms or conditions involved with preeclampsia will not surface. However, once started, there is some evidence which shows that hypertension itself can be improved with glyconutritional supplementation. [15]

As far as edema is concerned, physiologically, by about the sixth month of gestation, the baby's adrenal glands are formed and will begin to work. If the mother is stressed with work, family and lifestyle concerns or for any other reason, she will begin to utilize the baby's adrenal glands for support, which then depletes the baby. Since these glands secrete hormones that aid in utilization of proteins, fats and carbohydrates, when the mother attends her prenatal visit, edema might be noted and protein will be found in her urine sample. At this point, diet will be the key. Lifestyle, including rest and stress reduction, will also be addressed. Edema needs to be watched and treated as it might continue to be a problem throughout the rest of the pregnancy.

Glyconutrients, if added to the diet, will give the body the tools to facilitate intercellular communication. This means that all cell functions will be optimized, including repairing and rebuilding parts of the body with specific needs. The beauty of the body is that if you give it the tools, it will often heal itself. We do not have to decide what the body will take care of first. It will, in its infinite wisdom, do the job for us, according to its own priority system. In conjunction with the glyconutrients, phytogenins have also been beneficial to help modulate the hormonal function.

It is during the fourth to sixth month that mothers might also complain of **insomnia**. Usually the assimilation of proteins is inadequate and causes this condition. As the baby grows mom is also growing and showing, so she needs to make sure that she is digesting her proteins to maintain blood sugar levels. If mom cannot get to sleep, it could be that her adrenal glands are stressed. If she gets to sleep, but wakes up and can't go back to sleep, that might be a blood sugar issue. Usually the mother-to-be will state that she wakes up, gets up to go to the bathroom, then walks around until she finally ends up at the refrigerator for something to eat. After eating she goes back to bed and is finally able to fall asleep. This is classic low blood sugar. Mom is probably not digesting her foods properly and she may be experiencing hormonal issues as well. Glyconutritionals give the body the tools to modulate the blood sugar regulation.

Although there are more second trimester discomforts that can be discussed, we simply touched on a few of the important ones. As you can see, glyconutrient supplementation can help reduce the chances of any of these factors from even surfacing. Lifestyle, stress and what mom is eating are equally as important as supplementation. After all, supplementation is normally part of every pregnant woman's diet regimen.

Third Trimester

We now approach the third and final trimester of the pregnancy. If the first trimester was characterized by anxiety, the second by growth, then the third is clearly filled with excitement and anticipation. Everyone is watching and feeling the baby move. The baby is really beginning to grow. The prenatal visits are every two weeks and then quickly the visits are once a week. During the end of the third trimester the baby commonly grows a pound a week. The birth experience is now more eagerly anticipated.

This is the trimester when the pregnant woman may get **sugar cravings**. The reason for this is that the baby is now putting on fat. Everyone has heard of premature babies and how small they can be, especially if delivered more than three weeks early. This is because one of the last phases of the baby's growth is to put on fat. The fatty acids in the mother's blood stream may cause her to crave sugar. It is obvious that the baby's development is crucial now. Nutrition couldn't be more important. If the mother does crave sugar, it would make sense for her then to take in more of the healthy sugars, or glyconutrients. Remember, these are nontoxic at any level.

Part of the baby's development before birth includes **maturation of the lungs.** The baby can be delivered safely, in most cases, up to several weeks before the due date. But if born too prematurely, the lungs may not be completely developed and the baby might have to stay in a neonatal intensive care unit (NICU) until stable. That could take quite a while, which means the baby stays in the hospital with round-the-clock care and observation. That is not fun for anyone. Therefore, it is important that mom takes her naps, eats her good food, takes her glyconutrients and rests. Taking maternity leave during the seventh or eighth month, if possible, can be beneficial to both mother and baby.

A common problem that arises with the pregnant woman, which may cause her to deliver early, is **decreased amniotic fluid** levels. This can put her in the hospital if it happens too long before the due date. Over the years, there have been several anecdotal cases of restoration of these fluids. The cases were reported all over the United States, in women who began to take large quantities of the glyconutrient complex, along with several drinks a day that contained electrolytes. Effective restoration of the fluids in these women occurred within two to three days and allowed them to deliver at their due dates.

The beauty of the body is that if you give it the necessary tools, it will often heal itself.

One case to mention was a hairdresser who had two children. Both of her children were delivered by caesarean-section approximately three weeks early due to lowered levels of amniotic fluid. The babies were okay, but about six years later she got pregnant for the third time. She had the same obstetrician, ate the same foods and still worked as a hairdresser with the same hours. However, this time she added glyconutrients to her diet. She was actually taking the nutrients a few years before conception and continued through the pregnancy. The result was that the lowered level of amniotic fluids did not develop and she delivered vaginally - after her due date! She attributes this result to the addition of these nutrients to her diet. Not only is this a success story for her, but it also allowed her to save on medical bills because she delivered the natural way.

Labor and Delivery

Obviously, the pregnancy does not end here. The labor and delivery is the hardest part for both mother and baby. All the care, diet, supplements and prenatal visits lead up to the 12-24 hours of labor and delivery (the average time for first-time mothers). This is where "the rubber meets the road." There is only one safe way out of this pregnancy and that is birth! Hopefully, the new parents have taken their prenatal classes. The classes will reduce the fear that some couples have about the birth process. With parents educated and mom, baby and placenta in excellent health, the labor and birth should go well.

Another case to mention was a mom who was delivering her second baby. She had her first child at home and the second child was a home birth as well. She was a sensitive and frail person, and she generally had heavy bleeding during delivery. The general "rule of thumb" for these women is that if they bleed heavily during the first delivery, they will always do so. She had good health during her pregnancy and was very disciplined about eating well. With her first baby she bled heavily and her recovery after the birth took a very long time.

With the second baby, everything about the prenatal care was the same except that she had been supplementing with the glyconutrients from the beginning of the pregnancy. The first labor was about 26 hours, with about a three-hour pushing time. The second labor was about five hours and the pushing stage was minutes. She had just tablespoons of bleeding and after the delivery, she jumped off the bed and began walking around. She literally had no real recovery time. This was important because two things occurred. There was virtually no bleeding and recovery time was reduced dramatically. In obstetrics, inordinate bleeding (post partum hemorrhage) is a leading cause of complications and even death in labor and delivery. Since then, many anecdotal cases have been recorded in the glyconutritional practice with incredible recovery from labor and birth, along with decreased bleeding.

Conclusion

So, as can be seen, glyconutrients do provide great benefit for the pregnant woman. With the addition of these nutrients, what can be expected are better outcomes for mother, and also better outcomes for baby. With a good diet including glyconutrients, the tools for cellular communication, what is created is a healthy environment and optimal nutrition for the baby.

The difference in outcomes of mothers taking glyconutrients like I have seen, and those not taking them during their pregnancies, is dramatic. It is the opinion of this author and practitioner that practically **all pregnant women would benefit from glyconutrients**. Pregnant women cannot take anything that is toxic. These are nutrients that have a tremendous impact on both mother and baby and are nontoxic at any level.

Having cared for pregnant women for over twenty-one years, never before have I found any supplement that has benefited women every single time. But I must mention that the mother would also benefit from good chiropractic care. Such care, by a chiropractic doctor specially trained to treat pregnant women, is also recommended to keep them structurally and neurologically in balance.[16-20]

Thanks to glyconutrients, mothers and babies all over the world can have better health during this wonderful experience and better outcomes of pregnancy.

About the Author:
Victoria Arcadi, DC, DICCP

Dr. Victoria Arcadi has been a licensed chiropractor for over 20 years. She broke new ground with her first controversial and courageous studies and subsequent treatments of pregnant women. Dr. Arcadi went on to co-author a book with the famed and beloved Dr. Lendon Smith, who is known as "The Baby Doctor." She was the first to publish studies regarding the utilization of glyconutritionals with genetically damaged children and those with cerebral palsy. She has earned a Diplomate degree in Pregnancy and Pediatrics.

Editors Note:

As the newborn becomes detached from the mother's umbilical cord, it has to learn to cope independently. It needs glyconutrients for healthy growth and survival. If it gets them, you're going to be surprised by what can happen to even very sick children, as a result ...

Chapter 7

Glyconutrients for Babies and Children

Dr. Vicky Arcadi

Everyone needs glyconutrients, but our children are in the greatest need. Do you wonder why?

The world today is not what it used to be. Toxins are everywhere - in the water we drink, the air we breathe and the food we eat. For example, the notorious pesticide DDT has been outlawed in the United States, but it can still be detected in our rainwater. Earlier tests detected it even in human breast milk. Like the saying goes, "We are one world, one planet." These toxins are poisonous to all of us, but the most vulnerable are our children, born or unborn.

It is no wonder that children are born today with cancers. Some are born with congenital disorders never seen before. New syndromes and conditions are being described by clinicians every year. Genetic diseases are on the rise, both from inherited genes and mutated genes.

Our children are the most sensitive of any group in our society, which is why they need protection. They also need to be supplied with the necessary tools to allow their little bodies to grow and heal by themselves. This is what will be discussed in the following pages: how we can help our children by feeding them, among other things, some essentials that have been on our planet from the beginning of time - glyconutrients.

In the last chapter about pregnancy, we discussed some potential benefits of glyconutrients. We discussed why it is important to have the nutrients added to a pregnant woman's diet to enhance her own health and the health of her unborn fetus. Now it is important to discuss the benefits that these nutrients have on the generation of tomorrow - our children.

One of the most popular concerns regarding glyconutrients is their safety for babies and children. If you did a thorough study of what these nutrients really are, you will find that they come from foods. Glyconutrients are mostly from the plant kingdom and are non-toxic at any level. The problem is that we don't seem to get enough of these foods in our diets. They are just not available as such in the industrialized world. We cannot go to the market and buy them.

Why are these nutrients so important? They provide the necessary elements, or tools, for our cells to communicate. They provide the *glyco* - in glycoproteins which are indispensable to the structure and function of all cells. Without these nutrients, we most likely will function at less than optimal levels. We might not be able to fight off intruder microorganisms, such as bacteria and viruses, because the cell-communication lines that govern our immune response are not there. It is like trying to communicate without some vowels in our English language. We have **eight** glyconutrients that are necessary to communicate and, in most cases, we only get adequate amounts of **two** of these nutrients. As far as medicine is concerned, Glycobiology (the study of vital sugars in living systems) has been one of the most exciting new research fields in the past couple decades. More and more exciting and valuable studies on these nutrients are being reported each year.

So how can our children get all eight of these nutrients? *We must supplement* our basic diet, or perhaps move to the Fiji Islands and live off the land. Obviously, and happily, it is more practical to supplement, even though a trip to the South Pacific is always an attractive option.

Breastfeeding Is Best

You will be happy to learn that there is one safe food which contains most, if not all these nutrients. It is specially designed by nature for babies. This food is of course, human breast milk. It is no accident that the body of the new mother is designed to produce milk containing this rich nutrient source. A healthy newborn will search to find the mother's breast within thirty to ninety minutes after birth. This is an innate or instinctive action and clearly, the newborn's first priority. Not only does the breast milk contain most of the eight necessary glyconutrients (in the form of glycoconjugates, glycoconjugate sugars, simple sugars, glycoproteins, oligosaccharides, etc.), but it also contains various antibodies and the perfect balance of fats, amino acids, carbohydrates and water.[1,2,3] It never gets any better than this for babies. The Intelligent Design we find in nature is wiser than all human innovation.

The US Food and Drug Administration (FDA) recommends breast milk over cow's milk. In the October 1995 issue of *FDA Consumer*, Rebecca D. Williams wrote, "Cow's milk contains a different type of protein than breast milk. This is good for calves, but human infants can have difficulty digesting it. Bottle-fed infants tend to be fatter than breast-fed infants, but not necessarily healthier." She also added, "New parents want to give their babies the very best. When it comes to nutrition, the best first food for babies is mothers' breast milk." She goes on to say, "More than two decades of research has established that breast milk is perfectly suited to nourish infants and protect them from illness. Breast-fed infants have lower rates of hospital admissions, ear infections, diarrhea, rashes, allergies and other medical problems than bottle-fed babies." *Breast is best* is no longer a controversial issue, if indeed it ever was. All the experts today agree.

But the recent statistical history of breastfeeding in the United States is quite interesting. In 1958, just 20% of babies were breast-fed. In 1980, that number increased to 60%. Then, in 1990, an amazing 90% of babies were breast-fed! However, in 1993, that number dropped to only about 56%. That drop is of concern to some. And well it should be. The trend is now moving in the wrong direction.

The FDA, along with the American Academy of Pediatrics, is also tracking the length of time babies are breast-fed to determine immune function benefits. Ruth Lawrence, MD, Professor of Pediatrics and Obstetrics at the University of Rochester School of Medicine in Rochester, NY, and a spokeswoman for the American Academy of Pediatrics, states that the Academy recommends babies be breast-fed for six to twelve months. But it would seem to make sense that the longer the child breast-feeds, the healthier that child will be. It also stands to reason that the child will grow into a healthier adult.

Breast milk is well-suited for human growth and development because it is uniquely designed by nature for this purpose. Humans also have more highly developed frontal lobes. Breast milk contains all the nutrition and glyconutrients necessary to encourage and support the rapid brain development and growth of newborns and infants. There has never been an exact, synthetic duplication of breast milk and one will probably never exist.

The Intelligent Design we find in nature is wiser than all human innovation

Lars Hanson showed in his longitudinal study on breast milk, how breast-fed babies benefit later in life with "the transfer of immunity from mother to baby. Thus, it seems that breast-feeding might limit the appearance of certain diseases, such as allergies, autoimmune diabetes and celiac disease."[4] The point is simply that breast milk is the best food for babies. In fact, hypothetically, to consume breast milk as part of our diet each day of our lives would certainly benefit anyone, young or old.

Here's an interesting practical application. In clinical practice over the last 21 years, we have seen many babies who, soon after birth, contract all kinds of eye irritations and infections. This is not uncommon as the baby's immune system is very premature. After birth, the baby is exposed to our environment which is filled with numerous infectious elements. Rather than recommend an antibiotic drop or ointment for the eye, we have often recommended breast milk. Yes, breast milk can find natural application for topical use. After all, breast milk contains all the nutrients needed to help the baby's new body fight infection. So, we have often had the mother squirt breast milk into her baby's eye and it is not unusual to find that, sometimes within a day, the baby's body is able to take care of that infection. That's just one example of the healing power of breast milk.

As mentioned earlier, breast milk is known to contain most of the eight critical glyconutrients that all of us need in our diets for cellular communication and cellular function. Again, they provide the *glyco* - in glyco-proteins. Is it not a wise strategy for disease-prevention to then continue supplementing these vital elements found in breast milk, so that we can continue to get all the nutrients needed to sustain optimal health? It makes sense, especially since we know that they have no toxicity and the body recognizes them only as food. What could be better than breast milk? The answer? Nothing. However, a complex rich in the essential glyconutrients would be a close second.

> ***Nature is the source and the resource for all the body's essential needs.***

As a side note, one question that often arises with mothers is how to give these nutrients to their infants.

We discovered one way that worked very well with an eight-month-old baby who had severe cancer of both retinas of her eyes (called **retinoblastoma**). The baby had undergone the maximum of eight rounds of chemotherapy. Every month she had to be put under anesthesia so that the doctors could laser off the tumor in both retinas to hold off and reduce the tumor growth. The baby could not eat food. She could only breast-feed. The mother wanted to know how to give more of these nutrients to her baby. The best delivery system we thought, was to have the mother add large quantities of the glyconutrient complex to her diet every day to enrich and increase the concentration of the glyconutrients already in the breast milk. Interestingly, the baby soon started to get an appetite and she started to grow three teeth. Her tumors began to die and she began to eat more and more food. We were then able to add the nutrients directly into her own food. Her body was beginning to heal itself with cellular communication and her enhanced immune system continued to fight the cancer. It is remarkable that in almost every single case with this type of cancer, the eyes would have had to be removed. However, fortunately for this child, six years later and still taking these nutrients, she only lost one of her eyes. She never gets sick and she is doing very well in school. She is having a normal, healthy life.

If a mother would like to add these nutrients to an infant's formula or breast milk, that is something that is safe to do. Remember that the breast milk contains these nutrients already. But for children of all ages, they are safe and non-toxic. You would be simply adding nutrients that aren't available in the diet, to promote optimal health. If a child has a serious illness, these nutrients are still safe. However, it is advisable to consult with the pediatrician or specialist to at least monitor their medications, if any, and to follow the progress of the child. Remember: a sick child is always vulnerable, (the younger the child, the truer that is) and one should never presume in the face of any acute childhood illness.

Some Common Diseases in Children

Numerous children today are afflicted with serious chronic illnesses, some of which were never previously common in children. One such disease is **Diabetes** Type 2 which is also ironically known as "adult onset" diabetes or even more precisely, non-insulin-dependent diabetes mellitus. As of 2004, 1 in 500 children in the US have a diagnosis of diabetes, including both Types I and 2. We can compare this to 1945-1969, when a mere 1 in 7100 children had diabetes. Since 1958, diabetes in the United States has tripled to 16 million cases and is now the fourth leading cause of death overall.

Studies have shown some impressive improvements in patients with diabetes and its associated complications, after supplementing with glyconutritionals, with and without other nutraceuticals. The result was a 97% overall health improvement.[5,6] Up until the discovery and testing of these nutrients, there were never results such as these in diabetes studies, for any other form of dietary supplementation. More studies, especially with Type I (juvenile diabetes), are necessary. But there are indeed, some anecdotal cases of Type I diabetics reducing their insulin need through the use of glyconutritionals. However, please note, especially with diabetics, blood sugar levels must be monitored very closely.

But are these nutrients safe for children even if they are taking other medication? The answer is yes! These nutrients are foods - foods that we don't get in our diets anymore - and they are as safe as breast milk. However, it must be reiterated that **any child on medication must be closely monitored by their physician.** Medicines taken with glyconutritionals have been reported to work better in the body, even sometimes reducing the required medicinal dose for the same intended effect. These nutrients are believed to help cellular communication, affecting all levels.

Another disease on the rise with children is **asthma**. In 2004, nine million children in the United States were diagnosed with asthma. This is a dramatic increase compared to 1979 when only two million children suffered from asthma. In fact, asthma is now the leading cause of chronic illness among children in the United States. Asthma causes 500,000 hospitalizations and about 5,000 deaths annually. It is the sixth leading cause of death in children ages five to fourteen. The associated health care costs are in the billions each year, mainly due to the hospital visits and the numerous medications and inhalers asthmatics must use each day in order to breathe properly.

Difficulty breathing, with wheezing and sometimes more serious complications, are common presentations in most pediatric emergency wards. Of course, such attacks can indeed be life threatening. The classic *status asthmaticus* is a dire emergency. But that is serious stuff. It is late-stage intervention and management, when the young asthmatic can hardly get adequate air into their lungs. Long before that, children with reactive airway disease and hypersensitivity to environmental triggers need to be managed more proactively.

A study was done with fourteen asthmatics following a program of glyconutritionals, and glyconutritionals containing phytonutrients and phytogenins, for a period of three to thirteen months. The results showed an 86% reduction in the number of symptoms associated with asthma, with a 72% reduction in the number of other medications they had been taking.[7,8]

There has also been great success with chiropractic spinal adjustments in the management of asthma in children. Chiropractic care is highly recommended in the integrated approach with any child suffering from this disease. An article appearing in *The Journal of Vertebral Subluxation Research*, Vol.1, No.4, demonstrated the positive effects of chiropractic care on 81 children with asthma. Part of the approach, as with any disease, includes nutrition. It is well-known that better nutrition leads to better health. The nutrition of choice, from the research and results seen in clinical practice, overwhelmingly points to glyconutrients.[9] These children are deficient and the glyconutrients are known to be safe.

In the past, for conditions such as diabetes and asthma, our only treatment choices at best, were medications, vitamins, minerals and herbal remedies. There had never been anything available that worked at the cellular level. The monosaccharides, or glyconutrients, go inside the cell. The glyconutrients originate from foods and are classified in a new category termed "nutraceuticals." Nutraceuticals are food products, with no toxicity, that have pharmaceutical effects on the body, and are supported by science. Medications, vitamins, minerals and herbs have toxicities at certain levels. In both diabetes and asthma, the basic complication is that we are dealing with immune function issues. With the use of glyconutritionals, we are seeing immune function improvement as the body begins to heal itself, and with no known toxicity.

Some Rare Disease in Children

In 1997, we published the first Case Report utilizing glyconutrients with children who have a rare genetic condition called **Tay-Sachs disease.**[10] Children with this disease do not usually survive past the age of two to four years. It is a disease found in the Ashkenazi Jewish culture of Eastern European ancestry. Pregnant women of this heritage are screened in order to detect the gene in the fetus. If detected in the fetus, most often, a therapeutic abortion is recommended. There is no hope of survival for these children as they are missing an important enzyme.

This study was based on a Japanese child we saw who had to be fed through a nasogastric tube. The child was three years and nine months old and he weighed 16 pounds. All he could do was lie down. He was not able to move, he could no longer speak, or see, and he had limbs that were stiffened from the neurological damage associated with the progression of the disease. He had seizures and was deaf. He couldn't swallow and his head was oversized in proportion to his body.

The worst part of this disease clinically, can be the struggle of the caretakers with the constant respiratory infections and the extremely weakened function of the immune system. The child is compromised and sick all the time. The parents are burdened with weekly doctor's visits and numerous hospital stays. It is a very sad situation to experience.

These children most often succumb to pneumonia.

The results of this study were phenomenal. The glyconutrients were recommended as a supplement to the nasogastric diet. The complex of glyconutrients did not require digestion and therefore were quickly utilized without any extra energy expelled. This was very important because the child was literally starving to death. The results surprised all of us and demonstrated the safety of the glyconutrients, and also the power of the human body to heal itself. The child immediately started to gain weight and absorb his foods. From this study, we determined that better absorption was the first thing that happened. The second was that his immune system quickly became stronger. He stopped getting sick. The third thing that happened was that he began to feel better. As these positive effects began to take hold, his body, on its own priority system, began to heal itself. Remarkably his sight and hearing returned, his stiffness and spasms decreased and he had better digestive function. Within six months he gained fourteen pounds. He also received chiropractic adjustments two-three times a week. This was a case report, but no one in the attending medical community had ever seen improvement such as this in a case of Tay-Sachs disease.

This study launched more research and interest in adding these nutrients to the diets of other sick and dying children. There have now been significant numbers of children with genetic conditions responding well to glyconutrient treatment.

Another genetic Case report we published dealt with children who had Prader-Willi Syndrome. This is also a genetic condition where the children, with mental retardation and low muscle tone, eat themselves to death.[11] Then there was the case of cystic fibrosis, an inherited and fatal degenerative disease of the exocrine glands affecting the gastrointestinal tract and respiratory tract.[12] These Case Reports involved introducing glyco nutrients for the first time by simply adding them to the childrens' normal diets. In addition, other researchers looked at children with muscular dystrophy, specifically the FSH (or fascioscapulohumoral) type, which is also genetic. They also showed improvement when glyconutrients were added to their diets along with the use of a calcium channel blocker medication.[13]

What we are seeing in these children, after the addition of the nutrients to their diets, has been astounding and very rewarding. These children have benefited simply by improving the quality of their nutrition. The obvious way to benefit from improved nutrition is to add to any diet what is deficient in that diet. The glyconutrients were obviously deficient in such cases if they could not breast feed and/or stopped breast-feeding. **What we did with these children was to give them back what was missing.** The concept is so simple and so basic.

Another affliction that must be addressed with babies and children is the overwhelming number of cases arising within the spectrum of **autism**. Autism is usually manifested in the first year of life. These children show signs of extreme aloneness (lack of attachment, failure to cuddle, avoidance of eye gaze) They tend to insist on sameness (resistant to change, rituals, morbid attachment to familiar objects and repetitive acts). They have speech and language disorders (ranging from total muteness through delayed onset of speech to idiosyncratic use of language). They manifest uneven intellectual performance.[14] These children all have learning disabilities. Autism may actually be more than one disorder. Attention Deficit Disorder (ADD), Attention Deficit Hyperactivity Disorder (ADHD), Asperger syndrome, Angelman Syndrome and even Prader-Willi syndrome - just to name a few - are now also considered within the spectrum of autism. As of 2004, the experts consider 1 in 166 American children as being autistic to some degree. Again, we can compare this with 1970 when just 4 in 10,000 American children were autistic. That's another dramatic increase. Some experts are saying that autism is of epidemic proportions. There is usually very little hope for these children and many parents are forced to institutionalize their children.

Adding glyconutrients is another example of the body being empowered to heal itself.

However, there is good news. Glycosupplementation has been available for more than a decade and has been introduced to autistic children. We do have scientific documentation from studies which show that autism, and the afflictions associated with autism, can improve.[15,16] In addition, there have been many anecdotal cases reported from parents as well as from other practitioners.[17]

One such case that is worth mentioning involves another one of my patients, with **Prader-Willi** syndrome, who was ten-years-old and living in an institution. He was placed in the institution because he could not be handled at home. He had severe autistic behavior and had been living away from his family for years. His parents spent $4000 each month for his care. After only six months of glycosupplementation, his behavior improved so dramatically that his parents took him out of the institution! Not only did these parents get their son back, but they also will not be so burdened financially.

So what about children with permanent neurological damage, such as cerebral palsy (CP)? This neurological disease is a broad term for a syndrome whereby something happens developmentally to damage the central nervous system either during pregnancy, at birth or in the postpartum period. The child has impairment of involuntary movement that is characteristic of CP. The condition is static, non-progressive and requires a multidisciplinary, integrated approach to management. There is no medication or cure to reverse the syndrome. Most children eventually find themselves in wheelchairs. The occurrence is approximately two in every 1000 births, so it is a syndrome that is not uncommon.

One of my patients had **ataxic cerebral palsy**. We gave her the glyconutrients starting at 28 months of age. She had cerebellum involvement from the neurological tests and MRI studies and had been diagnosed with CP at 26 months at UCLA (University of California, Los Angeles). She had low muscle tone (hypotonia), with impairment of coordination and fine motor skills. She could not sit, stand or walk and she could not speak. After only six weeks on the glyconutritional supplementation, along with chiropractic adjustments, she was able to walk and began to talk. We published the Case Report, and today, eight years later, she is in a mainstream, full-inclusion school. Her neurological impairments have reversed and she has no problems walking or talking. She is not only riding horses, but is winning equestrian events.[18] With the return of the nervous system function, the pediatric neurologists at UCLA have no longer diagnosed her with cerebral palsy. She is continuing to flourish and is approaching a complete and full recovery and reversal of her affliction from birth.

One final note: there is also scientific evidence which shows that some children today are being born with a congenital inability to make glycoforms. They lack the mechanism for attaching the glyco- (or sugar), moiety to a protein. This dysfunction or disorder is otherwise known as a **congenital defect in glycosylation** (CDG), of which there are eight variants.[19] One of these syndromes is CDG-1b, an hepatic-intestinal disease. Without the oral administration of 1 of the 8 monosaccharides - mannose - the condition would be fatal. Dr. John Axford, an Immunologist of the Royal Society of Medicine in England states, "These diseases are characterized by multisystem abnormalities, but central nervous system defects predominate. New clinical entities continue to surface." He goes on to state, "Although eight defects in the glycosylation pathway have been identified, probably only the tip of the iceberg has been uncovered. A CDG should be considered in all patients, children as well as adults, who have any unexplained clinical condition."[20]

The Basic Principle

After treating these children, seeing the results and then writing the Case Reports, it became even clearer to us that these nutrients were eminently safe. It was also clear that all our adult patients should be taught about the glyconutrients so that they could make a choice for themselves and their children, i.e. whether or not they wanted to add them to their diets. To our knowledge, while actively using these nutrients on pregnant women and children over the last 9 years, every single patient has benefited from the improved nutrition.

What's the basic principle at work?

We believe that what made the body will also heal the body. Nature is the source and the resource for all the body's essential needs. If we give the body the tools, the body will often spontaneously heal itself. We take for granted that when we cut our finger, the body heals and repairs that defect on our finger often without a trace of it remaining. That's the body at work, healing itself. Repair of damage and disease is its normal or natural function. We're built that way. Adding glyconutrients is just another example of the body being empowered to heal itself. Don't you think that if the body perfectly heals something like a wound that we can see on the outside, the body could also heal from the inside in the same way? It is all cellular activity - cells defending cells, cells repairing cells, cells making new cells. In another way, we can say it is all cell-to-cell communication, cooperation and construction.

Hope

The experiences and stories regarding glycosupplementation are seen each and every day. It is incredibly exciting and rewarding to give hope to sick children all over the world. As a health care professional, I feel as though I have something I can offer parents for their children who otherwise had no hope. That is the big word - *hope.* Most parents of terminally ill children feel as though everyone with a supplement, or something that will be "a miracle" for their child, is approaching them. Parents often do not want to step over that line and begin to hope desperately but foolishly, when all along everything they have read and been told is dismal.

The message to you, if you are a parent with a very sick child, is that glyconutrients may not help your childs body to care itself, but glyconutrients will add to your child's quality of life. All the science and work done with children have indicated that, at the very least, glyconutrients will help to improve their digestion, their immunity will benefit and they will ultimately feel better as a result. That is really all we can promise. The future holds so much for these serious and unexplained symptoms of illness. Some of the top immunologists in the world have come to believe that glyconutrients will be a key factor in treating congenital conditions.

So, with the help of this book, more and more people will begin to understand how important these nutrients are for all of us. The fact is that we are all deficient. **Today's children are more deficient than we were at their age**, and we are more deficient than our grandparents were.

The science is there to show that there is great promise in the field of Glycobiology. Supplementation with these nutrients over time will gain more ground as more documentation and human studies are undertaken and completed. This science is only a few decades old. From the growing body of knowledge, we should hope that these nutrients will surely be part of almost everyone's diet and indeed, a recommendation by many an **informed and caring doctor.**

The most compelling issue to deal with is the fact that these nutrients are just food. This fact should cause the world to look at health from a completely different perspective. As we have used these nutrients in practice with many babies and children, it is rewarding to see how quickly they respond. They are the most sensitive to all things and these nutrients are no exception.

Conclusion

This chapter should help to make you aware of the great need for glyconutrients and the benefits they offer for a better quality of life. By taking glyconutrients, today's children can help prevent future diseases in themselves and their children. It would be to our advantage as adults, to take responsibility for our health by doing all that we can to optimize our own health and the health of our children.

In essence, the science of glycobiology has just been born. According to Dr. John Axford, "Most major diseases that afflict mankind (e.g., cancer, rheumatoid arthritis, heart disease, diabetes, infectious diseases and neurodegenerative diseases) directly involve glyconconjugates. The ultimate goal is to develop the science of glycobiology so that it can have a significant impact on our ability to define and support health, and to diagnose and manage disease."[20]

About the Author:
Victoria Arcadi, DC, DICCP

Dr. Victoria Arcadi has been a licensed chiropractor for over 20 years. She broke new ground with her first controversial and courageous studies and subsequent treatments of pregnant women. Dr. Arcadi went on to co-author a book with the famed and beloved Dr. Lendon Smith, who is known as "The Baby Doctor." She was the first to publish studies regarding the utilization of glyconutritionals with genetically damaged children and those with cerebral palsy. She has earned a Diplomate degree in Pregnancy and Pediatrics.

Editors Note:

In the next chapter, you will meet a doctor who really prides herself in being a super-mom. She will demonstrate some of what you learned in the past two chapters when she relates the birth of a glyco-baby. For her family with seven children and her patients, glyconutrients has become a living reality ...

Chapter 8

A Living Reality

Dr. Maria Mona

A few months after the birth of our fifth child in 1998, I received a call from a family member informing me of a new medical "breakthrough". She thought I would understand it because of my medical background. A stream of excitement came through her voice but I couldn't make sense of it. I showed little interest. The arrogance and pride I picked up in medical school showed their familiar colors. I resisted. However, she sent me some documents to read and I soon found out that the assembly of glycoproteins, which I vaguely recalled from medical school, are very critical for proper cellular structure and function and hence, the outcome of good health.

Questions came rushing through my mind.

Can carbohydrate or saccharide (sugar) molecules really influence extensively all biologic processes? How could that be? We were told a long time ago through 'educational texts' that sugars only provide energy. We were also taught that 'other sugars could only be made in the body from glucose' (glucose theory). It is now known that the assumption does not hold true.[1]

I wanted to discover more for myself what glyconutrients were and why it is critically important to know their significance. A Medline search on "glycoproteins" began. I noted a rapid growth of knowledge in a new field called Glycomics, which is the functional study of carbohydrates. In 1998, I saw references to more than 7,200 studies from all over the world. A tremendous amount of growing literature was revealing a common understanding on how cells use molecules with sugars to communicate. There are now about 20,000 articles published annually on the subject. Nobel Prizes for medicine in fields associated with these biologic sugars were astounding. There was apparent unity...the scientists were all saying the same thing. The new information was so wonderful and powerful. Yet questions still came to mind. *"Are these nutrients alive in us?" "Is this life-giving information?"* I knew that all scientific studies are not created equal. So I still proceeded with 'caution.'

A transformation had begun. I literally found myself being

translated out of a world of suffering and ignorance into an arena of health and enlightenment. I had known nothing about glycoscience until then. Indeed, it was a humbling experience.

Safety and Efficacy

Providentially, I read more information which convinced me that **even as a doctor, I could be free from the fear and shame of "not knowing**". Since I was nursing my fifth child then, I wanted to first investigate any literature regarding the safety and efficacy of glyconutrients. When it comes to research (medical or scientific), it should always educate us on these two guiding parameters: safety and efficacy. Here I was nursing a baby, an appropriate moment to reinforce the critical role of sugars/glyconutrients in the design of life! The vital sugars are found in human breastmilk but I could make no connection.

Besides the LD-50 studies on rats, I came across an earlier study that determined the potential for human cellular damage from the use of dietary supplements.[2] The study concluded that garlic, aloe and the three available multiple ingredient products containing glyconutrients were all non-toxic. There was no toxicity on the liver (cytochrome p-450 activity) or peripheral blood mononuclear cells. The study further noted the enhancement of the functional efficiency of natural killer cells and the capacity to reduce destructive processes by the increase in intracellular glutathione levels (antioxidant activity). As a result, there was a potential protection against microorganisms and even cancer. Because glyconutrients are non-toxic and plant-based, I realized that they are nothing but FOOD, yet with enormous capabilities "to perform an astonishing range of jobs" and not just act as a mere energy source.[3] Glyconutrients can fulfill that missing link in nutrition.

Plants are the primary factories for synthesis of saccharides/carbohydrates and in biological terms, they are the only living reservoir that can "capture" the power/energy of the sun. Therefore, plant food must be the best food. This foundational knowledge is the springboard for sustaining good health. The more I learned about glycoscience, the closer I came to understanding the real sustenance of life through its essentials. What a gift!

New Family Habits

With that blessed assurance, I started consuming glyconutrients along with five of my children back then. My husband was observing. It was comforting to know that the glyconutrient blend was providing the necessary food molecules to help supply the eight known saccharides required in cellular communication.[4] For further clarification, and to be more precise, a blend of glyconutrients can include four precursor saccharides (i.e. rhamnose, glucuronic acid, galacturonic acid and arabinose) to help make the more vital derivatives (i.e. N-acetylgalactosamine, N-acetylglucosamine, N-acetylneuraminic acid/NANA). In the biochemical sense, the acetylated forms would not be able to survive stomach acid, hence, precursors should be available so the body can manufacture the acetylated forms from them.

Supplementation is a common sense approach to bringing back the appropriate and expected nutrition to our deprived, stressed and often toxic bodies. Why supplementation? Because our 21st century diet does not provide enough necessary saccharides and we may fail to metabolize adequate quantities to support the necessary cellular defense, repair, regeneration and healing. All these require the normal structure and function of glycoproteins for effective cell-to-cell communication.[5] The whole process of providing the necessary saccharides requires several biochemical steps, which together require tremendous amounts of energy for enzymatic conversions and the presence of co-factors like vitamins and minerals.

It has been a real challenge to feed the family, including myself, all the necessary nutrients in terms of quantity and value for maximum health benefit. Who would think that eating ½ cup of spinach would suffice to support the needs of at least our basic functions? Cellular structure and functionality of our bodies are both compromised each day of our lives! Each family member has unique individual developmental needs. Their full potential to "blossom" in every stage of their life will be completely hindered, if they don't receive what is missing even before conception. I could picture a mother passing on "broken chips/genes" to her unborn child. In addition, it is not feasible to consume a huge enough volume of food to "raise the cellular synthesis rate to the maximal production level."[6] Who can eat a bucket full of oranges or brocolli all at one time? That's not practical, by any means. Thus, it would be prudent to supplement. In my situation it was an obvious necessity. It's up to you to recognize its significance.

These physiologically important carbohydrate molecules create a huge nutritional impact at the foundational level of the cells! This fundamental knowledge has been overlooked and ignored. It is not all about symptoms and disease and giving a drug to "fight" disease. Rather, it is about giving the body the appropriate food molecules to be in line with its original design to support its daily tasks. It's the ideal approach, the right and sound approach.

A total absence of these vital micronutrients would not allow any single biochemical or physiologic process to occur. Why? Because glycosylation could not occur. If we consume only a fraction of what is required, or if we overload on only some (i.e. our current diet is overloaded with glucose and fructose ie. table sugar), then deficiency and disease would be encouraged. In other words, without an attached sugar (glycosyl) moiety, many vital functions won't be carried out efficiently. We are designed to eat the right building blocks of foods - called macronutrients. (i.e. proteins, fats and carbohydrates). We are built from, repaired and fueled by these substances found in the diet. We also cannot forget the very important micronutrients which consist mainly of vitamins, minerals and other antioxidants. As mentioned earlier, the ones that are missing are the most valuable and important. We stumble over the same problem of not knowing what our cells need primarily. We consciously or unconsciously deny this simple fact. In turn, this repetitive act leads us into feeding our bodies inappropriately with improper molecular forms of food. This potentially invites our early demise.

Our bodies preferentially require dietary sources of glyconutrients. Once again, it's part of the supreme design. To emphasize this preference, our intestinal tracts have been found to have specific "pumps" or transporters for these glyconutrients.[1]

The Mystery Unfolds

It amazes me that glyconutrients could fill the "big piece of the puzzle" in the arena of natural health and nutrition. They are indeed **the missing link in nutrition.** They are fundamental to health and disease and the key to wellness. In my entire time in medical school and training, I have no recollection of anyone discussing the indispensable connection between diet and disease per se. Rather, nutrition was more or less taken for granted. But the evidence is now available and the explosive growth in glycobiology I described earlier makes it an issue for every doctor to reckon with - sooner or later!

The July 2002 issue of *Scientific American* presents a refreshing portrait of glycoproteins, and of the *glyco-* (sugars) in particular, "*so ubiquitous are these molecules that cells appear to other cells and to the immune system as sugarcoated.*"[3]. Dr. Ajit Varki of Scripps Research Institute describes it simply, "that every cell in the body is covered by this coating of sugars."[7] What powerful descriptions! We are born with these sugar molecules, forming several thousands of glycoproteins already known, but with more to be identified. They appear in and on cell membranes, inside every cell (in organelles: mitochondria, ribosomes, the Golgi apparatus and of course, in cytoplasm), and in the extracellular fluid.

The mystery is portrayed in an article in *Acta Anatomica, "Although numerous glycoprotein glycans have been characterized, we do not know what the principles are that guide their formation, nor the reasons why they have been selected by nature out of the billions of structures of similar sizes..."* [8]

The presence or absence of these vital sugar molecules determines whether the operating genes can transcribe messenger RNA (ribonucleic acid) and in turn communicate instructions for the proper synthesis of molecules to influence the maintenance, regulation and restoration of systems within the cells and tissues, to attain the normal state of physical being. That's just the way we're supposed to be. However our functioning capabilities have been dampened by our lifestyles, time after time, to produce a reflection of our "limping" cellular structures and our weak physical foundation. We have this potential, but we often don't allow it to manifest itself.

Everyone is a product of the beautiful union of two cells, the egg and the sperm. Have you ever thought of how this union came about? Now we know that cellular communication is the key to this union.[9] I never had the right perspective from the beginning. The wonder of it all is captured in a single sentence by J. Hodgson in the 1990 Bio/Tech issue, *"Almost without exception, whenever two or more living cells interact in a specific way, cell surface carbohydrates will be involved."*[10] Dr. Varki echoes the same in the October 2001 article "$34M Sweetens Area's Research Coffers, Scripps", adding *"glycosylation has a big effect in how interactions occur."*[7] From these statements, we see a great take-off after the union of sperm and egg described, in an article of *Acta Anatomica* entitled, *"Glycocoding as an Information Management System in Embryonic Development."*[11] The title alone mirrors an evolutionary process equipped with a precise biological information management system. The saccharides represent an alphabet of biologic information with unsurpassed coding capacity. The guiding principles are operative through the ability of carbohydrates to direct other molecules in a supreme orderly fashion despite the "extraordinary structural variability of sugars".

Then I came across much more in *Acta Anatomica*. The 1998 issue was solely dedicated to Glycoscience. It is very informative on the signaling pathways before the manifestation of cellular responses. Since the sugar units store information and establish an 'alphabet' of life, a deciphering process by receptors has to occur. An array of both qualitative and quantitative aspects of such expression is revealed. In this process, the message is decoded and then transduced by several signaling pathways.[12]

I was enlightened by the word "*decoded*". The word decoded simply means 'converted from code to plain text.' The glyco-code is transmitted and communicated through cellular responses and then transcribed as physical realities!

Super Mom

As I mentioned earlier, I started consuming glyconutrients in late 1998, after learning of its safety and efficacy. At that time, I was already experiencing joint pains and developing a soft growth on the dorsal aspect of my right wrist. Every morning I would experience stiffness and pain in my feet. It would take quite a while to "settle down" so I could start my day. After the first week on the glyconutrients, I was able to get up from bed refreshed and without pain. My energy level had increased and I noted a deeper sleep as I was not being awakened by light sounds as before. What a blessing that was to a mother of small children. I was also a lot more peaceful as weeks went by. The growth on my wrist was totally gone after a few months. When I came down with a cold after the first six months of use, I increased my intake because of what I had learned by then. My body recognized the "food"! In 24 hours, I was able to get rid of the cold. This was somewhat of a surprise to me, since it would usually take at least a week for me to get over my persistent cold symptoms.

Because of these early physical experiences, I concluded further that perhaps every part of my body could possibly be corrected and nourished. I now realized there was hope. I had had several years of antibiotic therapy since I was born. This included the "sentence" to be on antibiotics when I came down with rheumatic fever and a Grade 1 heart murmur. That meant approximately 5-6 years on Penicillin G and the development of *Streptoccocus B* in one of my pregnancies. That was not to mention the many different types of antibiotics that were also prescribed. More drugs were administered for my allergies. I also had two surgeries. My body was toxic and malnourished. Being underweight was a great issue for me and I would feel dizzy all the time. Despite all these problems, I managed to have several babies. However, I was literally a walking survivor and not a "healthy" camper. I was not well, much of the time. I kept thinking, "*Physician, heal thyself*".

Recall that I was nursing my fifth child when I first started on glyconutrients. I noted that she was a lot "happier" and more content compared to the others. Her first year was without an ear infection, even though I supplement-fed her with formula that I used as a crutch back then. This was notable since the others had experienced at least two or three episodes of respiratory problems. My other children were with my mother after I gave birth. They were introduced to a glyconutrient blend with phytonutrients in the form of convenient gummy bears by another family member. None of them experienced any physical ailment while away from home. This was great, since nursing a new born was taking a lot of time and I didn't have to worry about them.

It wasn't long before I became pregnant again with our sixth child. I was confirmed pregnant around 17 weeks gestation and didn't know 'til then. The first trimester was a breeze. Imagine, I did not experience any nausea or vomiting at all this time. I was eating better and maintained a good weight. My past records for the first 5 children show pre-term labor and delivery. I always experienced premature contractions and I would be on "bed rest" from around 26 weeks until I delivered around 35-36 weeks. To be on complete bed rest for two months in the hospital was a horrific experience. Once you have a pre-term baby, you tend to have successive pre-terms. However, the sixth child was only a few days short of term and was heavier than the average of 5.5 lbs. Premature contractions were not as frequent or severe and I was able to hold on a little bit longer than the previous one.

My husband started noticing the changes and started taking glyconutrients himself. Before I share the best pregnancy, the seventh, I would like to remind you that I was still actively researching and learning more about glyconutrients on a day to day basis. For this, I was being prepared through my own experiences.

I managed to share the excitement of what was happening in my family with some groups of people early in the year. In the course of one of my travels, I came down with an upper respiratory infection. My aunt told me to try taking "other" supplements. As soon as I added some phytonutrients and phytosterols to the glyconutrients, the coughing stopped within a few hours and I noted a "painless" menstrual period just before I boarded the plane. This was the opportunity for me to learn about synergistic nutritional relationships.[13] Notably, the "complex and intertwined biological events require specific and orderly factors and co-factors." Hence, "one is required for the metabolism of the other". I also found myself looking on a deeper level at how our five body systems (i.e. immune, defense, energy, endocrine and elimination) are interrelated. It also became more obvious that modulation and balancing of these different systems is critical. Once cellular communication is enhanced, regardless of the amounts of glyconutrients taken, other needs of the cells will become exposed. An interplay of biochemical and physiological support is expected through the harmonious relationship of specific bio-active substances found naturally in plants. The report on the "augmented" optimal health system study by Dr. Gil Kaats, et al was an eye opener.[14] The researchers added phytonutrients and phytosterols and the study revealed the reversal of ten bio-markers for aging. That impressed me, so I started taking the synergistic nutrients and more changes started happening.

Meanwhile, I started receiving chiropractic treatments for the severe scoliosis of my back. I was "bone on bone" in two areas of my neck and two in my lower spine.

I recall a quote from Albert Schweitzer, MD, a Nobel laureate and medical missionary who had said, "*Each patient carries his own doctor inside him. We are at our best when we give the doctor who resides within a chance to go to work.*" Those are great words!

My body quickly responded and after three months, my vertebral discs seemed to be like new! I experienced a higher level of function for I was able to take deeper breaths and I no longer experienced numbness and tingling on my right arm. Apparently, the glyconutrients were able to reach the nutritionally deprived areas.

A Glyco-Baby

In late 2001, we conceived our seventh child. I was using a complete line up of glyconutritionals for at least a year before conception. I was able to finally incorporate some regular physical activity by juggling around family time. I was now much better "equipped" with the right nutritional building blocks for a healthier pregnancy, labor and delivery and of course, a healthier baby. My metabolism was more stable and I no longer had 9-1-1emergency calls. Larger serving sizes of glyconutrients, along with phytosterols, phytonutrients, vitamins and minerals in a whole food matrix, were all taken to ensure a healthy pregnancy and a healthier baby. Once again, the first and second trimester went by fast, with more "happy" days devoid of nausea and vomiting and no fatigue. I had more sleep than ever. There was no development of new "striae" on my abdomen, since I actively used a topical glyconutrient-phytosterol complex to nourish my skin. The baby was more active in the womb compared to the previous six children. The entire pregnancy was normal, with no premature contractions. I did not have to depend on friends and family to bring dinners since I was "up" and "about" and able to prepare healthy meals before labor.

Labor went faster, with stronger contractions. I declined any intravenous line and any medications and totally depended on glyconutrients. My husband kept on pouring "a lot" of glyconutrients into my sports bottle. Delivery was "comfortable" and more enjoyable. Another topical glyconutrient product was used as the baby's head was coming out. There was no vaginal tear and swelling. Women who have had several pregnancies have the risk of hemorrhaging, but not in my case. The amount of post-partum bleeding was less. I had regular "menstrual-like" flow about four hours after delivery. My whole body was not fatigued after the event. The baby reached term, weighing six pounds, eleven and a half ounces, the heaviest of all. She was more alert and aware of her environment. As she reached out for my finger to latch on, I thought that was a symbolical reminder that sugars speak in a "language of touch". What a blessed sight! My post-partum recovery was excellent. I had more energy than ever. I nursed the baby in the first few days without being dependent on codeine for uterine cramps. I was able to nurse for a whole year. The baby was a picture of good health. To crown the experience, both my attending obstetrician and post-partum nurse witnessed all the events and eventually they started on glyconutrients for themselves and their families.

> *"We are at our best, when we give the doctor who resides within a chance to go to work."*
>
> -Albert Schweitzer, MD

My children were exhibiting vibrant health, year after year. One of the kids' commented, "Mommy, we are enjoying all the holidays now...we also don't have to buy "nose" tissue all the time!" We were receiving complements from others, despite our initial reservations. In time, we no longer had urgent care visits for ear infections and other typical pediatric problems. Previously, I remember the nights I had to "recall" what I had learned from medical school..."what now? what bacteria, what virus is involved this time?..." It had been "mental" torture and the sickly experiences had taken a toll physically on me as the mother. Then I stumbled into Louis Pasteur's quote at his deathbed in 1885, "I have been wrong. The germ is nothing. The 'terrain' is everything." The terrain is our body. This confession emphasizes the importance for the body to have all the essential tools to defend and heal itself. Glyconutrients are certainly among them. The physical evidence is demonstrated through our "built in clocks" in the Golgi apparatus, a cellular organelle. "Glycosylation in the Golgi includes coding for a timer and address to determine how long the complex molecule lasts and where in the body the moiety is to be sent."[6] That's real necessary information.

For a busy mother with a growing family, this "freedom" through glyconutrients was priceless. The introduction of healthier and nourishing foods at the table was an easy transition for the young ones since the cravings for "junk" lessened. The first three children and my husband started to follow along. The whole family was now committed to building the foundation of wellness. There was more discipline deeply ingrained in daily living. The children were growing with a nourishing foundation. They were being nutritionally prepared for their next phase of growth and development.

During the course of my studies in glycoscience, our son, eight years old at that time and now eleven, became amazed by the cover of *Science* magazine.[15] He came up with his own rendition of the sugar molecules with the DNA-RNA helical structure using different colored balloons. What a thrill of protection he discovered! He intentionally popped the "blue" balloons that he named as the sugar coated molecules. He further explained that the "DNA is now exposed to danger!" That was for me, Glycoscience 101 from the mouths of babes! Learning wellness and its foundation through the family's daily experiences was an exciting addition to our home school curriculum.

Sharing the Benefits

We were approached by a lady one day who wanted to know what I was giving my children. She noted that they were healthy. She wanted her son to be healthy too. The family doctor wanted to introduce Ritalin for the diagnosis of ADD/ADHD. After telling her of the benefits and allowing her to educate herself, she decided to put her son on glyconutrients in gummy form. After three months on the glyconutrients, he had better concentration and became well behaved and later received a "blue" award from the principal. His grades of "F" and "C" were moving up to "B" and "A". A well-rounded glyconutrional program was introduced months later and the child was able to "graduate" from a private special education school for learning disabilities to a regular public school. This transition saved the family the high cost of schooling that was $600 per month! His motor skills and reading skills were all markedly improved. The teacher took note of his "beautiful" handwriting. His height and weight improved from fifty percentile to ninety percentile. In addition, he had infrequent doctor visits. The parents were ecstatic over their son's dramatic improvement. The nutritional foundation of the boy had just begun.[16,17]

A young man in his late twenties was suffering from a skin disorder, allergies, and seizures. He was sick throughout his whole life. His wife related the times when he would have to go home from work and end up in the emergency room or urgent care, at least once a month. She was taking over household responsibilities since he couldn't function well. Both husband and wife were desperate to find a solution. The blend of glyconutrients and other glyconutritionals were introduced. Initially, his body showed more rashes but his seizures came under control. As time went by, his skin improved. It would seem that in the simplest of terms, the body has an internal priority list. Since the glyconutrients may act like zip code addresses in some way, these nutrients knew where the problem of highest priority was.[7] In this case, it was the neurologic system of this man's body. He became happier and was able once again to assume household responsibilities. He could now spend more time with his family and enjoy the children. The wife was so grateful for her answered prayers.

Another nice elderly lady showed up in one of my presentations. She was very skeptical. However, as a lung cancer survivor and having other active issues, she decided to give glyconutrients a "try". I took pains to emphasize that the body usually needs some time to heal, especially after years of insult. I also emphasized the different life spans of cell types in the body, especially the typical four months for the red blood cells in particular.[18] There was little apparent change by the fourth month, just on typical maintenance quantities. Financial constraint was another issue but I encouraged her to stick with the program. When the funds came in, she was able to feed her body the appropriate amounts and in turn, physical responses started to appear faster. Her cholesterol level which had been in the 300's, dropped in a few months.[19] Her allergies were relieved and she was able to get out of her house more often. Her body is now actively healing and she is seeing more changes. Her doctor is aware of the glyconutrients she has been taking and has approved of them. She is now seventy and glowing radiantly with good health.

Another lady with whom I shared glyconutrients was desperately wanting to get off her anti-depressants. She was typical of so many in our modern industrialized society. She was longing for a better life, after her unfortunate bout with esophageal cancer. Laboratory results revealed that her thyroid was not producing adequate hormones due to the radiation treatments. That's a well known side effect. No wonder she was depressed all the time, for we know that depression is also clearly associated with hypothyroidism. Within just a few months on glyconutrients her thyroid actually started to function better. Phytosterols were added later and she blossomed into a new happy person. Her outlook in life changed and her spirits were up. She was no longer on anti-depressants!

In August 2003, I received a call from my own obstetrician regarding the case of a young mother in her early 20's who was on life support in a comatose state. The patient had an unremarkable labor and delivery and was discharged with her baby after three days. But then, a few days after discharge she fell ill and fluid accumulated rapidly in her lungs . All allopathic means were tried and failed. The introduction for her of a newly FDA-approved drug was costing our state a tremendous amount of money. Her team of doctors believed that she would not be able to make it through the weekend. Since this was a life and death situation, I decided to seek encouragement from another doctor who had an experience with this type of scenario.[20] I commend him for his big heart. Through a 3-way phone conversation, my obstetrician was able to gain the confidence to introduce glyconutrients. The risk/benefit ratio was clearly in favor of trying a new intervention. Scientific information was immediately presented to the other doctors in the team. My obstetrician has a giving heart that led her to offer the patient a fifty gram tub of powdered glyconutrients, while waiting for more supply. That same day, after the intermittent infusion of twenty-five grams of glyconutrients through a feeding tube, the patient stabilized within a few hours for the first time. She regained consciousness and was off the ventilation support after just a week. While the patient was recovering, the attending obstetrician appealed to the medical director of the state insurance and emphasized that a hundred dollar product is "peanuts" compared to the high cost of medical care! I commend my obstetrician for her compassion and her persistent efforts for the sake of her patient. She was truly looking after the needs of her patient. The patient came home to her newborn after three weeks! What a life-giving event.

For some reason in December 2003, I insisted on informing my dad of the cost of being sick. I had deep concern regarding his overall lifestyle, in particular - his eating habits. My mom had informed me of his excessive eating habits. I let him know that if there are "hindrances" or "anti-nutrients" in the picture, it would take a longer time for his body to achieve optimal health, even though he had already started taking glyconutrients. The warning was ignored. Sad to say, in February 2004, he had a stroke. He lost his speech (became aphasic) and developed weakness in his right upper extremity. He had access to the best medical advice and care, but I knew that traditional medicine would not offer him the best hope for recovery and better quality of life. I had to appeal to dad's attending physician for him to officially include glyconutrients in the management of his care. He resisted, even with all the science behind glyconutrients. The information available in the PDR (Physicians Desk Reference) for Non-Prescription Drugs and Dietary Supplements was not enough either.

Fortunately, my dad was appointed a new case manager who gave us the encouragement to pursue the appeal. She informed us of her own magnificent recovery from breast cancer when she incorporated glyconutrients. Then came a nutritionist who had the duty to examine the information on the glyconutrients and I had the chance to educate her on them. She understood. However, a waiver letter had to be submitted to expedite the approval. Dad's recovery speeded up after the doctor approved the protocol I had written. Larger serving sizes of glyconutrients and other synergistic nutrients were administered through a naso-gastric tube. More progress was noted when dad was transferred to a skilled nursing facility. Again, I had to deal with a new staff that was feeding him the same foods that contributed to his toxic and congested body. One of the tests showed that he had had a silent myocardial infarction. I thank God that he had received some protection through glyconutrients, even before the stroke.

I persisted.

The nurse coordinator wrote my dad off the chart, believing that he would "end up just like the rest." Dad's wonderful recovery defied her stubborn uninformed belief. He was discharged walking in strides, not in a wheelchair. The coordinator at the facility got on glyconutrients for herself and her family. I am so happy to report that to date, Dad is regaining his speech steadily, learning his fifth language, regaining his motor function, breathing comfortably and eating well. He now prefers eating vegetables! A lot of his friends noted that he started to 'look younger' and complemented him on his glowing skin. Mom now has more incentive to remain healthy. My dad is alive and has a better quality of life compared to other stroke victims. For this, I give thanks!

*"**I** have been wrong.*

The germ is nothing.

The 'terrain' is

everything."

-Louis Pasteur, 1885

Conclusions

In our modern society, people tend to depend on others to take care of their own bodies. Too many of us have forsaken the responsibility to take care of ourselves. In time, the ability to listen to our own bodily responses is lost. To do that might be a difficult task in the beginning, but it's worth every effort to learn and understand when the body speaks. The experience that my family and I have had with glyconutrients have been most rewarding. I hope that this chapter and the entire book in fact, will enrich and encourage you to try these supplements and then to stay on the course to wellness with glyconutrients.

About the Author:
Maria N Mona, M.D.

Dr. Maria Mona found her calling in the "true" field of wellness. She earned the degree Doctor of Medicine from Far Eastern University in Manila, Philippines in 1988. She is currently pursuing her second and third post-doctoral degrees in Natural Health. She is a certified member of the American Nutraceutical Association.

Editors Note:

Glyconutrients are important in health but they also influence disease. So we turn next to the leading cause of death in the industrialized world - cardiovascular disease. Much of this is preventable. Can glyconutrients make a real difference? Let's find out ...

Chapter 9

Glyconutrients & Cardiovascular Disease

Dr. Luis Romero

Cardiovascular disease is a very broad and widely-recognized category that includes all conditions that affect the heart and blood vessels. In this chapter, we want to review some basic concepts about cardiovascular diseases, the associated risk factors and the apparent implications of using glyconutrition as nutritional health support.

#1 Killer

To begin, let's just consider some alarming statistics from the Center for Disease Control (CDC) in Atlanta, Georgia:

- Heart disease and stroke - the principal components of cardiovascular disease - are the first and third leading causes of death in the United States, accounting for more than 40% of all deaths.
- About 950,000 Americans die of cardiovascular disease each year, which amounts to one death every 33 seconds.
- Although heart disease and stroke are often thought to affect men and older people primarily, it is also a major killer of women and people in the prime of life.
- About 61 million Americans (almost one-fourth of the population) have some form of cardiovascular disease.
- Coronary heart disease is a leading cause of premature, permanent disability among working (productive) adults.
- Stroke alone accounts for the disability of more than 1 million Americans.
- Almost 6 million hospitalizations each year are due to cardiovascular disease.

Needless to say, cardiovascular disease is a huge burden on society in terms of death and disability. That's a major concern. In addition, its economic effect on the U.S. health care system grows larger as the population ages. In 2003, the cost of heart disease and stroke was projected to be $351 billion: $209 billion for direct health care expenditures and $142 billion for lost productivity from death and disability.

What are the so called cardiovascular diseases? They may be broadly sub-divided into two main groups:

A) *Heart (cardiac) diseases* - which include, disorders of the heart per se, as the cardiovascular pump, as well as diseases of the coronary blood vessels surrounding and supplying the heart itself.

B) *Vascular diseases* - which refers to diseases of the blood vessel system (arteries, capillaries, veins) within a person's entire body, supplying organs such as the brain, eyes, kidneys, arms and legs, etc...

Cardiovascular diseases, in general, also have common risk factors and changes within the body's arterial - capillary bed. The risk factors are those scientifically confirmed to be related to, or are able to induce, develop or aggravate these diseases. They include some physiological characteristics or conditions as well as important lifestyle/behavior patterns that can clearly be modified.

RISK FACTORS
For Cardiovascular Disease

Physiological	**Lifestyle**
Hypertension (elevated blood pressure)	Cigarette - Tobacco Smoking
Hypercholesterolemia (elevated cholesterol levels in the blood)	Sedentary Living (Lack of Exercise)
Hypertriglyceridemia (elevated triglyceride levels in the blood)	Obesity
High levels of homocysteine in the blood	Poor Nutrition
Diabetes Mellitus	
Infections with "Stealth Pathogens"	
Post Menopause	
Stress / Anxiety	
Genetics (Family History)	

Atherosclerosis

It is now widely accepted that although cardiovascular diseases have multi-factoral "inductors", they all contribute to the development of the main anatomical and functional disorder that constitutes the base of most of these diseases - ***Atherosclerosis.***

The process of atherosclerosis is characterized by a hardening / thickening of the arterial - capillary walls. This pathological process is initiated by some sort of damage to the intima, which is the inner layer of our arteries and capillary vessels. The damage is characterized by abnormal physical changes within the endothelial cells which turn the characteristic normal "smoothness" of the endothelium into a rough surface which allows molecules and cells to adhere to that damaged area.

When atherosclerosis begins, another phenomenon soon occurs at the damaged endothelial surface. **Cholesterol** and other molecules start to deposit there, leading to the creation of an intra-vessel plaque. This process continues and the sequential deposit of cholesterol creates a progressive reduction of the vessel lumen, thereby reducing the blood flow that normally passes through that area of the vessel.

The atherosclerotic process leads to 'fatty streaks' and 'fibrous plaques' which contain more than just cholesterol. Other fats, mainly including triglycerides, also precipitate on the plaque, sometimes along with platelet cells, heavy metal deposits and other toxic molecules, as well as bacteria, viruses, fungi - all of which have been demonstrated in autopsies.

Platelets are blood cells indispensable to the coagulation (clotting formation) process. These cells start to aggregate (stick together) and by doing this, contribute to the progressive narrowing of the blood vessel lumen.

The progressive narrowing could eventually end in the total obliteration (occlusion) of the affected vessel. If that happens, blood flow through the artery or capillary ceases. Any tissue dependent on blood flow for oxygen and nutrients would die, resulting in what's known as infarction. In the case of the coronary arteries surrounding and supplying the heart, this leads to a **heart attack** or **myocardial infarction**. When the blockage of the artery occurs in a vessel supplying the brain, this will lead to what is called an **ischemic stroke**. Cutting off the blood supply to other organs or limbs in this way can lead to different serious consequences. Other complications of the atherosclerotic / cardiovascular process may cause secondary hemorrhagic (bleeding) event, which shows up in the affected organ or tissue.

Today it has also been demonstrated that three other factors are involved in the generation of atherosclerosis. One is *inflammation* and the second is, the presence of *pathogens* (bacteria, viruses, fungi) - in some medical research, they are called Stealth Pathogens. The third factor is *abnormal angiogenesis*. The term 'angiogenesis' refers to the formation of new blood vessels, which can predispose to atherosclerosis if there are underlying abnormalities.

By all means, atherosclerosis is a very complex, multi-factoral process that can lead to the development, progression and complications of cardiovascular diseases. Because of its importance as the main killer in modern times, the general population should know that **atherosclerosis is a very preventable disease**. We can prevent it and we can change not only the occurrence, but also the course of its evolution, and therefore, its end-points: namely, the costly complications to healthcare and the primary and secondary deaths related to it.

Risk Factors

Almost all cardiovascular risk factors are ***identifiable, controllable and reversible***. Therefore, we can intervene and change the bothersome statistics, which are unfortunately worsening.

Physiological Risk Factors

Hypertension

Hypertension corresponds to a well-defined cardiovascular risk factor. Long-term hypertension (above the normal limits 140/90) causes the natural elasticity of the blood vessels to deteriorate, as well as it favors endothelial intima damage, thereby inducing atherosclerosis. As such, hypertension alone can trigger any acute cardiovascular event, such as a heart attack or stroke.

Hypertension is generally a controllable cardiovascular risk factor. Control involves achieving the proper lifestyle (especially nutrition and exercise) and good medical management.

Dislipidemia: High Cholesterol and High Triglycerides

The word *dislipidemia* means, a disorder of the lipid content within the blood stream. Lipids include cholesterol and triglycerides which are "indispensable fats" that form structural molecules within all our cells and are also normally present within the blood stream. These fats are attached to other molecules (proteins) for transport, forming complexes called lipoproteins.

There are four main types of cholesterol transported in the blood as lipoproteins. The two very important and well known types are named low density lipoprotein (LDL), commonly referred to as the BAD cholesterol carrier; and the densest one, named high density lipoprotein (HDL), also referred to as the GOOD cholesterol carrier.

Research studies have shown that elevated LDL is a definitive risk factor for triggering, developing and complicating atherosclerotic / cardiovascular diseases. The higher the level above the considered upper limit of normal (100mg/dl) progressively worsens the process and prompts the person with this elevated BAD - cholesterol (LDL) to develop the progressive disease and become potentially exposed to suffer an acute event. On the other hand, research studies have also shown that, the higher the level of the GOOD - cholesterol (HDL) which should be above 50 or even 60mg/dl, the more protected that person will be, preventing the progression and any potential acute cardiovascular event. Total cholesterol should be below 200 mg/dl, while triglyceride levels should be below 150 mg/dl.

All of us need to know the indispensability of keeping our blood levels of cholesterol and triglycerides within normal limits, with low fat and high fiber diets, exercise and supplementation. In this way, we will be closing doors to these significant cardiovascular risk factors.

High Levels of Homocysteine

Homocysteine is an amino acid related to the metabolism of cysteine, which converts to glutathione (the cells super antioxidant). For many years, the scientific literature has pointed out the correlation of high blood levels of homocysteine and the development of atherosclerosis, by damaging the inner lining of arteries and promoting blood clots.

Inadequate intake of folic acid and other B-vitamins is correlated with progressively higher levels of homocysteine in the blood stream. It is not surprising that blood levels of homocysteine have progressively increased over the last 30 years, and correspond with the increasing incidence of atherosclerosis. Why? It reflects common characteristics of the modern USA diet: high in calories, high in (bad) fats, with lots of preservatives, but also, very poor in vitamins, including folic acid and many other indispensable micro-nutrients.

Normal homocyseine levels were considered to range from 5-15 micromoles/lit. But levels above 6.3 have been shown to cause a steep, progressive risk of heart attack. People with high blood levels of homocysteine should be advised to get enough folic acid and vitamins B6 and

B12 in their diet. They need to include green leafy vegetables and grain products fortified with folic acid in their diet.

Diabetes Mellitus

Diabetes Mellitus (or just, diabetes, for our purposes) is a group of metabolic disorders with one common manifestation: hyperglycemia (high blood glucose levels). Chronic hyperglycemia causes damage to the eyes, kidneys, nerves, heart and blood vessels.

Diabetes Mellitus is classified in two Types - 1 and 2. In the first case, diabetes that is characterized by absolute insulin deficiency and relatively acute onset, usually starting before 25 years of age, corresponds within the new classification (1997) as Type 1 diabetes mellitus. On the other hand, Type 2 diabetes mellitus (formerly called adult-onset or non-insulin dependant) is characterized by insulin resistance in peripheral tissue and an insulin secretion defect of the beta cells within the pancreas. This is the most common form of diabetes mellitus (90% of the diabetic population are - Type 2) and is highly associated with a family history of diabetes, older age, obesity, lack of exercise, and more prevalent in Blacks, Hispanics and Native Americans. It is more common in women, especially women with a history of gestational diabetes (during pregnancy).

Any patient with two fasting plasma glucose levels of 126 mg per dl (7.0 mml per L) or greater, is considered to have diabetes mellitus.

Uncontrolled diabetes can develop very serious complications. Therefore, we need to prevent this disease in the first place, or if we already have established diabetes, we need to maintain the best possible metabolic control. Medical management is indicated but in addition, the most important lifestyle resources for achieving good metabolic control of diabetes mellitus are:

- Correct **diet** - meal plans such as that proposed by the American Diabetes Association, ie. low fat, balanced protein intake and abundant green vegetables and some fresh fruits;
- Physical activity - **exercise** on a regular basis is recommended, if not mandatory;
- Good **hydration** - water is best. Avoid America's favorite beverages: soda pop, coffee and alcohol;
- Effective **weight management** - this can be affected by the previous three factors.

We should all focus on prevention strategies, the only affordable approach for coping with the spiraling burden of this costly and bothersome disease.

Inflammation, Infections and "Stealth Pathogens"

This is a previously unrecognized risk factor but a growing body of research cites blood vessel inflammation as a major independent risk factor for cardiovascular disease. Researchers at University of Iowa, Iowa City, report that very small amounts of an endotoxin (a substance present in bacteria) can cause blood vessels to swell. According to associate research scientist Lynn Stoll, "With chronic infections, like smoker's bronchitis or periodontitis [infection of the gums], small amounts of bacteria can intermittently get into the bloodstream where they don't belong. Often, these infections are just sort of smoldering there without major symptoms. They are not severe enough to require treatment. But these types of infections can linger for months or years, causing inflammation that can, over the long term, potentially contribute to blood vessel blockage."

In her book about *Stealth Organisms, Cell Wall Deficient Forms: Stealth Pathogens*, Dr. Lida H. Mattman presents a long list of stealth pathogens implicated and found during autopsies and microscopic and immune tests of the cardiovascular atherosclerotic lesions, as well as others attacking the blood cells. They include bacteria like *chlamydia pneumoniae, helicobacter pylori, porphyromonas gingivalis,* and viruses like cytomegalovirus (CMV), herpes simplex virus 1 and 2, enteroviruses and hepatitis A virus.

Post - Menopausal State

In women, hormone production by the ovaries from the first menstruation to the last one, is a protective factor against the development of cardiovascular diseases. However, in the peri-menopause and more so, within the post-menopausal period, declining hormone production and its physiology becomes a real risk for developing cardiovascular disease. In addition, post-menopause favors the development of high blood pressure, elevates the bad (LDL) and total cholesterol and reduces the good (HDL) cholesterol, among other undesirable consequences. This last consideration is the main reason for the continuous (though cautious) recommendation for hormonal replacement (HRT) in post-menopausal women. But numerous studies have also shown that conventional HRT could lead to developing future malignant diseases.

Post-menopausal cardiovascular disease and stroke can account for a large percentage of all adult female deaths. The increased risk after menopause is 1 in 50 in the 45-65 age groups, and rises to 1 in 3 above 65 years of age. However, the good news is that published studies show effectiveness, with no side effects, when phytohormones are used in post-menopausal women, to control symptoms and reduce the increased risk for having cardiovascular events.

Genetics

We have 50% genetic information from each of our parents, which makes us either more prone to, or more resistant to, developing certain diseases, including the cardiovascular ones. It is a well recognized risk factor. If you have a close relative who suffered from heart disease or stroke, you are more likely to develop a similar condition. However, this is a relative risk and not an absolute one. It is not an inevitable consequence. In fact, more and more scientific studies have shown that we can 'override' our genetics, with nutrition, with exercise and adequate lifestyles. More recently it has also been shown that we can also do this by using certain phytonutrients as well.

Lifestyle Risk Factors

Now we turn from physiology to **behavior**. The emphasis is now on personal choices and lifestyle habits that can have just as important an effect in causing cardiovascular disease as any of the more internal issues we just covered. The obvious first consideration is that of smoking.

Smoking

It is widely recognized and published in the medical literature that cigarette smoking is the single most alterable risk factor contributing to premature development of cardiovascular disease, as well as many other chronic illnesses like respiratory disease (asthma, emphysema), cancer, complications of diabetes, gastrointestinal disorders, skin (premature wrinkles) and more recently a focus on neurological chronic degenerative illnesses like multiple sclerosis. This all leads to smoking-induced deaths, accounting for approximately 430,000 deaths annually in the United States.

In the inner layer of the blood vessels (the endothelial cells), smoking induces cellular mechanical changes that will alter the indispensable smoothness of the intima which precipitates atherosclerosis and all its horrendous consequences. Smoking also triggers and aggravates hypertension (high blood pressure) thereby facilitating and accelerating blood vessel hardening and other damaging alterations.

In many publications, a warning equation is referred to that is summarized as:

Smoking + High Cholesterol + Hypertension = Cardiovascular Time Bomb

What to do when we smoke? *Did you ask the question*? **You need to QUIT as soon as possible**. Smoking cessation programs have been shown to effectively reduce the damaging effect of this risk factor for cardiovascular disease.

Today, there are so many proven methods that no one who wants to quit has an adequate excuse. You can use a pill, a patch, gum, hypnosis, laser, psychology, group therapy, and the list goes on. The addiction is a habit that can be broken. Nicotine dependence and withdrawal is now well understood and can be effectively managed. So, speak to your doctor TODAY and if you can't find help, for whatever reason, get on the phone, talk to a friend, go to a pharmacy ... just do whatever it takes. It will save you money, and prevent bad breath, the inability to savour the taste of good food, alienation, body odor, home odors, dental bills and even premature wrinkles. But most of all, **it could save your life!**

Sedentary lifestyle

Modern life is crowded with all kinds of gadgets and things that require less and less physical effort. That makes it easier to be lazy and yet be comfortable going about our daily life. Between the automobile to take us everywhere, elevators and escalators to take us up and down floors, television to entertain us without any sweat, office jobs that demand a computer and little more, home appliances and furnishings that wash, clean, vacuum and do almost everything else ... who ever needs to use personal energy. Electricity is cheap, machines are everywhere and there's always an excuse for the lazy alternative. Despite all the ads, videos and workouts on television, Americans have become more like couch potatoes in each successive decade since the last world war. We are paying a huge price for this new sedentary lifestyle. And we're not alone. It's the plague of contemporary, affluent societies.

A new study reported in the South China Morning Post, which was conducted by the University of Hong Kong and the Department of Health in Hong Kong, suggested that "*living a sedentary lifestyle is more dangerous for our health than smoking*". In light of this recent scientific report, it is mandatory to broadcast the alarming, life threatening situation about sedentary living, and to emphasize that the more you move and physically use your body, the healthier it will become.

Particularly, with respect to cardiovascular diseases, moderate exercise strengthens the heart muscle. The exertion of the heart at increased demand strengthens the muscle fibers just like any other muscle when used under stress or physical exercise. It also increases the growth of small collateral vessels that improve coronary blood circulation around and into the heart. It favors increase in good (HDL) cholesterol and reduces bad (LDL) cholesterol. It improves weight management, reduces hypertension and reduces complications in diabetics, with improved sugar control. Again, moderate exercise (increased heart rate within limits for 20-30 minutes, for 3 - 4 time periods each week) is an all-win situation. Even the less demanding activities like walking and swimming can help and be somewhat protective.

If you cannot afford to go to a gym; if you have no home apparatus or equipment for daily work out; if you cannot walk or jog for half an hour, three or four times per week, for any reason ... then please *dance at home to fast music,* 30 to 45 minutes 4 to 5 times per week, at your most convenient time. *Get a skipping rope* or just *step on and off a common kitchen-step.* Any of these will do the trick. Now, if you have any physical disability, *exercise with the healthy part of your body,* but please *move, move and continue moving your body* to provide it with a better level of health prevention and good health maintenance, thus preserving your cardiovascular system and prolonging your healthier life.

Obesity

This risk factor is a real big one (no pun intended), not only because obesity is a major contributor to cardiovascular diseases, but also because of its dramatic growth statistics in American society.

The American Heart Association (AHA) has identified obesity as a major risk factor. Almost 70 percent of diagnosed cases of cardiovascular heart disease is related to obesity. According to experts from the AHA, a gain in weight of 20 excess pounds actually doubles the risk for developing cardiovascular disease.

Animal studies have documented that increasing the body fat tissue above normal, alters the myocardial (heart muscle) fatty acid metabolism and its working efficiency. Several other studies have demonstrated that obesity triggers and complicates cardiovascular diseases and because of this, the alarming statistics make this a national epidemic. In fact, this is not a singular effect, because obesity unfortunately is now proven as a risk factor for developing the majority of all chronic degenerative illnesses.

Obesity is linked to a metabolic syndrome called *Syndrome 'X'* in which sufferers have obesity combined with high blood pressure and high blood fats (cholesterol and triglycerides). Another unhealthy metabolic state is, *hyper-insulinism*, referring to high blood levels of insulin. The fat tissue tends to block the insulin receptors on the cell membranes leading to an increase in blood insulin levels.

Obesity today is a major public health problem. The US Surgeon General has labeled it as a national epidemic that includes all ages. Obesity among children has tripled over the past 30 years. Many obese children have high cholesterol and high blood pressure levels. Children and adolescents have shown an alarming increase in the incidence of Type 2 diabetes, ironically known as adult-onset diabetes. To compound this further, overweight adolescents have a 70 percent chance of becoming overweight or obese adults. Today we are seeing more and more overweight - obese adolescents with early evidence of cardiovascular disease.

Hippocrates wrote 360 years B.C. about lean people having a lower incidence of sudden death than obese individuals. Yet, here we are in the 21st century A.D. and obesity is causing hundreds of thousands of premature deaths in the most affluent nation that the world has ever known. It's time for the nation to discard this excess baggage which is an albatross of our own making.

Weight management is truly health management!!

Poor Diet

The problem of obesity reflects the serious problems with the typical diet in North America today. We eat far too much high calorie, high fat, and low fiber, over-processed, extensively-preserved, fast and convenience foods. Libraries are filled with all the books written about cooking and baking on one hand and about losing weight and looking fit on the other. But introduce the fast pace of modern life, the changing family structures and roles, the massive advertising and promotion of convenience foods, and the industrialization of the entire food supply - and you have the perfect recipe for a generation to carve its own graves with its own teeth.

Most of the risk factors for cardiovascular disease we discussed earlier have a strong dietary component. We know that diet can affect hypertension, diabetes, dislipidemia and homocysteine levels for sure. In fact, good management of any of these conditions demands that dietary intake become a central concern of both patient and doctor.

Just as a guideline for the reader, here is a simple summary of what you ought to remember as you seek to maintain a healthy diet:

- Eat small, regular and varied meals. (Make each one look more and more like a rainbow in color).
- Drink 6-8 glasses of fluid daily. Preferably, more water, fresh fruit juice and milk, and less pop, coffee and alcohol.
- Decrease salt and refined sugar intake - seen and unseen.
- Run away from fats before your very eyes.
- Increase fiber intake (whole cereals, grains, fresh fruits and vegetables).
- Shop for health (you will eat what you buy)
- Supplement your diet - especially with GLYCONUTRIENTS!

Prior to the scientific discovery of the eight necessary and vital sugars referred to as glyconutrients, many molecules present in the inflammation cascade were already recognized, but the "*code*" of cell-to-cell communication was not clear. It has now been demonstrated that this code depends on these eight sugars (monosaccharides). They combine with proteins to form glycoproteins which thereby acquire many different shapes. By doing so, they are able to form letters of an alphabet with which cells can communicate with each other. Of these eight necessary sugars, only two are commonly available in the normal western diet. Supplementation with the complete range of these vital nutrients will therefore make good sense and a host of benefits have been shown to be derived in both health and disease.

Now we want to address the value of such glyconutrient supplementation to the prevention and management of cardiovascular diseases in particular.

Underlying Mechanisms

We have seen in the description of the cardiovascular risk factors that they have a common denominator of abnormal cellular and organ responses that all directly or indirectly derive from changes at the molecular or structural levels and which favor the initiation and exacerbation of cardiovascular diseases. These common denominators for all cardiovascular disease result in some characteristic changes which can be summarized as follows:

- Inflammation (the body's response to any injury)

- Abnormal enzymes present at the site of inflammation (swelling)
- Abnormal cellular metabolism inside cells in the local area
- Presence of stealth pathogens and their toxins (tissue and blood)
- Abnormal capillaries in the swelling site-abnormal angiogenesis

These underlying mechanisms are at the heart of cardiovascular pathogenesis. In other words, they critically influence and even determine how the diseases originate and propagate. If we could influence these important determinants, we could, in principle, alter the incidence of cardiovascular diseases and their burdensome complications.

The good news is - that's where glyconutrients come in.

Inflammation

Any significant injury or insult to the body causes a primary event that triggers some white blood cells (neutrophils) which become attracted by the alarm-signals coming from the inflammatory (swelling) site. Neutrophils will come away from the blood stream, traverse the blood vessel wall and will arrive at the 'exact swelling tissue' zone. This process is meditated by several molecules, including the most important cytokines. This initial step is followed by the arrival of other specific immune cells which are drafted and put into action to arrest the injury and reverse damage. This entire coordinated process requires specialized cell-to-cell recognition and communication and that's where glycoproteins and hence, the glyconutrients become very important.

Glyconutrients are essential players in all the complex mechanisms involved in the inflammation cascade. They govern early changes at the intima, lining blood vessels, and are linked to almost all the actions of immune system cells. Thus, they are definitive markers for connecting information needed in communicating messages, recognizing sites for action, and for signaling cell surface receptors and molecules inside cells to act or re-act. This is a clear example of cell-to-cell communication in which glyconutrients provide the key.

Glyconutrients can help to prevent or block this early inflammation and can contribute to repair or reverse its consequences. For example, in laboratory animal models, mannose was shown to prevent an inflammatory crisis. Glyconutrients have direct actions on cytokines, enzymes and cells that are characteristic in the inflammation process/site. It appears that these "healing sugars" were designed in nature to be able to block many of these same molecules and cells to inhibit the abnormal changes that occur in the inflammatory (swelling) process. At the risk of oversimplification, glyconutrients have a definitive anti-inflammatory biological action and in this way, they become very beneficial to people at risk or suffering from any kind of cardiovascular disease.

Enzymes on swelling site:

At the local site of inflammation (swelling), abnormal enzymes appear to enter into a vicious cycle within the inflammation process. This cycle facilitates a number of metabolic abnormalities within cells. The inhibition of abnormal enzymes is another beneficial implicit action of these healing sugars. When glyconutrients inhibit these abnormal enzymes, they provide an essential anti-inflammatory effect.

Anti-Infectious Agents effect

We now know the overlooked risk factor in cardiovascular disease related to the presence of infectious agents (stealth pathogens) and their endo-toxins. Fortunately, glyconutrients have an interesting broad spectrum action against microbial agents of different types.

Let's briefly review some of these.

Microorganisms, including bacteria, viruses, fungi and parasites, gain access to our body and they use some molecule-receptors called *adhesins* that bind to the cell surface sugars and so become able to attack those very cells. Some of the recognition and molecular interaction between the microorganisms and the host cells have been studied and have shown the presence of mannose on both sites (the invaders and the hosts). Other interactions are not yet well demonstrated, but knowing the importance of glyconutrients in cell-to-cell communication functions and their ubiquitous role in the immune system reactions, it is reasonable to presume that glycoforms are involved in any microorganism invasion, recognition and retaliation as well. In this particular case and other biological cell-to-cell interactions, vital sugars (carbohydrates) are utilized as cell defense protectors and covers. When microorganisms attack, cells get coated with molecules like "mucins" (cf. mucus) for blocking the attackers' entry, and these molecules are mainly, carbohydrates.

Studies performed using glyconutrients have shown the "antimicrobial effects" of these healing sugars. By knowing this, we can conclude that glyconutrients should be used when cardiovascular diseases are present or when prevention of related ailments is desired.

There is one remaining process that increases the risk for cardiovascular disease but which has only recently received attention.

Abnormal Angiogenesis

Angiogenesis is a biological process by which cells and tissues get nutrients and oxygen provided by the blood coming through the tiny capillary vessels. This process when nourishing a normal cell / tissue is called, *normal* angiogenesis, and when it is involved in feeding an abnormal cell /tissue, it is called *abnormal* angiogenesis. The indispensable biological response in each cell's life is coded and mediated by molecules called growth factors, which also contain sugars (glycoproteins) and this is another important fact when considering this next function of glyconutrients.

Angiogenesis has been studied in different research centers around the world. One of the most important is at Harvard University where a group of researchers headed by the world renowned Dr. Judah Folkman. Since the early 70s, Dr. Folkman was able to show that abnormal angiogenesis was present in all inflammatory processes, and he also pointed out that, if abnormal angiogenesis could be blocked, the inflammation could be controlled and by doing so, would contribute to control and perhaps reverse the underlying associated process.

Researchers have shown that some other sugar-containing molecules (glycans) involved in the formation of the abnormal capillary vessels are different from those participating in the normal angiogenesis. This fact is very important, because the main role of glyconutrients in cell-to-cell communication, takes on additional significance in combating abnormal capillaries (abnormal angiogenesis) and by doing so, combating inflammation as well.

Glyconutrients have also been found to have anti-growth factor blocking activities at the site of formation of these abnormal capillaries, and by doing so, abnormal angiogenesis is further inhibited.

Conclusion

In summary, the biological actions of glyconutrients are extremely important in the presence of cardiovascular diseases, because they have beneficial effects in preventing the deleterious consequences of all the common denominators found in these diseases. As such, they exert biological effects that are:

- Anti-inflammatory,
- Anti-abnormal blocking (ectopic) enzymes,
- Anti-microbial (stealth pathogens) and
- Anti- abnormal angiogenesis.

Each of these underlying influences is involved in the development, exacerbation and complications of all cardiovascular diseases. Therefore, there is clear benefit for controlling and even potentially reversing cardiovascular disease by:

- Identifying the proper risk factors;
- Controlling and even potentially reversing their negative pre dispositions, by making healthy lifestyle choices, and, by
- Using nutritional supplementation, especially GLYCONUTRIENTS.

About the Author:
Luis R. Romero, MD

Internist, Cardiologist, Clinical Pharmacologist. Post-Graduate from Harvard University and University of Massachusetts. Professor of the Fisher Institute for Medical Research. President of Humanitas International Foundation. Vol. Associate Professor at the University of Miami MILLER School of Medicine. National and International lecturer on Health Education, Health Promotion and Holistic approach to healing.

Editors Note:

Cardiovascular disease is the #1 killer in industrialized societies. But it is followed closely by cancer. This remains a challenge today, threatening at least one in three adults. Chemotherapy, surgery and radiation are not the only options. Let's explore next, a natural intervention that at best may favor prevention, but at least will enhance adjuvant therapy. It's all about the feared 'C' word ...

Chapter 10

Glyconutrients and Cancer

Dr. Emil Mondoa and Mindy Kitei

In April, 1978, I was in my second year of medical school. Having completed a year and a half of intensive schooling in the basic sciences that underlie medicine, I had just started seeing my first real patients. Word came to us about a rare phenomenon occurring in the wards of our teaching hospital. The effects of the experience have remained with me ever since. Indeed, I remember it as if it were yesterday.

An elderly woman had been admitted to our hospital with a diagnosis of thyroid cancer. But within a few days, and with no treatment, one of the residents noted that the patient's tumor had begun to shrink. Without chemotherapy, without radiation, without medical intervention of any kind, it continued to get smaller. Within a few weeks there was no trace of the malignancy that had brought her to the hospital.

What was most gratifying was that the patient experienced no vomiting, no weight loss, no hair loss, no opportunistic infections - none of the unpleasant complications associated with the treatment of cancer. Although the woman was not my patient, I was among the steady stream of young medical students and doctors who shuffled up to the fourth floor to catch a glimpse of the miraculous lady. The mother of one of our internal medicine professors, she - and her son - were overjoyed at the outcome and as intrigued as everyone else by this unexpected event. Hers was a case of spontaneous remission of cancer, one of many medical terms for, "We don't know why this has happened, but we're glad that it did."

Close To Home

Fast-forward eight years to October 1986. It is 2 a.m., and I am with my own mother, who is dying of breast cancer. I try to ease her pain, placing my hands on her swollen belly and hugging her as best I can. She had been treated two years before with surgery and radiation, but now the cancer has spread everywhere; her doctors have told me that there is nothing more they can do. Deep down, I know it is hopeless, but I keep trying to find hope. Tears pour down my face in the semidarkness of the hospital room. I feel helpless like a child by my mother's side. I don't know how to help her except in the most basic, human way - by showing her that I love her.

Doctors come face to face with death and often develop a defensive professional attitude to it. Other physicians had warned me that it feels different when your own family is affected. The most painful emotion for doctors is helplessness. That helplessness becomes a constant companion when we are unable to do anything of lasting value for many of the patients we encounter. When we help relieve someone's symptoms without addressing primary causes, the nagging feeling of having not done enough always remains. **There is so much more of what we don't know than of what we do know**.

As I stood by my mother's bedside I remembered the woman who experienced a spontaneous remission, and I wondered why it doesn't occur more often. Why wasn't my mother getting well? What prevents the immune system from waking up and taking care of business, as it ought to? Why do our bodies so often seem to function at a fraction of their intelligence? Do cultural blinders prevent us from seeing obvious and natural solutions? Is it just a matter of shifting focus?

My mother was not as lucky as the woman I encountered in medical school. She died on November 1, 1986. Since then, as I have gone about my business as a doctor and a student, I have kept one eye open for the secret of spontaneous remission. I know that its potential is within us and is innate to our bodies, but we remain blind to it somehow. Perhaps the elements of fear and desperation in our approach to treating cancer aggressively cause us to miss something obvious. The hope that we will discover what triggers these remissions has kept me in medicine.

Fighting Cancer Daily

The key to understanding spontaneous remission in cancer is appreciating that while it looks to be a highly unusual event, a miracle, it isn't: it is the rule. Every day normal people develop dozens of abnormal cells. Sunlight, viruses, bacteria, toxic chemicals, free radicals, poor nutrition, and genes all contribute to their development. Thousands of cells become malignant every year, but the body's vigilant immune system destroys them before they become full-blown cancers. When cancer develops, it means that some malignant cells have eluded detection and have established themselves. But even people with damaged immune systems generally do not end up with dozens of tumors of different kinds.

Cancerous, or neoplastic cells have within them genes that fail to respond to normal restraints. The cells these genes inhabit divide on and on to form a tumor and eventually break free and spread, or metastasize. By the time we pinpoint the trouble with screening techniques, such as a mammogram in the case of breast cancer, the process has been ongoing for months or years and there are already billions of abnormal cells busily replicating.

Support Players

The most efficient roles for glyconutrients in the diet are as broad-spectrum prevention, as nutritional protection, and as a means to increase the body's ability to sustain its structures and keep its identity intact. But when saccharides are added to the diet, it's been demonstrated that they can increase the efficiency of immune cells, whose job it is to scan the body for cancers and destroy them directly or call on other agents to assist.

If a cancer is already established, glyconutrients can, in some cases, arouse the immune system sufficiently to regress the tumor. **You should always consult your doctor before trying glyconutrients if you have cancer.** Some mushrooms and pectins have blood-thinning effects, and some cancer patients are vulnerable to bleeding problems, both from chemotherapy and from the cancer itself. However, my searches of the Chinese and Japanese literature did not reveal any studies or cases of abnormal bleeding resulting from the use of these mushrooms. **You should never try to use glyconutrients as a sole treatment for your cancer. Glyconutrients are nutritional supplements that work well with traditional therapies to help your body heal.**

Glyconutrients tend to work better in preventing problems than in treating them.

When embarking on glyconutrient supplementation for cancer, start slowly, and build up gradually over a few weeks. Take glyconutrients with a glass of water about a half hour before meals. If you experience cramping or diarrhea, cut back on the dose and build up more slowly; also consider taking the glyconutrients with meals. There is some evidence that supplementing with vitamin C (500 to 1,000 milligrams in divided doses) helps diminish gastrointestinal side effects. Those in remission should continue taking glyconutrients (see later in this chapter for information on which glyconutrients have been studied for particular cancers) to support the immune system, although the dose may be cut by 25 percent after the first year of remission. For patients being treated with radiation or chemotherapy, adding glyconutrients to the mix improves both the odds of recovery and the quality of life. See below for more on curbing the side effects of traditional cancer treatment, followed by information on specific cancers and the foods and extracts that have been used in clinical trials to treat them.

Chemotherapy

Polysaccharide P

Chemotherapy - the use of powerful drugs to kill cancer cells - is often highly toxic because it's not selective about which cells it kills. Many innocent, normal cells die along with the cancer cells. Glyconutrients enable the body to recover faster from the debilitating effects of chemo. Polysaccharide P, from the mushroom *Coriolus versicolor* and a close cousin of polysaccharide K, has been found to protect patients against the unpleasant side effects from chemotherapy and radiation as well as to relieve many of the same symptoms - pain, nausea, fatigue, cold sweats, and poor appetite - caused by the cancer itself.

The glyconutrient has proved successful in ameliorating side effects from several kinds of cancer in humans, including stomach, esophageal, and non-small-cell lung cancer.[1]

Maitake D-Fraction

According to an expert at Kobe Pharmaceutical University in Japan, maitake extracts and maitake D-fraction not only inhibit cancer and its spread in cancer patients, but the glyconutrients also significantly reduce cancer pain and the side effects of chemotherapy.[2,3,4] In one trial of 165 participants with different, often advanced, cancers, 83 percent of those taking maitake reported a lessening of pain, and 90 percent reported a lessening of chemotherapy symptoms, including vomiting, nausea, reduced appetite, hair loss, intestinal bleeding, and lowered white count.

Lentinan

5-Fluorouracil, better known as 5-FU, is a powerful drug used to treat many kinds of cancers, including breast, ovarian and colon cancer, as well as other neoplasms of the digestive tract. One of its side effects is to shut down the bone marrow, preventing the production of the white cells, including neutrophils, macrophages, and lymphocytes - all critical to a healthy immune system. In mice, Japanese researchers found that intravenous lentinan (from the shiitake mushroom) promoted the rapid recovery of the white blood cells in the marrow and in the bloodstream.[5]

Radiation

Active cells are killed easily by radiation, and as a general rule, cancer cells are active. But the process of killing cancer cells also damages or destroys normal tissue in the irradiated area. Radiation suppresses bone-marrow production and spleen function, leading to anemia and low white-cell counts - and thus to suppression of the immune system. Although the radiation itself is painless, the cancer patient may feel very sick in the days and weeks following the treatment as cells begin to swell and die and their contents break up into the body, which then endeavors to sweep up the damage.

Glyconutrients, including reishi and Aloe vera, have been found to decrease radiation sickness in animals and to help them recover faster.[6,7,8] Animals given these glyconutrients along with radiation gained weight faster and were less nauseated, and their blood counts returned to normal faster than did the counts of controls that were irradiated but did not receive glyconutrients. Topical preparations have also proved to be helpful. In one double-blind study on mice conducted at the renowned M.D. Anderson Cancer Center in Houston, Texas, a topical gel containing acemannan from aloe reduced skin reactions to radiation significantly.[9] The glyconutrient also increased the amount of radiation required to inflict skin damage. Researchers found that the gel was most effective if applied daily for at least two weeks immediately after each radiation treatment. The scientists found that the aloe didn't work if it was applied before irradiation or beginning one week after irradiation.

Cancer Types

Bladder Cancer

Japanese researchers have found that whole edible mushrooms, including shiitake, maitake, and oyster - not just their extracts - are protective against bladder-induced cancers in mice caused by a chemical toxin.[10]

In a small human study, oral administration of 3 grams of polysaccharide K to patients with bladder cancer daily for seven days prior to surgery resulted in an increased ability of killer white cells to eradicate cancer cells in five of the ten patients studied.[11] In addition, some animal studies indicate that polysaccharide K enhances the effectiveness of the chemotherapy agent carboquone, resulting in less weight loss and increased inhibition of both tumor growth and spread to the lungs (where bladder cancer often metastasizes).[12]

Breast Cancer

Studies in humans with breast cancer suggest that polysaccharide K may convey additional benefit to standard chemotherapy, radiation therapy and endocrine therapy with tamoxifen, an estrogen blocker, used to treat the disease.

Polysaccharide K seems particularly helpful when a tumor protein marker called HLA B40 registers positive in the breast tumor. (HLA stands for histocompatibility locus antigen.) When breast tumors register a particular HLA antigen called B40, it usually signifies a more favorable prognosis. Researchers at Gumma University School of Medicine in Japan found that when B-40-positive patients took standard chemotherapy plus 3 grams of polysaccharide K a day for two months a year for five years, the 10-year survival rate was 100 percent.[13] That's in contrast to the controls, the B40-positive patients who received only standard chemotherapy: Their survival rate was 84 percent.

While the B40-negative patients didn't fare nearly as well as either of the B40-positive groups, those on polysaccharide K did do better over ten years. However, at five years, those on chemotherapy alone did marginally better: the survival rate was 82 percent on chemo alone versus 76 percent for those on chemo plus polysaccharide K.

Part of the problem with using saccharides to treat breast cancer, or indeed any cancer, is that saccharides aren't tried until other measures have failed - they tend to be used in desperate, last-ditch efforts, and by that time the cancer is advanced and more resistant to treatment. Earlier intervention in cancers, as with most other serious illnesses, generally yields more favorable results. Breast-cancer studies with C3H/OuJ mice, a breed that develops breast tumors spontaneously, support this fact. In a Japanese study, these tumor-prone mice were divided into two groups of forty. Both groups received a normal diet, but one group had polysaccharide K added to its feed. Within fifteen weeks, both tumor incidence and number were significantly lower in the polysaccharide group, as compared with controls, and survival rates also improved.[14]

Along similar lines, in another Japanese study, researchers fed female rats a cancer-causing agent called DMBA. Some also received polysaccharide K daily in addition to the cancer-causing agent. It took significantly longer for the polysaccharide K-fed rats to develop breast tumors than for the control rats.[15] Just as important, response to treatment with tamoxifen significantly improved in those rats that received polysaccharide K.

Maitake D-fraction has also proved significantly helpful in animal studies on breast cancer. In one study, researchers at Japan's Kobe Pharmaceutical University implanted breast cancer cells in young mice; the tumors were later removed.[16] Then the investigators injected half the mice with maitake D-fraction daily for ten days, while the controls received a placebo injection of saline. After twenty days, 100 percent of the control group had developed breast tumors and metastasis, whereas only 8 percent of the maitake mice had breast tumors and 7 percent had metastasis.

Colon Cancer: A Patient's Success

I first met seventy-five year old F. at her rural farmhouse in the spring of 1997. A few months earlier, she had had surgery for colon cancer. Unfortunately, F's cancer was caught very late, and surgeons were able to remove only some of the tumor and perform a colostomy. The cancer had also spread to the liver, where colon cancer usually travels first. F. had been employed as a school administrator for many years but was too ill to continue working at the school she loved. But the day I met her, she was sitting up and receiving phone calls from students and teachers, still helping them resolve problems. They welcomed her sensible advice and her kind, reassuring voice. F. has a strong will and a sharp wit.

But her body was failing her. F. was already real thin, and her cheeks were sunken. A hospice patient, she had the wasted look common in people with advanced cancer. F. had opted against chemotherapy or radiation. She had had a full life, she told me, and didn't want to suffer more from the treatment than from the disease itself. She did agree to pain medication and gentler alternative measures, including nutritional supplementation, massage therapy, and a therapeutic-touch method of healing called Reiki. Without chemotherapy and radiation, her life expectancy was about two months.

I suggested to F. that she add a mixture of arabino-galactans and a stabilized aloe extract in powder form to her regimen. Over a week or so, she gradually upped her dosage to 3 grams daily in divided doses. About a month after starting on the protocol, her appetite began to perk up and she gained weight. In all, she gained about 30 pounds. Her sunken cheeks filled out, and her energy improved. She was able to take care of her own grooming needs and cook an occasional meal - a significant improvement in her quality of life. F. continued doing well for eighteen months; she died in her sleep in her own bed at the age of 77. Did glyconutrients account for her improved, longer-than-expected life span? Studies suggest that the saccharides may indeed have contributed.

Colorectal and Stomach Cancer

Promising Japanese studies on colorectal cancer suggest that polysaccharide K may improve the chances of survival. In a study at the Kyushu University School of Medicine, after two groups of patients totaling 111 had surgery for colorectal cancer, one group of 56 patients received polysaccharide K (3 grams a day for two months, then 2 grams a day for two years, then 1 gram a day thereafter), and the other group of 55 patients received a placebo.[17] The study was double blind - meaning that neither the scientists nor the patients knew who was getting the glyconutrient and who was getting the dummy drug. Patients had advanced disease, stages III and IV. (In contrast, in stages I and II, the cancers are caught earlier and are less invasive.) Both groups were followed for eight years. Of the polysaccharide K patients, 40 percent survived, versus 25 percent of controls. The glyconutrients also affected the disease-free period of time: 25 percent of the polysaccharide K patients were disease-free at eight years, compared with only 8 percent of controls.[18,19]

In controlled studies on humans, adding 1 milligram of intravenous lentinan twice weekly or 2 milligrams of IV lentinan once weekly to traditional treatment protocols showed impressive results in increasing survival rates and improving the quality of life of people with advanced and recurrent stomach cancer and colorectal cancer.[20,21,22] Researchers found that T cells and macrophages mediated the glyconutrients' antitumor effects.

Lentinan is better absorbed and more effective intravenously than orally. Obviously, using IV lentinan must be done with your physician's approval and administered by a qualified health professional. Serious side effects have occurred with IV lentinan, and they include fever, chills, back and leg pain, elevated liver enzymes, and anaphylaxis - a serious and potentially fatal allergic reaction. Doses must be calculated by your doctor according to your weight and health status.

Esophageal Cancer

Researchers at the Cooperative Study Group for Esophageal Cancer in Japan followed 158 esophageal cancer patients for five years.[23] Patients were placed in one of four groups. One group received chemotherapy, the second group received chemotherapy and 3 grams daily of polysaccharide K, the third group received only polysaccharide K, and the fourth group served as the controls. Patients on polysaccharide K and chemotherapy had a significantly better survival rate at five years than did those on chemotherapy alone.

Leukemia

In a 1981 study at the School of Medicine at Tokai University near Tokyo, researchers administered polysaccharide K along with standard chemotherapy to fourteen patients with acute leukemia; 14 other patients served as the controls and received only standard chemotherapy.[24] The scientists found that complete remissions were longer in the polysaccharide K patients. In addition, the average survival time for those on polysaccharide K was twenty-one months, as compared with twelve months for the controls. Only one of the controls is still alive, as compared with three polysaccharide patients. Of course, standard chemotherapy for leukemia has come a long way since this 1981 study, conducted today with the more advanced chemotherapies plus polysaccharide K.

Liver Cancer

Liver or hepatic cancer is one of the fastest progressing and most virulent cancers. Active hexose correlated compound (AHCC), derived from the shiitake mushroom, increases survival times and quality of life for people with liver cancer caused by hepatitis C, a common cause of hepatic cancer.[25] In a 1999 Japanese study of 126 patients, forty-four received 3 grams of AHCC daily, while eighty-two received a placebo after surgery. After one year the AHCC patients registered a significantly higher survival rate than the control group. In addition, key blood markers indicated that liver damage dropped, while white-cell and red-cell counts rose. Patients also reported an increase in appetite. However, whereas survival, blood work, and quality of life improved in the AHCC group, tumor recurrence did not decline. Curiously, although the AHCC patients with hepatitis C did survive longer, those who didn't have hepatitis or those with hepatitis B (another cause of liver cancer) did not experience better survival rates.

Other liver cancer studies involving people have been less optimistic. In a study at Hirosaki University School of Medicine in Japan, researchers found that Polysaccharide K and lentinan in combination with the standard chemotherapy drug 5-FU provided no additional benefit in prolonging life or the quality of life over the 5-FU alone.[26]

A professor at Kobe Pharmaceutical University has focused a great deal of animal research on maitake D-fraction's ability to prevent liver cancer. In one study, he injected liver cancer cells into mice. One group of mice then received maitake powder in their feed, another group received maitake injections, and the third group served as controls. After thirty days, the scientist found that 100 percent of the controls had developed liver cancer, as compared with 19 percent of the maitake-fed mice and 9 percent of the maitake-injected mice.[27]

Next the professor added the chemical N-nitrosodi-n-butylamine, which induces liver cancer, to the diet of three groups of mice. Again, one group received maitake powder orally, another group received maitake injections, and the third group served as controls. Results were similar to those in the first trial: One hundred percent of the controls developed liver cancer, versus 22 percent of the maitake-fed mice and less than 10 percent of the maitake-injected mice.[28]

In another study, the professor investigated the effects of maitake D-fraction injections in combination with the traditional chemotherapy drug Mitomycin C.[29] After injecting liver cancer into mice, he divided the mice into two groups: the Mitomycin-only mice versus the Mitomycin-with-maitake-D-fraction mice. Following ten days of therapy, he found that the D-fraction potentiated the Mitomycin significantly. About half of the Mitomycin-only mice developed metastasis, versus only 13 percent of the mice that received both Mitomycin and maitake D-fraction.

The key to efficacy may be in the timing. As stated earlier, glyconutrients tend to work better in preventing problems than in treating them. When, for instance, scientists administered polysaccharide K to hamsters before injecting these lab animals with a liver cancer-causing agent called Thorotrast, the cancer incidence was reduced by about half - and the lives of the hamsters that developed cancer were prolonged.[30]

Lung Cancer

Lung cancer is one of the deadliest cancers, and it's often not caught until late in the disease process. Five-year survival studies conducted at Gunma University School of Medicine in Japan on lung-cancer patients after radiation therapy resulted in complete or partial shrinkage of the tumor. Of the 225 patients in the study, 170 had squamous cell lung cancer. Half of the group was randomly assigned to receive 3 grams of polysaccharide K in cycles of two weeks on and two weeks off, while the other half, the control group, received a dummy drug. Survival in the polysaccharide K group was significantly longer than in the control group.[31] Patients in the study were classified as stage I-II or stage III. (Again, in stage III, the disease is more advanced than in stage I or II.) The five-year survival rates of patients on glyconutrients with stages I-II and stage III disease were 39 percent and 26 percent, respectively, while the controls' rates were 17 percent and 8 percent. In the world of oncology, that's a big difference.

Lymphoma

Lymphomas are solid tumors of white blood cells called lymphocytes. Jacqueline Kennedy Onassis and King Hussein of Jordan both died from a form of the disease called non-Hodgkin's lymphoma. Viruses have been implicated in causing lymphoma in humans and we know viruses can cause the disease in animals. Laboratory mice infected with certain viruses, for instance, develop lymphomas quickly. Colleagues at Hebrew University-Hadassah Medical School in Jerusalem showed that polysaccharide K delayed the onset of lymphoma in mice inoculated with a lymphoma-causing virus.[32,33] Although it couldn't protect the mice from the disease, polysaccharide K did slow down the progression of the lymphoma and caused infected cells to die. In addition, the glyconutrients also increased activity of cytotoxic T cells, which in turn destroyed the abnormal cells.

Nasopharyngeal Cancer

Nasopharyngeal cancer is cancer of the pharynx, which is located directly behind the nasal passages. In a 1989 study conducted at Machay Memorial Hospital in Taipei, thirty-eight patients with nasopharyngeal cancer received radiation and a course of standard chemotherapy. Next, investigators gave patients either 3 grams of polysaccharide K or a placebo daily. Survival for the polysaccharide patients was 28 percent after five years, as compared with 15 percent for controls. [34] These findings echo those of an earlier study by some of the same scientists.[35]

Prostate Cancer

Prostate cancer used to be a subject that men shied away from discussing. But as prominent men - including actor Sidney Poitier, Senator Bob Dole, retired general Norman Schwarzkopf, junk-bond king

Michael Milken, New York Mayor Rudy Giuliani, and comedian Jerry Lewis - have begun opening up about their own experiences with the disease, the stigma has slowly lifted. Prostate cancer is the second most common cause of cancer death in men, after lung cancer, and is more prevalent in blacks than whites. Prostate cancer can be slowly progressive or virulent; the latter scenario occurs more often in younger men, with the disease claiming the life of musician Frank Zappa at age fifty-three and actor Bill Bixby at fifty-nine.

I've heard two compelling anecdotes of patients with prostate cancer who've benefited from glyconutrients. In April 1996, P., a sixty-five year old art professor, began experiencing difficulty urinating. His family physician referred him to a urologist, who found a large tumor on physical examination. A blood test called a prostate specific antigen (PSA) test confirmed the diagnosis of prostate cancer. He had a particularly aggressive form of the disease, and his tumor was too large to remove. Instead, he was immediately started on radiation and chemotherapy, but the tumor continued to grow. Seven months later, he decided to start supplementing with rice bran, rich in alpha-glucans and the polysaccharide arabinoxylane, which has been shown to promote natural killer cell activity in test-tube studies.[36] P. took 1 gram three times a day and within four months, the tumor had shrunk sufficiently to be removed surgically. A year after surgery, he halved his rice-bran intake and has remained on it and in remission for four years.

When forty-nine year old E. went for his annual physical exam, his doctor felt a small nodule on his prostate gland. His initial PSA reading was very high at 112 (0-5 is normal). Distraught because he had a young family and a peaking career and couldn't face dealing with the possible consequences of his illness, including impotence and urinary incontinence, E. decided against traditional medical treatment and instead, after conferring with a friend, tried glyconutrients. He took 3 grams of powdered aloe extracts daily. Four weeks later his PSA was 11; six weeks later it had dropped to 3, and, on examination, the nodule had disappeared.

While E.'s story had a happy ending, not everyone responds to glyconutrients, and in any event, we can't be sure that E. did respond directly - his could have been the rare case of spontaneous remission. Furthermore, glyconutrients often work synergistically with traditional therapy. It should not be a matter of choosing one over the other. Human studies using Aloe vera or rice bran to treat prostate cancer have not been done, so I can't recommend either P.'s or F.'s protocols until more is known.

To help improve immune functioning, however, supplementing with aloe extracts or rice bran is a good idea. Read rice-bran labels carefully; doses vary. To enhance flavor, some manufacturers add sweetener, which diabetics and those watching their weight should avoid.

Animal studies do indicate that glyconutrients can be effective in treating prostate cancer. National Institute of Health Swiss athymic mice (they have no thymus gland) are a breed of laboratory animal that lack T cells - white blood cells vital to immune system functioning. At the University of North Carolina at Chapel Hill, researchers found that polysaccharide K reduced the rate of growth of human prostate cancer cells injected into these mice, particularly when the cancer was caught early.[37] Polysaccharide K also increased host survival and decreased the incidence and number of cancerous lesions in the lung, to which prostate cancer often spreads.

Glyconutrients often work synergistically with traditional therapy.

These researchers also tried polysaccharide K on athymic Beige mice. Unlike the Swiss mice, Beige mice are deficient in natural killer cells as well as T cells, and unfortunately, the Beige mice did not reap the same benefits in the study. Despite glyconutrient supplementation, the cancers spread rapidly. **This finding suggests that natural killer cell activity is critical in fighting tumor growth and metastasis - and glyconutrients also boost activity of these cells.**[38-41] In another prostate cancer study at the University of North Carolina, this time on rats, researchers found that although polysaccharide K didn't reverse prostate cancer on its own, it did enhance the effects of standard chemotherapy by improving survival, retarding growth locally, decreasing metastasis and prolonging life.[42] Moreover, the researchers postulated that polysaccharide K may enhance the effects of standard chemotherapeutic agents in resistant prostate cancer.

Like polysaccharide K, pectins reduce prostate-cancer metastasis in animals. In one study, rats with prostate cancer that received pectin had significantly fewer lung metastases than did control rats.[43] In addition, urologists at New York Medical College recently reported that a beta-glucan extract of maitake mushrooms killed prostatic cancer cells in the test tube, an effect potentiated by vitamin C and the cancer drug carmustine.[44]

Sarcoma

Several glyconutrients have been tested on sarcomas - malignancies that spring from cells of connective tissue, including muscle, cartilage, and bone. In fact, there are more than fifty articles on the medical computer database Medline that address the use of saccharides to treat sarcomas - many with promising results. Following in the footsteps of Dr. William Coley a hundred years before, Texas researchers in 1991 injected acemannan from aloe straight into the tumors of 43 cats and dogs.[45] Of those animals, twenty-six showed evidence of their immune system attacking the tumors, and twelve showed significant clinical improvement, assessed by tumor shrinkage, tumor necrosis (meaning the tumor shriveled up and was destroyed), and prolonged survival. Five of the seven animals with fibrosarcomas, which arise from the fibrous connective tissue, were among the twelve that improved.

Japanese researchers at Tokyo's National Cancer Center Hospital demonstrated that extracts of sarcodon and reishi mushrooms are also effective against sarcomas in animals.[46] Other researchers suggest that polysaccharide extracts of reishi and murill mushrooms as well as Aloe vera are effective against sarcomas.[47,48,49] When scientists tested an aloe polysaccharide on melanoma and sarcoma tumors in mice, they found that it effected cures only in fibrosarcoma tumors. However, the growth rate of other tumors slowed down in the treated mice, unlike in the controls.[50]

Skin Cancer

G. is a fifty-year old lab technician who presented in 1999 with a bleeding malignant melanoma, the most serious form of skin cancer, on his back. Tests revealed that the cancer had already metastasized to distant lymph nodes, skin and bone, and that the tumor was particularly aggressive. After the local tumor was surgically removed, he was started on chemotherapy and placed on interferon to help jump-start his immune system. The interferon made him very sick and he asked to be taken off the drug. Besides, it wasn't working: The melanoma continued to grow. (Many melanoma patients do not respond favorably to traditional chemotherapy.) On his doctor's advice G. decided to try glyconutrients, including aloe extracts (12 grams daily) and yeast beta-glucans (100 milligrams daily). After one month the metastases began to shrink on CAT scan. A year later he was in remission and taking 4 grams of aloe extracts daily, plus the yeast beta-glucans. He went back to work feeling healthy and well.

Recent animal studies suggest that glyconutrients may improve survival and inhibit the metastasis of melanoma in mice by increasing T-cell and macrophage activity against the melanoma cells.[51,52] In one study, researchers at Tokyo Women's Medical College discovered that by increasing neutrophil action, polysaccharide K decreased the size and the number of liver-cancer cells that spread to the lungs in mice.[53] In another study, polysaccharide K suppressed, both *in vitro* (in the test tube) and *in vivo* (in the organism), melanoma metastasis in mice.[54] Cordyceps is also effective. In one study, IV injections of cordyceps extract into mice with melanoma resulted in an increase of natural killer cells, key players in the immune response, and a decrease in metastasis to the lungs.[55]

Stomach Cancer

Stomach cancer is far more common in Japan than in the United States, and Japanese scientists are focused on uncovering the causes of this disease. Published in the journal Lancet, a 1994 Japanese study of 262 patients with stomach cancer concluded that the five-year survival rate of the group given 3 grams of polysaccharide K plus chemotherapy was significantly higher than the rate for those on chemotherapy alone.[56] The five-year disease-free rate was also substantially greater in the polysaccharide K-treated group. In general, the more advanced the gastric cancer, the lower the patient's immunity. Other studies indicate that cell-mediated immunity is restored if the patient receives polysaccharide K or lentinan.[57,58]

In another study, researchers treated stage III stomach cancer patients with polysaccharide K or placebo after surgery.[59] Although polysaccharide K extended the disease-free period over eighty months, survival was not significantly extended. The self-critical researchers chastised themselves for their tentative dosage of 3 grams daily for the first two months, then 2 grams daily for up to fourteen months, followed by 1 gram daily for the remainder of the trial. Had the dosage remained at 3 grams daily, the scientists theorized, results would have been more encouraging. No significant side effects were observed, except for a darkening of the fingernails in four of the seventy-seven patients.

In Brief:
Other Human Cancer Studies Using Glyconutrients

Polysaccharide P

In a review article, a 1992 double-blind Chinese trial is described in which 274 patients with stomach, esophageal, or lung cancer received chemotherapy and radiation plus either 3 grams of polysaccharide P or shark liver oil daily (another immune booster, shark liver oil is rich in omega-3 fatty acids, the active component in fish oils).[60] Effectiveness was calculated on improvement in blood profiles, including white count, and significant increase in weight or the ability to care for oneself. At the end of the six month trial the scientists broke the code and found that polysaccharide P was effective 82 percent of the time, versus 45 percent for the shark liver oil.

Bovine Tracheal Cartilage

Rich in saccharides, bovine tracheal cartilage has shown efficacy in several types of hard-to-treat cancers, including those of the brain, pancreas, lung, and ovary. Animal and human studies at Hershey Medical Center and elsewhere suggest that the glyconutrient may improve the immune response against many kinds of solid tumors, particularly kidney cancer, which is usually resistant to conventional treatment once it has spread.[61,62] In particular, the glyconutrient has been shown to shrink metastases in the lung, to which kidney cancer often spreads.

Aloe Vera

In a 1998 study conducted in Milan, Italy, twenty-six patients with advanced solid tumors (including cancers of the breast, gastrointestinal tract, brain, and lung) who hadn't responded to traditional therapy were treated daily with 20 milligrams of melatonin, which has been shown to induce some benefits in untreatable metastatic cancer patients. Another twenty-four patients received 20 milligrams of melatonin daily plus a tincture (alcohol-based liquid) of Aloe vera, 1 milliliter twice a day.[63] A partial response was achieved in two of the twenty-four patients treated with melatonin plus aloe, whereas none of the patients treated with melatonin alone improved. In addition, the cancer stabilized in fourteen of the aloe patients, compared with only seven of the melatonin patients.

Conclusion

Glyconutrients can improve both the odds of recovery and the quality of life in cancer patients. Glyconutrients also enhance standard chemotherapy and radiation and ease their debilitating side effects.

Although hundreds of studies have pointed to the efficacy of glyconutrients in treating many kinds of cancers, it's important to note that **glyconutrients are just one part of effective treatment**. Whatever treatment a cancer patient undergoes, good nutrition is essential. That is a tall order even at the best of times, given our food supply as it is and contemporary lifestyle patterns. Of course, it's tough to eat right when radiation and chemotherapy are making you sick. Again, that's where glyconutrients are beneficial.

About the Authors
Emil I. Mondoa, MD and Mindy Kitei

Dr. Emil I. Mondoa is a practicing, board-certified pediatrician affiliated with Our Lady of Lourdes Medical Center in Camden, New Jersey; South Jersey Medical Center in Vineland, New Jersey; and the Alfred I. duPont Hospital for Children in Wilmington, Delaware. He also holds an MBA from the Wharton School, with a focus on health-care management.

Mindy Kitei is an editor, writer and instructor who contributed to the Philadelphia Daily News, Philadelphia Magazine, TV Guide and Applause magazine. She has a BA in Communications from the University of Pennsylvania and a Masters in Journalism from Northwestern University. She has taught at Temple University.

This chapter is adapted from the book
Sugars that Heal, by Emil I. Mondoa, MD and Mindy Kitei,
published by Ballantine Books NY (2001) and is used by permission.

Editors Note

Cardiovascular disease and cancer may be the big killers but there are a number of chronic diseases that impose a huge burden of morbidity in the population. The next chapter explores the role of glyconutrients in a select few of these diseases. There might be something for you there ...

Chapter 11

Glyconutrients in Chronic Disease

Dr. Blaine Purcell

I have had the privilege of observing first hand, some of the remarkable benefits that people experience when glyconutrients are added to their diets in both sickness and in health. As a physician practicing general Internal Medicine, my daily routine involves seeing people with ailments. Usually, these ailments are chronic degenerative diseases. They include diseases like diabetes and its many complications, hypertension, elevated triglycerides, low HDL, obesity, both rheumatoid arthritis and osteoarthritis, other autoimmune conditions such as asthma, lupus and MS (just to mention only three of the 87 known autoimmune conditions).

This chapter contains scientific reviews devoted to areas of compromised health in which the known necessary dietary sugars have shown promise. The abundance of quality data already available regarding immunomodulatory activities of the necessary glyconconjugate sugars is very impressive. Please remember that **the information included here is not intended under any circumstances to substitute for a doctor's care or any other form of proven therapy.**

In western allopathic medicine, we treat symptoms or groups of symptoms that we call a disease, but with dietary intervention with glyconutrients we support systems and normal physiology at the cellular level. The author of Breakthrough in Cell-Defense put it eloquently: **"The best self defense is cell defense!"** In practice, I reach for the 'best of the best' which results in an integrative approach to health and disease. I, like others who have checked into glyconutrients, find them to be as old as life itself.

In my effort to share this information, I have had the good fortune of collaborating here in Las Vegas, Nevada with Dr. Bud Hawkins in weekly Nutrition Briefings. There Dr. Hawkins stresses to the audience that we have choices and options. The body can *build, defend, repair, regenerate, regulate, reproduce* and *heal* itself. He has often asked the rhetorical question: "Why does the body have a problem doing this?" It is further explained that the origin of health challenges come from environmental toxins and insults, stress, medications and poor nutrition.

Again, what the body needs for fuel and maintenance, besides oxygen, is protein in the form of essential amino acids; essential fatty acids in the form of omega 3, 6 and 9; vitamins, minerals and water. The catalysts for interactions of these fuel components are enzymes which are critically needed in small amounts for any reaction to take place. The missing link is super sugars (necessary monosaccharides). Many sugars are synthetic (e.g. high fructose corn syrup, Aspartame, Splenda, maltodextrin, Sucralose, Equal and Saccharin) The body does not know how to metabolize these chemicals and in fact, turns high fructose corn syrup, for example, into triglycerides that essentially become fat! Each of the others has documented negative side effects.

In my practice, glyconutrients benefit everyone who decides to add them to their diet. While no minimal daily intake of glyconutrients has been established by the federal government, I have observed the body's ability to heal when glyconutrients are added to one's diet. Glyconutrients have done more good for more people than many of the pharmaceuticals that I am authorized to prescribe.

The Fires Within

The common thread that I have found in the pathophysiology of all chronic degenerative diseases is Inflammation. Let's discuss the recent research and observations about this broad category, highlighted recently on the cover of *TIME* magazine. Reporters Gorman, Park and Dell wrote the cover story entitled "The Fires Within". Their topical summary states:

"Inflammation is the body's first defense against infection, but when it goes awry, it can lead to heart attacks, colon cancer, Alzheimer's and a host of other diseases."

Nutrition affects every aspect of health, including how the body will respond to the numerous environmental insults it encounters each day. Unfortunately, in our fast-paced society, proper nutrition has become a low priority. Clearly, good nutrition enables the body to deal more effectively with many pathologic conditions, including inflammation. This concept is supported, for example, by the recent research of

D. L. Lefkowiz, in which administration of mannose, or polymers of mannose, prevented arthritic flares in rats.[2] Also, mannose as well as N-acetlyglucosamine, inhibit radical production of neutrophils. This implies that sacccharides can limit tissue damage.

Inflammation has suddenly become one of the hottest areas of medical research. Hardly a week goes by without the publication of yet another study uncovering a new way that chronic inflammation does harm to the body. Just to illustrate, it destabilizes cholesterol deposits in the coronary arteries, leading to heart attacks and potentially even strokes. It chews up nerve cells in the brain of Alzheimer's victims. It may even foster the proliferation of abnormal cells and facilitate their transformation into cancer. In other words, chronic inflammation may be the engine that drives many of the most feared illnesses of middle and old age.

This concept is so intriguing because it suggests a new and possibly much simpler way of warding off disease. Instead of different treatments for, say, heart disease, Alzheimer's and colon cancer, there might be a single, inflammation-reducing remedy that would prevent all three.

Figures A and B demonstrate the cell-to-cell communication facilitated by carbohydrates to instruct the neutrophils where to slip out of the blood stream as they migrate into the tissue to the site of inflammation.

Figure C then shows the perpetuation of the cellular infiltration associated with inflammation because of the cross talk between the neutrophil and the macrophage. The communication signal between these cells is the mannose of the myeloperoxidase. This demonstrates the immunoregulatory effects of saccharides.

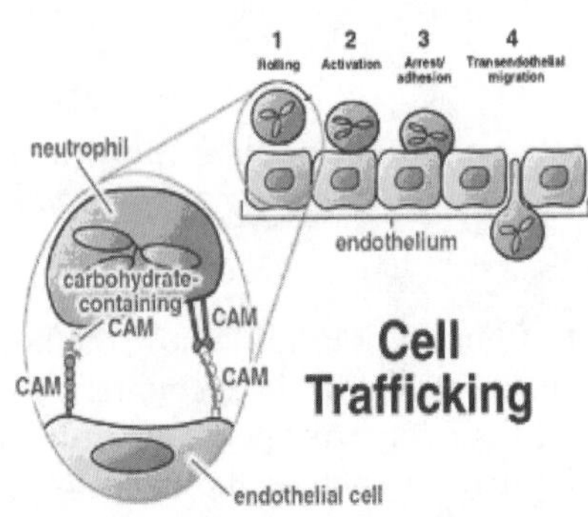

Figure A - Glycoscience.org ©

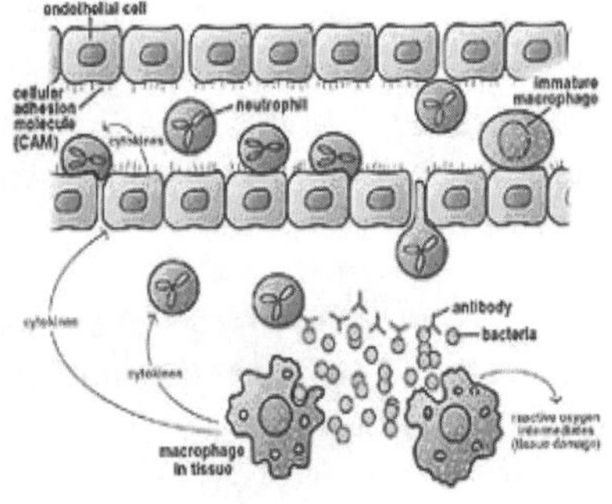

Figure B - Glycoscience.org ©

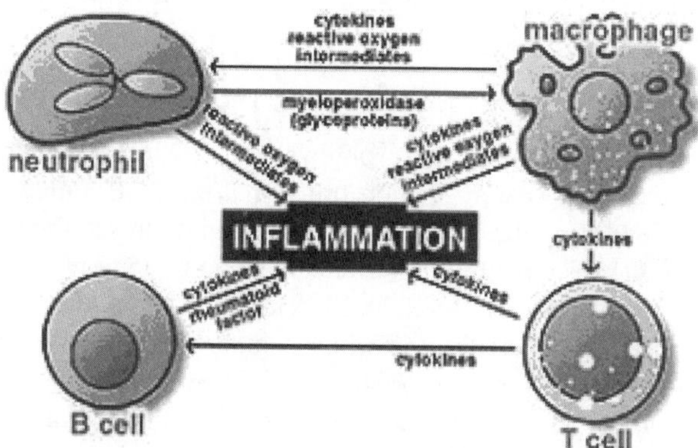

Figure C - Glycoscience.org ©

As a localized inflammatory response proceeds, a systemic aspect of the inflammation occurs concurrently. Soon, wave after wave of immune cells flood the site, destroying pathogens and damaged tissues alike -- there's no carrying the wounded off the battlefield in this war. It's therefore no wonder that the ancient Romans likened inflammation to being 'on fire.'

In medical schools across the United States, cardiologists, rheumatologists, oncologists, allergists and neurologists are all suddenly talking to one another, and discovering that they're looking at the same thing. Just a few years ago, "nobody was interested in this stuff," says Dr. Paul Ridker, a cardiologist at Brigham and Women's Hospital who has done some ground breaking work in the area. Dr. Ridker identified a marker for inflammation in heart patients. It is known that half of all heart attacks occur in people with normal cholesterol levels. Not only that, as imaging techniques improved, doctors found much to their surprise, that the most dangerous plaque was not necessarily all that large. Something that hadn't yet been identified was causing those deposits to burst, triggering massive clots that cut off the coronary blood supply. In the 1990s, Ridker became convinced that some sort of inflammatory reaction was responsible for the bursting plaques, and he set about trying to prove it.

He discovered that a simple blood test could serve as a marker for chronic inflammation. He settled on C-reactive protein (CRP), a molecule produced by the liver in response to an inflammatory signal. By 1997, Ridker and his colleagues had shown that healthy middle-aged men with the highest CRP levels were three times as likely to suffer a heart attack in the next six years as were those with the lowest CRP levels. Eventually, inflammation experts determined that having a CRP reading of 3.0 mg/L or higher could triple your risk of heart disease. The danger seems even greater in post menopausal women than in men. Conversely, folks with extremely low levels of CRP, less than 0.5mg/L, rarely have heart attacks.

Extinguish the Fire

A recent small pilot study published in the "Proceedings of Fisher Institute for Medical Research" demonstrated that the CRP could be reduced in patients who added a mixture of 8-10 known glyconutrients to their diet. This is profound since these simple micronutrients have no toxicity when consumed in any quantity. In contrast, in late 2004, Merck pulled Vioxx off the market as it was causing increased heart disease when compared to placebo, in a study to testthe effects on intestinal polyps. Likewise, Pfizer finally disclosed to the public that in its study done in 2000 there was a similar risk when high doses of ____ drug was consumed for 2 years or more.

For many other chronic conditions affecting different systems of the body, inflammation is the heart of the problem. That inflammatory response is modulated when glyconutrients are consumed, because the vital sugars impact the important synthesis and deployment of glycoproteins inside and on the surfaces of cells involved in the process. That is one plausible explanation for the results we have been seeing when these micronutrients are added to the diet.

Another promising explanation deals with Stem Cells. Dr. H.R. McDaniel contends that recent research literature supports the proposition that was observed more than 25 years ago by himself and by veterinarian Dr.Robert Carpenter. At the time they did not know what these cells were that they were observing, several days after treatment of animals with a pharmaceutical grade of poly-mannose.[3] They called them G-Cells but now it is believed that those cells were Stem Cells with a full complement of glyconutrients ready to repair organs, including the brain.

Now, let's look at the relevance of glyconutrients to some of the most prevalent chronic diseases of our time. Space will only allow us to cover a few of them here.

Diabetes

Most Americans still have no clue about how to avoid disease and weight issues with a truly healthy diet - primarily because they're trapped in the dangerous paradigm of "health" fostered mostly by the pharmaceutical industry.

The allopathic paradigm has people convinced that there is a pill for all their health problems, or one coming soon, and they need not worry about preventing or overcoming their disease or other disorders. The current public perception is that there are cures. In truth, for many chronic conditions, doctors merely patch over the symptoms while the underlying cause continues to fester and grow.

The best example is diabetes with all its complications and related conditions. Consider these statistics:

- There are 18 million diabetics in the US, and 1 million pre-diabetics
- Diabetics spent 25.3 million hospital days in 2002.
- One third of those born in 2000 will develop diabetes in their lifetime.
- The $132 billion total annual cost of this disease consists of $92 billion direct medical costs and $40 billion indirect costs.
- Workers lose 8.3 days per year per person, compared to 1.7 days for non-diabetes workers.
- Diabetes patients' HC dollars are 3.5 times higher than non-diabetics. ($9,493 compared to $2,604each year).
- In 1997 there were 55 million diabetic disability days.

Blood sugar levels linked to cancer and death risk

Findings from the Korean Cancer Prevention Study published in the January 12, 2005, issue of the *Journal of the American Medical Association* (JAMA), revealed an association between having elevated blood sugar and diabetes, and the risk of developing and dying from cancer, as well as mortality from all causes.[4]

Assistant Professor of Epidemiology Sun Ha Jee and colleagues, followed 1.3 million Koreans aged 30 to 95 (64% men and 36% women). The participants were followed for ten years, during which the incidence of cancer and deaths associated with the disease were tracked. Individuals who had diabetes or those without the disease whose fasting blood sugar levels were elevated, had a greater risk of developing or dying from cancer than those with normal blood sugar. Subjects whose glucose was greater than or equal to 140 mg/dl had more than double the rate of death during the study period compared to subjects whose blood sugar was lower than 90 mg/dl.

The authors explained that glucose intolerance could be one way that obesity increases cancer risk. Dr Jee commented, "This study provides more information on glucose intolerance, an emerging cause of cancer. It points to increased cancer risk as another adverse consequence of rising obesity around the world."

In adult onset Type 2 and juvenile onset Type1 diabetes, the most important intervention is lifestyle modification. Dietary intervention is the most important lifestyle modification. Glyconutrients have proven to be a critical missing link as a dietary intervention. Later in the chapter we will illustrate with discoveries from observation of patients. For now, I would like to share early scientific validation and pilot studies that have been published as case reports.

On January 31, 2005, the *Boston Globe* declared "Researchers find Diabetes Trigger, Possible Fix". The researchers, from Joslin Diabetes Center in Boston, discovered a genetic "master switch" in the liver that is turned on when people become obese. Those researchers found that once turned on, this switch produces low-level inflammation, which disrupts the body's ability to process insulin, causing Type 2 diabetes. Since we are speaking of inflammation as you recall from earlier in this chapter, and since glyconutrients modulate it, then the fix lies in turning this switch off. The researchers are studying some drugs related to aspirin for doing this job. I would propose that they look at glyconutrients for doing that same job, since we have already seen some similar results in the case studies described next.

Autoimmune Diseases

In 2002 several of my patients with autoimmune diseases and I were interviewed by Barbara J. Noseh, a writer with the *Nevada Woman Magazine.* Her subsequent article was entitled "Manna from Heaven -Families find Relief (and miracles) for Autoimmune Disease from a Nutraceutical."

According to the American Autoimmune and Related Diseases Association, Inc., autoimmune disease is now the third major category of illness in the United States and many other industrialized countries. This follows cardiovascular disease (Ch. 9) and cancer (Ch.10). Autoimmune disease is a category of diseases that includes more than 80 serious, chronic illnesses that are triggered when the body's immune system mistakes its own tissues as foreign and then attacks itself, causing various diseases that can involve almost every human organ system. Following are some of the more familiar diseases thought to have an autoimmune component:

- Allergies
- Antiphospholipid syndrome
- Asthma
- Autoimmune hepatitis
- Cardiomyopathy
- Chronic fatigue syndrome
- Crohn's disease
- Fibromyalgia
- Graves' disease
- Hashimoto's disease
- Diabetes (Usually Type I)
- Juvenile arthritis
- Mixed connective tissue disease
- Multiple sclerosis
- Myasthenia gravis
- Pernicious anemia
- Psoriasis
- Rheumatoid arthritis
- Scleroderma
- Sjogren's syndrome
- Systemic Lupus Erythematosis
- Ulcerative colitis

Observations Of Patients

Myasthenia Gravis

My own father, Graham Purcell, was diagnosed with myasthenia gravis (MG) in 1994. MG is an autoimmune condition that affects the weakest muscles in the body. It is manifested at the eyelid and the diaphragm at the acetylcholine receptor site (the neuromuscular junction). In 1996 when I was introduced to glyconutrients, my dad started on them at the suggestion of one of the early scientists and researchers in the field. Veterinarian Dr. Robert Carpenter had been my classmate at Texas A&M University, College of Veterinary Medicine. After his Air Force career and on becoming a Director of Laboratory Animal Medicine, he consulted with private industry. He is one of three scientists listed on the original patent of a single glyconutrient called Acemannan (Polymannose) developed for veterinary medical use in feline leukemia, fibrosarcoma in dogs and as a vaccine adjuvant. The patent actually lists many other properties.

After consideration and upon learning that the principal effects of the full complement of glyconutrients were in immune modulation, I decided to recommend this to my dad who was taking large doses of prednisone at the time. Since he had previously experienced an exacerbation of the MG after weaning totally off prednisone by an expert in this condition, he was reluctant to go below 10 mg every other day. By 2004, however, he had started to wean further down, with monthly blood tests for the blocking antibody for acetylcholine. Experts from NIH and other tertiary centers suggested a weaning protocol that we implemented to slowly wean down by 0.5mg per month. At the time of writing, dad is presently down to 8.0 mg (a 20% reduction in the deadly debilitating drug, prednisone) and with no withdrawal effects or complications. He takes an entire array of micronutrients in an optimal health program.

Asthma

A symposium took place at the Baylor Dental School, Dallas, Texas, and was published as Supplement No. 1 - August 1997 of the Journal of the American Nutraceutical Association. I was invited to present two case studies on asthma which demonstrated with objective data, improvement in the peak respiratory flow of two patients, following dietary supplementation at 30 days and 6 months. This was the first time that objective data in the form of peak respiratory flow was followed in patients on glyconutrient supplementation. Peak flow is a simple patient-friendly means that replicates the forced expiratory volume for one second. A much larger prospective study was later done, supporting these earlier findings.

One of the two subjects I reported on was K., a 67 year old female, who suffered from life-threatening asthma. I introduced glyconutrients to her in the acute care setting, soon after learning of this technology in 1996 and after all drugs had failed to give her relief from severe asthma. First, it allowed me to discharge her from the hospital. In 30 days, her peak flow had improved by 300% and stayed that way for 6 months (to the end of the study period). The most important thing was that she substituted these economical, non-toxic and harmless in any amount, plant extracts for a $1,500 monthly expense. This expense included her drugs, frequent doctor visits and emergency room visits.

She was able to return to work in a smoke filled casino without interruptions or medical emergencies. She feels good. She feels strong. K. says she was reborn, not only into life itself but, even better, into a brand new healthy life.

Systemic Lupus Erythematosis

D. was a basically healthy adult when she was overcome with a serious illness in January 2000 that would remain a mystery until June of that year. She was then diagnosed with Systemic Lupus Erythematosis (SLE), one of the most destructive autoimmune diseases.

For D., almost that entire year was marked by migraine headaches, red and swollen joints, angina, mouth sores and unbearable, full-body pain that reached a climax on November 28, when she wrote in her journal, "can't move, everything hurts." She was referred to me by her aunt in Iowa. That day she saw me in my office and the next day she was started on an optimal health program similar to my dad's, but with extra bulk glyconutrients.

Twenty-four hours later, there was less pain and her mouth sores had diminished. Her journal records ups and downs, good days and bad, but steady progress. Finally, on January 2, 2001, her journal trumpets, "Woke up pain-free!" After that, some pages are empty because "I'm too busy living", but January 18, she documents "more energy every day, no aches, no pains, no sores." As long as she includes these micronutrients in her diet, she does fine. (Leaving them out of ones' diet, sometimes for as little as 24 hours, can cause a return of previous symptoms).

Multiple Sclerosis, Muscular Dystrophy and Myasthenia Gravis

L., a 49 year old female, had multiple diagnoses. She had been to some of the medical centers many consider to be the "Ivory Towers or Meccas of Medicine." They all disagreed on her diagnosis and had as many of those as the specialists she had seen. Diagnoses included multiple sclerosis, muscular dystrophy, myasthenia gravis and or combinations of neuromuscular pathologies. She had been told she had less than 2-3 months to live. Then she read a success story, in the *Nevada Woman Magazine* about another lady who enjoyed a dramatic response to glyconutrients, having been partially paralyzed and confined to a wheel chair.

L. could not hold her head up when her husband, M., rolled her into my exam room. She could not flex her hips (not even raise her knee 6 inches vertically to touch my hand). She was taking between 30-60 mg. of prednisone daily. That's high. If she tried to wean off prednisone, she ended up on life support (on a ventilator) because of respiratory failure.

She too, was started on the same optimal health program, again with extra glyconutrients. I went to the house of one of her friends 10 days later, to explain what these micronutrients were and why she needed to take them. There was this woman who greeted me at the door … thirty feet inside the entry way, she told me her name. I could not believe it. Another miracle, it appeared. In thirty days she was stronger. Two years later, L. is living life to it's fullest but must remember that she still has these diagnoses and can get tired and unsteady if she overdoes it. Most importantly, she will not be leaving her 10 year old son without a mom.

It is generally not advisable to change medical treatment programs abruptly and independently.

Diabetes Mellitus-Type 2

A. is a 28 year old Latin male who presented with a blood glucose level of around 550mg%. That's very high. Normal is less than 140 mg%. He was rescued with insulin and hydration as patients are usually extremely volume depleted with this situation. He was started on oral medication and had formal instruction on personal care and diet by certified diabetic educators. He started on the same optimal health program plus extra glyconutrients and a product that has quick release phytogenins and chromium used in sports recovery. In one month his sugars were under 140mg%, usually around 90mg%, on no medications at all, but continuing on the micronutrients described above. The patient had stopped his medicines against my advice.

That's just the bare facts. It is generally not advisable to change medical treatment programs abruptly and independently. Patients with known medical conditions or who have taken regular prescription medications, should always consult their personal physician before making such drastic changes to their management and care. That is the wise approach. Some have gambled and won, but life definitely should not be reduced to gambling.

Diabetes Mellitus and Kidney Failure

W. is a 52 year old male, born in Dominica. He works at a job that would be terminated if he went on dialysis. He was diagnosed with Type 2

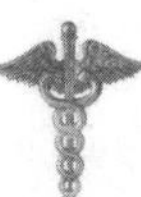

Diabetes but required insulin in the 1970's and experienced kidney failure around the year 2000, due to diabetes. As a consequence, he also has serious high blood pressure. He came to see me in July of 2004.

Before seeing me, he had inquired about having a kidney transplant. He was told that he had to lose 50 pounds. He started on glyconutrients and the rest of the same optimal health program I have used, excluding the vitamin/mineral supplement which contains minerals such as magnesium. His insulin requirements immediatly dropped in half. At the same time, he drastically changed his food program. His blood creatinine level was around 6 and it dropped to 4 and then to 3.2. These lower creatinine values imply improved kidney function. But, his calculated creatinine clearance placed him off the list for immediate dialysis. About this same time, we changed his medications and took him off one that protects the kidney but which can raise the potassium and creatinine levels.

The best news is that he lost 40 of the necessary 50 pounds, which then replaced him on the transplant list. His potassium is still in the normal range. The main point of this case is that diabetics on insulin or secretogogue drugs (like Glipizide or Glyburide, etc.) must be very careful and increase their glucose monitoring. Additionally, I generally recommend that they cut their insulin requirements by 50% on the first day. We also see reductions in the protein (albumin) being lost in these diabetic nephropathy (kidney disease) cases.

Pemphigus vulgaris

S. became my patient officially only around 2000, but I observed her miraculous recovery from Pemphigus vulgaris in 1997.

"In early 1997 it started with a few blisters in my mouth that filled with blood. When each blister's delicate surface broke, the remaining open sore was slow to heal. One morning I awoke with what felt like razor blades in my throat. Two doctors saw nothing! Even a biopsy did not indicate a clinical condition. Within a few weeks my entire mouth and throat blistered; I couldn't eat - even drinking water was extremely painful!

"Many tests and two hospitalizations finally led to a diagnosis of Pemphigus, a rare immune disorder. By early September, I was taking 90 mg of prednisone and 110 mg of imuran daily; plus other drugs to treat the 'side effects'. I lost more than 50 pounds. Circulation to my fingers decreased so severely that my right thumb was in danger of being amputated. Neither a heart specialist, dermatologist, immune specialist nor internist was able to help. Every day I became more ill.

"In October 1997 a friend told me about a nutritional discovery that 'might' help. I tried the "natural" products only because I had nothing to lose. Living to see 1998 was improbable. Within two weeks of taking a relatively small amount of the glyconutritional supplement, some healing was evident.

Within another two weeks, in early November, I was able to start reducing the drugs. The first real food I was able to eat in 1997 was on Christmas Day: a little turkey & sweet potato!

"By the end of March 1998 I was free of all drugs. The doctors were astounded by the rapidity of my improvement. Beginning January 1998, I began to add other supplements such as vitamins, phytoestrogens and something for intestinal support. Each added supplement seemed to accelerate my healing and the elimination of the drugs from my system.

"I no longer suffer from blisters and open sores in my mouth or on my body. Osteoporosis, diagnosed as serious in 1999, is gone. I see no specialists. I now enjoy a complete sense of wellness and I no longer live in fear of the destructive disorder, Pemphigus."

Hypertension, Lipids and much more

Dr. B. is a 76-year-old retired optometrist who had hypertension and dyslipidemia - low (good) HDL and high (bad) LDL cholesterol. He started on these micronutrients in 1997. He resisted then and now, taking pharmaceuticals. He insists that the pharmaceuticals treat symptoms only, while nutrition and micronutrients treat systems of the body to move towards normal physiology. He suffered from a myriad of complaints including hypertension, dyslipidemia, osteoporosis, allergies, prostate cancer, solar keratosis, halitosis and more. Almost all his clinical variables improved with micronutrients and today he's a very 'happy camper'. The doctor states: "It doesn't take a study to convince me that these micronutrients work. Folks, just look at the results from all the various systems; this is incredible." His comprehensive record-keeping even documents how his onchomycosis (stubborn, hard-to-treat toenail fungus) cleared up.

Conclusion

I recommend only the best of the best; that is to say, we want the best micronutrients (nutraceuticals) as a foundation for optimal health and the best pharmaceuticals, when needed on top of a solid nutritional foundation.

The recent cover story in *Newsweek*, (January 17, 2005) was entitled "Diet and Genes: The New Science of Nutrition and Aging." A single quotation sums up what this chapter has been all about. "It isn't just what you eat that can Kill you, and it isn't just your DNA that can Save you - it's how they interact."

This underscores the new science of nutritional genomics. I take these functional foods and recommend them to everyone including my patients and family. We have seen positive results in over 50 gene-mediated conditions. What was discussed in the *Newsweek* article is the argument that we need to make diagnosis based on genotype, so we can go beyond trial and error. But I have observed that it does not matter much what the diagnosis is when nutrition is the focus and better health is the goal. I have personally seen so many conditions positively impacted.

It is the most exciting times for those interested in offering an integrative approach to health with the Best of the Best. I feel that the complete mixture of glyconutrients offers significant relief for much human suffering and I predict you will be hearing much more about all this in the years ahead. That's my prognosis!

About the Author:
Blaine S. Purcell, MD, JD, DVM

Dr. Blaine Purcell received his medical degree from the University of Arkansas. He did an internal medicine residency at the University of Nevada where he trained in cardiac rehabilitation. He received his undergraduate and doctor of veterinary medicine degrees from Texas A&M University where nutrition was emphasized. He received his J.D. from the University of South Dakota. Dr. Purcell integrates conventional medical treatments for chronic diseases with complementary nutritional and anti-aging therapies. He has more than 20 years internal medicine experience helping patients prevent and reverse chronic disease. He is on staff at six Las Vegas Valley hospitals.

Editors Note:

You've noticed the central role of inflammation in chronic disease and clearly that demands even more attention. And that's what it will get in the next chapter. But it might get a bit heavy and technical too, so if you get in too deep, just jump ahead to, the lighter subject of fitness and sport, in the chapter that follows it ...

Chapter 12

Glyconutrients and Inflammation

Dr. Shafina Thawer

Dr. John Demartini, made me deeply aware of something I had not consciously realized before. In the entire universe, there has been no greater species discovered than the human. No greater miracle has been witnessed than the process whereby two cells come together to form a unique human being, whose magnificence is unparalled. And up to today, all the books, in all the libraries, in all the world, have still not captured the essence of all the miracles that take place in every cell, in every human body, in every moment of time. Each moment of this life is generated by trillions of processes, occurring through trillions of nerve impulses and trillions of biochemical reactions such that every thought, emotion or action causes a universal change in the physiology of the human body. You get the point? This is called '*Innate Intelligence*'.

This life force strives at all times to keep the body in balance. We call this, *homeostasis*. However, in today's world we are constantly subject to numerous insults, stresses and toxicities. In fact, at this moment there's not a single human being who is not surrounded by some form of toxicity. It could be microorganisms, cigarette smoke, air pollution, water pollution, pesticides, herbicides, car exhaust, processed foods, radiation, pharmaceutical and recreational drugs, physical trauma, child abuse, emotional abuse, neglect, slander ... and the list goes on and on. In such a toxic environment our body has to forever work to keep up the unceasing battle.

In these stressful times, it is more important than ever to ensure that your body is as close to optimal function as possible. It is vital that your immune and nervous systems are at their best. This means constantly striving to eliminate any physical, emotional or chemical causes of interference to maximize your body's innate ability to heal itself. This is called Innate Immunity.

Let's briefly outline each category of interference.

Physical (structural)

The first stage of development in an embryo is the central nervous system (CNS). According to Gray's Anatomy, the brain, spinal cord and spinal nerves control and coordinate all organs and structures of the human body. It is therefore essential that there is no physical interference in the pathway of the central and peripheral nervous systems. Any interference could cause a disruption in the electrical nerve impulses with resulting consequences. In order to ensure that all systems of the body are functioning optimally, including the immune system, we must ensure that there is no 'interference' with the nervous system. That is the purpose of chiropractic care.

Emotional

It is clear that emotions produce changes in physiology. An obvious example is stress. Just think what happens to you in times of stress, or fear, or love. Today, the power of mind-body medicine is being investigated actively and the application of these findings is already producing results. It brings in the science of quantum physics and non-linear dynamics, along with studies of electromagnetic and nerve impulses. Current methods of detecting emotional interference widely use the science of behavioral and clinical kinesiology. It is important to remove any emotional roots that could cause chronic 'fight or flight' physiological changes.

Chemical

Human biochemistry is like an abyss of endless chemical reactions. Its complexity is baffling and its depths - fathomless. That is, if you look at it from its parts. But what is most fundamental to all these chemical reactions? Until recently it was thought that the 'protein' code was the real magician behind all life processes. Now we know that there's another key player. Fundamental to all cell-to-cell communication is a 'carbohydrate' code derived from the eight vital sugars that spell out the 'language of life.' These sugars combine with the proteins to increase specificity and enhance diversity.

Glycoprotein molecules coat the surface of every cell that has a nucleus in the human body. So as you can imagine, they're constantly involved in all those 'endless biochemical reactions' we were just alluding to. Therefore, it must be important to have an abundant supply of these essential building blocks. Herein lies the problem. Of the eight necessary participants, only two are found copiously in our diets - glucose and galactose. This generally drives the body into further stress response costing energy and ultimately - life and death issues.

We will now go on to focus on the role of carbohydrates in the cell biology of inflammation in particular, and discuss some associated findings in inflammatory diseases.

Inflammation

Inflammation is an essential part of the immune response which may be initiated due to trauma, infection, chemicals, heat or any other tissue injury. In response, the local tissues release dozens of chemicals to signal for help and initiate the inflammatory response. In the process, numerous white blood cells are channeled toward the affected area to aid in the immune response.

Let's elaborate a bit more on the process of inflammation itself.

This process is as familiar as a sprained wrist or ankle. Such injury has likely resulted in the ligaments, tendons and musculature being stretched into their elastic or plastic zones, and some associated findings are edema, tenderness and a local heat response. Classically, there is *color* (heat), *dolor* (pain), *rubor* (redness), and *tumor* (swelling), plus or minus *functio laesa* (loss of function). In all this, there is a most elaborate process taking place beneath the skin.

First line of Defense: advance Marines

There are macrophages that are already present in the tissue affected. Known as histiocytes in the subcutaneous tissue or alveolar macrophages in the lungs, or microglia in the brain, among others, they immediately begin their phagocytic (pac-man like) actions. Nearby sessile macrophages become mobile and move into the area as a line of first defense, but the numbers are not great. The cells enlarge along with their vacuoles, and the phagocytic action ensues.

Second line of Defense: declare War

While the macrophages begin the battle, the injured tissue sounds off an alarm (via secreted cytokines) that attracts circulating neutrophils to the affected area by a process called chemotaxis. These neutrophils penetrate the endothelial wall in stages. (i) they constantly travel through the blood stream, (*circulation*); (ii) when summoned, they slow down to a roll and close in to the periphery of the blood vessels (*margination*); (iii) there, they flatten against the wall (tight *adhesion*) and are ready for (iv) *transmigration*: ie. the endothelial gates between cells open willingly to allow the neutrophils to continue on their journey to the site of injury. At the same time, inflammatory products travel the blood stream and eventually get to the bone marrow where the neutrophils are born and bred. These also trigger the capillaries to open their floodgates and let the neutrophils pour out and make their way down the same path as the previous ones. This acute elevation of neutrophils is called "neutrophilia".

Third line of Defense: call up Reserves

Through the same process, circulating monocytes (significantly less in number compared to neutrophils) also enter through the capillary walls. Once at the tissue site, they transform to macrophages that can consume five times the amount of bacteria that neutrophils do. Although macrophages are much more powerful phagocytes, they are far less in number and therefore it takes time (days to weeks) before macrophages become the dominant phagocyte.

Fourth line of Defense: institute the Draft

Just in case the battle turns into a full-scale war, the bone marrow begins to increase production of granulocytes and monocytes, which after four days of development are ready to be released for action. This line of defense can be employed for years generating 20-50 times the normal amount of production.

Glycoproteins Everywhere

The role of carbohydrates in human biochemical processes is now known to be vitally necessary. Let's now explore how this applies to inflammation.

The endothelium of the blood vessels at the site of inflammation expresses cellular adhesion molecules (CAMs) which bind to the carbohydrate portions of other CAMs on the surface of the neutrophil. A group of glycoproteins called **selectins** have been found to participate in neutrophil rolling (*margination*). They are classified as E (endothelial), P (platelet) and L (lymphocyte) selectins. The interaction between the neutrophil glycan and the E selectin glycoprotein is what causes adhesion of the neutrophil to the endothelial wall. Take note: the structure of that glycan contains four of the "big eight" sugars.

In the next stage, tight *adhesion* is caused by interaction between glycoproteins known as **integrins**, and other glycoproteins that mediate the firm adherence of neutrophils to the inner walls of the venules. Platelet-endothelial cell adhesion molecule (PECAM-1) is also an important glycoprotein on the endothelial cell that is involved in *transmigration* of the neutrophil. Think of PECAM-1 dancing with the glycoproteins on the surface of the neutrophil. The cell wall now joins the excitement, parting between two cells to allow the neutrophil passage.

Thus, glycoproteins are involved at each stage of neutrophil passage through the endotheial cell wall. Lymphocytes and monocytes also use surface specific carbohydrates to determine where to exit the blood.

There are two relatively uncommon genetic disorders that both seriously impact the body's inflammatory response resulting in recurrent infections.17 Both are affiliated with alterations in glycoprotein structure. There is first leukocyte adhesion deficiency type I (LAD-I) wherein there is a deficiency in the synthesis of the integrin glycoproteins that play a role in tight adhesion of the neutrophil. Then there is leukocyte adhesion deficiency type II (LAD-II) caused by a lack of fucose. Fucose forms part of the normal structure of the same glycan on the surface of the neutrophil that interacts with the E-selectin on the endothelial wall in the process of rolling. The fact that deficiencies of these vital sugars can yield serious consequences underlines the importance of adequate supply and accurate synthesis of these important glycoprotein molecules.

Let's pause and briefly take a moment to frame this in context. Of the entire process of inflammation, we have discussed only a fraction. That's just the phenomenon whereby the neutrophil penetrates the wall of the blood vessels to the site of tissue injury. At each small step we saw how ultimately, glycoproteins on one surface interact with glycoproteins on another surface. In each one of these "conversations," there is continual use of eight recurring 'vowels', for without these "vowels," the language wouldn't exist. If just one of these is missing, there would be a miscommunication. Just as that slip leads to a myriad of problems in human relationships, this same principle creates havoc in the intercellular language. There are literally billions of such conversations going on in your body just as there are billions of interpersonal communications going on in the world right now. Having the right amount of vowels (vital carbohydrates) is indispendable in your alphabet soup of biochemical life processes.

And that's not all. Sugars continue to be involved throughout the entire inflammatory response. Let's go back to that now.

The release of pro-inflammatory cytokines by the macrophage is what attracts more neutrophils into the area. However, it is the neutrophilic myeloperoxidase (an enzyme) released from already present neutrophils that interacts with the mannose sugar receptor on the macrophage to initiate the release of those cytokines, including tumor necrosis factor (TNF).

As the *local* inflammatory response continues, an acute-phase systemic response is also initiated. This causes a shift in the proteins produced by the liver and positively affects mannose-binding protein whose primary function is to bind carbohydrates. Why? Because mannose binding protein binds to mannose residues on certain pathogens and facilitates phagocytosis. It also initiates the so-called complement cascade which further helps to bind bacteria to either neutrophils or macrophages.

The macrophage has at least three different receptors that bind mannose. The purpose of these receptors is to receive the mannose residues protruding from the cell surface of the pathogens to detonate phagocytosis. After the initiator of inflammation has been cleared out, more macrophages move into the area to clean up. Their responsibilities include the chore of eliminating dead neutrophils. Dead neutrophils are recognized by carbohydrates expressed on the cell surface. Semi-professional phagocytes and fibroblasts eat up dead neutrophils once again through carbohydrate recognition of fucose or mannose expressed on the cell surface of the neutrophil.

Mannose also participates in the resolution of inflammation, by inhibiting certain neutrophil functions, particularly the production of free radicals. Free radical damage to the already injured tissue would create more damage and leave the inflammatory process unresolved, or would initiate another round. Chronic inflammation is a key factor in many autoimmune disorders. It is therefore essential that the inflammatory process is communicated correctly through the cells, for if not, it may result in an unresolved inflammatory process which may have further damaging consequences. So we see that glycoproteins once again play a critical role in not only the initiation of the inflammatory response, but also in the resolution of inflammation, primarily through recognition of mannose molecules on the cell surface.

It is now undeniable that glycoprotein and other carbohydrate interactions play a key role at the most detailed intermediate stages of inflammation and the immune response - from beginning to end.

Chronic Inflammation

Rheumatoid Arthritis

Rheumatoid arthritis (RA) is a connective tissue autoimmune disorder that can affect any synovial joint in the body. The hallmark findings from x-rays are soft tissue swelling, thinning of adjacent bone, joint space narrowing and marginal erosions. The distribution of findings is so diverse that the symptoms have been said to be only 80% accurate.

Neutrophils are again present in RA afflicted joints in all stages of disease. Macrophages and other immune cells cooperatively cause the release of cytokines, plus free radicals and enzymes that all play a dominant role in the destruction of the affected joint. Cytokines, particularly TNF, play a significant role in destroying the joint. The majority of cytokines are released by the macrophage. The influence of these cytokines is most notable in their ability to initiate the "cytokine cascade" that is evident in clinical disease. The recurring stimulation of the inflammatory process goes on to cause tissue destruction. Tissue destruction is also a result of free radical production and secretion of enzymes by the neutrophils. However, as we saw above, mannose derivatives act on neutrophils to prevent free radical production, as does another of those vital sugars, N-acetylglucosamine.

Examining rheumatoid arthritis gives us insight as to the serious destructive and damaging effects of chronic, unresolved inflammation. It therefore becomes evident how important it is for the inflammatory process to be working 'right' from onset until resolution, and we now know that glycoconjugates play an essential role in ensuring that this is case.

Producing IgG

The term IgG refers to a class of immunoglobulins that are crucial to the inflammatory response. They serve as a kind of ID tag that protects 'friendly' cells, while otherwise labeling the target enemy for final destruction.

Individuals suffering from RA have been found to have structural variations of their IgG molecules. Findings indicate that there may be a lack of one or both terminal galactose 'sugar' molecules on IgG. The variances have been defined as G0- for no galactose molecules, G1 - for one galactose molecule, and G2- indicating that both galactose molecules are present. There have been numerous studies of the link between abnormal glycoforms of IgG and the severity of symptoms of patients hosting RA. Significant findings indicate that G0 patients experience the worst symptoms. Why? The explanation seems simple enough. Under normal circumstances the galactose would be transferred and added to the preceding N-acetylglucosamine molecule as a final step in the synthesis of the IgG molecule. When the galactose molecule has not been added, it leaves the previous sugar (N-acetylglucosamine or

GluNAc) exposed. Mannose-binding protein can then combine with the GluNAc which in turn results in activation of a pro-inflammatory cascade of proteins in the blood.

Let's go even a bit deeper. We'll find more 'sugar' activity yet.

As you might expect, galactose is added to N-acetylglucosamine via a catalysed reaction. The special enzyme (a glycosyltransferase) transfers galactose from elsewhere to an N-acetylglucosamine acceptor making the sugar chain longer. This enzyme is brought to the intracellular membrane and can be localized to the Golgi apparatus (GA), but may also be found in a soluble form in milk, amniotic fluid, cerebrospinal fluid, saliva, urine and serum. Dr. John Axford, and his colleagues have demonstrated a significant defect in that same enzyme which results in a profound change in the galactosylation of IgG. These changes have been integrally associated with the pathogenic mechanisms associated with inflammation in RA. It is not yet known what causes expression of a defective enzyme. However, it has been found that each of the rheumatic diseases has its own 'sugar print' which is characterized by its own variation in the IgG variants. It is suggested that each disease has its own specific rise to the resultant faulty glycolysed IgG molecule.[20]

Interesting information on the pathology of an afflicted RA joint lends to the following extrapolations. It has been found that there are neutrophils present in an arthritic joint at every stage of the disease. These neutrophils increase joint destruction through the release of enzymes and production of free radicals. However, it has also been found that both mannose and N-Acetylglucosamine 'sugars' inhibit neutrophil production of free radicals. Studies have shown that injecting arthritic rats with mannans (polymers of mannose) helped to prevent arthritic flares. It would be reasonable to assume that if the body had an adequate or abundant supply of mannose then it could possibly prevent the onset of arthritic flares, thereby enhancing the quality of life of the afflicted individual by reducing symptoms and perhaps even 'undoing' the pathology of the disease.

What Causes Arthritis?

Although the exact cause of RA is unknown, it is suspected that it may be related to certain bacterial (streptococci) and viral (Epstein Barr) origins. In order for bacteria to invade a cell, it must first attach to the target cell. In many cases this occurs due to a reaction between proteins acting like adhesives on the bacteria and sugar chains (glycans) on the surface of the cell membrane glycolipids and glycoproteins.

For example, *H. Pylori* attaches to the stomach epithelial cells by at least two glycans: Neuraminyl-galactose (containing NANA and Galactose) and Lewis-b substance (containing Fucose, Galactose and N-Acetylglucosamine). Essentially, this demonstrates that **bacteria attach to cell surfaces via glycoproteins and glycolipids on the target cell membrane. Administration of essential sugars would compete with the bacteria for the attachment site, and prevent the penetration of bacteria.** This could stress the relationship between adequate sugar supply and enhanced immune function, which in turn would prevent the onset of disease in the first place.

The role of IgA, a different class of immunoglobulins in breast-milk is another great example. IgA found in mothers' breast milk binds microbes and other antigenic materials to prevent them from reaching mucosal membranes, where they might cause infections or deposition of toxins on intestinal epithelial receptors. All this suggests that even if the eitiology of RA is bacterial or viral, the entrance of the invading microbe may be preventable in the first place.

A study conducted by Dr. Axford investigated whether the changes in sugar content affect the binding ability of Rheumatoid Factor (RF). Because IgG GluNAc is missing a galactose enzyme (G1), it makes the molecule more mobile[25] which may have something to do with the fact that five of the 16 monoclonal rheumatoid factors bound better to IgG that was deficient in galactose.[20] This establishes a correlation between the IgG structure and symptomatic expression of RA.

Another study investigated the relationship between lymphocytic GTase activity and serum agalactosylated immunoglobulin G levels (G0). It was found that defective lymphocytic GTase in RA patients is associated with abnormal G0 changes. Therefore GTase activity in RA is reduced and may cause problems with galactolysation of IgG.[25] It is suggested that normal cells have a feedback loop which stimulates the release of GTase in the presence of G0 molecules, however it is predicted that this positive feedback loop is disrupted in RA resulting in increased serum concentrations of G0.[20] RA has been associated with GTase Iso-enzymes that may be less reactive because of an increase in their sialylation. It would be of interest to find the causes of the defective enzyme and if those causes can be eliminated or remedied.

A study group of 23 pregnant patients with RA was conducted. Eleven (11) of them experienced spontaneous remission of symptoms, while 12 did not. The group that did not was further divided into unchanged and relapsed disease activity.[20] Findings indicated that the remission group had statistically significant decrease in IgG GluNAc levels (missing galactose molecule(s)). A remarkable finding showed that there was significant negative correlation (-0.80) in the remission group in direct contrast to the positive correlation of the relapse group (+0.87).[20] This once again establishes a relationship between normal IgG structure and expression of RA symptoms.

It would be interesting to establish a relationship with the patients above who had been breastfed with those who had not. The findings could help support current research which indicates that breast-fed babies have less incidence of inflammatory bowel disease, autoimmune diseases, chronic infections, and respiratory and food allergies.[22] Breast milk contains most of the necessary glycoconjugate sugars and the array of resulting glycoconjugates serves in the most vital processes that are necessary for proper child development such as nerve development and immune function.[22]

C-reactive protein, and anti-nuclear antibodies are not found in healthy individuals. Patients with positive results for both tests were sampled from an internal medicine practice and given 650 mgs of glyconutrient complex daily and the results for the re-test indicate that glyconutrients can have anti-inflammatory and immune enhancement qualities.[24]

As we have discussed previously the structure of the glycoform is directly related to its function, therefore it is crucial that they are synthesized correctly. Glycosyltransferases are the enzymes responsible for putting the individual sugar pieces together to create what we call the 'sugar code' of life. Most glycosylation is conducted in the golgi apparatus (GA) of the cell. It is the site of glycan elongation and termination.[20] The highly ordered and sequential action of the glycosyltransferases evidences the complexity and specificity with which glycans are built.20 The elegant biosynthetic glycan-processing pathway in the cell allows, in principle, the same oligosaccharide to be attached to quite different proteins without having to code the information into the DNA of the individual proteins. However, the orientation of the attached oligosaccharide with respect to the polypeptide may greatly affect the properties of the glycoproteins[26], and the story of IgG is a prime example.

What Can We Do?

So these are the findings, but the pressing question is WHY? What is the root cause? If we don't have the basic factors needed for life expression, how can we expect to express life fully?

It seems that if our bodies were functioning at 100% we would be able to prevent the onset of many disease processes in the first place. Study after study illustrates that when the body is supplied with the necessary raw materials, it has an innate ability to orchestrate normal functions.

There is discussion on how or why a deficiency of isoflavones is observed in cancer (prostate, breast, colon) and coronary heart disease and how or why their presence seems to prevent osteoporosis.[30] It's better to prevent cancer, heart disease, diabetes or any other disease, than to treat it. I heard somewhere once: "an ounce of prevention is better than a pound of cure", and today I can think of no better way to prevent disease, dysfunction and disorder than through a healthy nervous system, and to promote healthy body chemistry than through proper supplementation of vitamins/minerals, glyconutrients, phytohormones and antioxidants. Let's focus on prevention!

> ***Most major diseases that afflict mankind directly involves glycoconjugates.***

Oligosaccharides (glycoconjucates) from human milk remain intact through the digestive process (soluble fiber) to act as ligands that protect the baby from pathogens. The glycoprotein IgA comprises 70-80% of the antibodies in human milk. Cytokines play a role in cell-to- cell communication and immune system activation, and these are also glycoproteins. Glyco-sphingolipids of human milk are important in the development of the nervous system and gangliosides are glycolipids important in brain development.[22] The point here is, that not only are these glycoconjugates available in human milk but that glycoconjugates are an integral part of life from the beginning, they are the roots of life. It is now understood that there is a 'sugar code' in biological structures that relates to both health and disease.[31]

Understanding this new and developing glycoscience is essential to our understanding of disease processes and their management.[31] Most major diseases that afflict mankind (e.g. cancer, rheumatoid arthritis, heart disease, diabetes, infectious diseases and neurodegenerative diseases) directly involves glycoconjugates. The ultimate goal is to develop the science of glycobiology so that it can have a significant impact on our ability to define and support health, and to diagnose and manage disease.[31]

Conclusion

When you get right down to it, it's all about conversation. Everything manifest in our world is through communication; buildings, events, celebrities, laws, religions, relationships. Everything. Think about how many conversations are going on in the world right now. In the same sense, **your body is a world, the chemistry is conversation, the glycoconjugates are the language, and the essential sugars are the vowels. It's that deep, that intricate, that involved. There's chemistry to** everything in life: love, pregnancy, sports, movies, sex. How functional is your chemistry? How functional is the chemistry of those diseased? How functional is the chemistry of your baby, if you have one? How functional, I asked. Remember, it's all about function.

Glycoscience means hope. It breathes life. It causes transformation:

- From "ill" to "well".
- From sickness to wellness.
- From outside-in to inside-out.
- From disease and disorder to health and life.
- From treating sickness to preventing disease.

Yes, This Science means life. Are you ready to live?

About the Author:
Shafina Thawer, DC, FICPA

Dr. Shafina Thawer, graduated from Los Angeles College of Chiropractic (LACC) at Southern California University of Health Sciences (SCUHS). She is also certified by the International Chiropractic Pediatrics Association. She currently practices in Encino,CA

Editors Note:

Clearly the body knows exactly how to cope with inflammation. But we must still do our part - adequate nutrition and supplementation, including glyconutrients, plus moderate physical activity. There's a synergy there in both conditions of fitness and injury. Let's see ...

Chapter 13

Glycoproteins in Fitness & Sports Injury

Dr. Frank Bredice and Spice Williams-Crosby

Looks can be very deceiving. Just because someone looks good on the outside does not necessarily mean that he or she is healthy on the inside. In our practices, we've seen strong power lifters and endurance athletes who have died suddenly of heart disease or succumbed to cancer before the age of 40. Fitness level cannot and should not be based simply on how someone looks.

We believe fitness is a state of being wherein all systems of the body are operating at *optimal wellness*. This includes cell-to-cell communication, endocrine homeostasis, gastrointestinal integrity, maximum nourishment (with reserves), cardio endurance, musculoskeletal strength with flexible muscles and tendons. We speak of reaching a goal that requires patience, focus, and for most people, a complete change of lifestyle --not some quick and easy designer pill that does it for you magically while you sleep.

For true fitness, you need to do the work. You need to strive for Limit Strength, Starting Strength, Explosive Strength, Agility, Flexibility, Static Balance, Dynamic Balance, Strength Endurance, Local Muscular Endurance, Speed Endurance, Cardiovascular and Cardiorespiratory Endurance, High Muscle Mass, Low Percent Body Fat, Freedom from Stress, Freedom from Disease or Injury, and Preventative Lifestyle. It's a complete package - possibly overwhelming in total, but certainly achievable in increments.

The major stumbling block that holds most people back from optimal fitness/wellness is their diet. The American diet is so severely deficient in nutrients, that it's a wonder any of us is still standing tall or strong. It is our belief that a large section of people who have been diagnosed with ADD, OCD, ADHD and a lot of other D's (for disorders), are actually suffering from what we call NDD (Nutritional Deficit Disorder). That's often their underlying disorder. They lack the very state of wellness and fitness that we speak of. Not only do Americans consume more saturated animal fat and fried foods than any other country in the world, the average American takes in over 100 pounds of white, refined sugar every year. And if that's not bad enough, we now have fad diets that are erroneously telling us that carbohydrates are the real bad guys. The truth is not that carbohydrates as a whole are bad - in fact, they are necessary for optimum health - but rather where the carbohydrates are coming from. There is a big difference between sixty grams of carbs from organic whole-grain cereals and sixty grams of carbs from processed commercial cereals. We know it must be confusing and difficult for the real truth-seekers who are constantly trying to settle into the kind of comfortable lifestyle that doesn't always require the counting of calories, fats, carbohydrates and proteins to stay healthy. They are fed up with the fads.

Changing Times

According to a recent article in the Journal of the American Medical Association (JAMA), an estimated 40% of Americans are turning away from the traditional use of drugs and are now searching for alternative products to treat their medical problems. As of 1997, out-of-pocket expenditures relating to alternative therapies were conservatively estimated at $27 billion. We're happy to say that the reasons most given for this change were that conventional drugs are (1) too toxic, (2) too expensive, and (3) too unreliable. Of course, the FDA, recognizing the growing trend of people looking elsewhere for cures and good health, began stepping up their enforcement efforts to control or eliminate any products that made "off label" health claims (their position being that any product that professes to provide any type of healing benefit is technically a drug). This is rather ironic since every manufactured 'drug' has to have an LD_{50} level which measures its own toxicity!

Let's explain a bit further.

The LD_{50} or colloquially, the 'semi-lethal dose' of a particular substance is a measure of how much constitutes a lethal dose when taken internally. In toxicological studies of various pharmaceutical substances, tests are conducted whereby drugs are administered to lab animals in varying doses until 50% of them die, ergo the term LD_{50} or "Lethal Dose, 50%." Well, the multi-billion-dollar nutritional industry spoke out (actually they cried out) in protest, and the subsequent stand-off between the nutritional industry and government culminated in the 1994 passage of the Dietary Supplement Health and Education Act, otherwise known as the Hatch-Harkins Bill, named after its sponsors. This new law (aka the DSHEA law) created an entirely new category of products called "nutraceuticals" -- natural food products that carry what were once considered 'illegal' label claims. In general, the criteria for qualifying as a nutraceutical will be scientific studies showing safety, stability, and proven effects.

One of the first patented formulations to emerge under this new law was a glyconutrient complex that utilized a combination of eight vital monosaccharides (sugars) that aid in the body's cell-to-cell communication, and we might add, are necessary for optimum health. Saccaharides, by the way, are the good 'sugars' found in the body. In fact, for people with diabetes, these eight monosaccharides are a must. Other chapters in this book have already addressed this. We could say that in the last century we had essential amino acids, vitamins and minerals but in the 21st Century we're going to pay attention to these vitally necessary monosaccharides.

Glycoproteins

Scientists now know that there is a language of cellular communication encoded within the body's molecular structure. In order for the body to work at its optimum, that structure must have all the letters of its "alphabet" in place if the cells of the body are going to communicate properly with each other. If not, the language of the cells gets garbled and proper communication begins to break down. When saccharides bond with proteins they form "glycoproteins" (glyco meaning sugar and protein meaning amino acids) whose carbohydrate content is significant, ranging from 1% to over 85% by weight.

Scientific knowledge concerning the importance of glycoproteins in cell-to-cell communication is relatively new. Proteins, which are made up of various combinations of amino acids, were originally thought to be the primary communication molecules of the body. In fact, what we know as The Biotech Revolution began as an attempt to create new drugs based on proteins. However, we are finally beginning to realize that the structural simplicity of the protein molecule limits the number of possible configurations it can make in combination with other molecules, the bottom line being that the body performs many more functions than those that can be attributed to the molecular configurations possible with proteins.

However, in contrast to the simpler proteins, many more molecular configurations are possible with the more structurally complex carbohydrate molecule, which has two isomeric forms and six bonding sites. The resulting oligosaccharide chains of glycoproteins have many functions, both inside and outside the cell:

- They affect proteolytic processing of precursor proteins to smaller products.
- They are involved in biological activity of human chorionic gonadotropin (hCG).
- They manufacture enzymes (the tools the body uses to build the glyco-portion of glycoforms).
- They encode all biological information.

Monosaccharides representing letters of this 'sweet language of biological information' are similar to amino acids and nucleic acids, but with a coding capacity that is unsurpassed.

Forty percent of Americans are turning away from traditional use of drugs

It was Alexis Eberendu, Ph.D., who isolated and identified mannose from Aloe vera. He wrote a dissertation entitled "A Method for Determining the Molecular Structure of Carbohydrates" that was done at North Texas University, Denton, Texas. This unique technology and methodology eventually led to the creation of a glyconutrient complex including all eight vital sugars (monosaccharides). On a late night hunting for other information in the medical library, Reginald McDaniel, M.D. (member of the assembled research team put together at Carrington Laboratories by Bill McAnalley, Ph.D. toxicologist,) accidentally found an article in *Annual Reviews of Biochemistry (*1985) by R. Kronfeld and S. Kronfeld that explained why mannose is so important in cellular synthesis. Shortly thereafter, Dr. McDaniel began pilot studies in AIDS patients with formal FDA research exemptions in August 1985 and observed how aloe juice was improving clinical symptoms and laboratory values caused by the retrovirus.

Eventually, a team of scientists was formed and their research yielded more positive results in the fight against lupus, scleroderma, cancer, rheumatoid arthritis, diabetes, myocarditis, mixed connective tissue disease, fibromyalgia (pain in muscles, swelling, inflammation, etc.), and many more autoimmune diseases when glyconutrients were incorporated into the diet of some of these patients. As Dr. McDaniel has so poignantly stated, "In a nutshell, genes in the center of every living cell constitute instructions for conducting life, and the programs coded in the genes are expressed in cellular synthesis. Each cell assembles from nutrients and elements supplied in the diet, bioactive structure and function compounds essential for good health and productivity. We have found that there is virtually no condition that cannot benefit to some degree by enhancing the supply of nutrients that are used in biochemistry, i.e., the "chemistry of life."

Many of our patients ask how much and what kind of carbohydrates does one have to eat in order to have an adequate supply of the necessary monosaccharides and to protect themselves from the perceived consequences of their deficiency. Well, you can either eat a lot (and we mean a lot) of good wholesome natural grains, vegetables and fruits somewhere on a mountain top where the air is free from chemical contaminates, or you can use a daily supplement of a glyconutrient complex that carries the eight vital monosaccharides that will give you the protection you need.

The raw materials that are needed to make glycoprotein molecules all come from plants. The plants capture the sun's energy and then they in turn produce the carbohydrates or the sugars that the human body requires. The sugars found in these plants are vital for good health. The body breaks down the plant carbohydrates, restructures them into small saccharides, then uses those saccharides to build the glycoproteins required for accurate cellular communication. It's that simple!

Most Americans get way too many simple sugars and consume all the wrong kinds of carbohydrates. The next time you see a TV commercial advocating the use of a candy bar to enhance your creativity or sports ability, turn the channel! It's lying to you and you're buying into their misinformation, if you believe them. In fact, processed food like that will destroy your ability to perform correctly and show up in long-term damage. True complex carbohydrates in a natural state are what we need, and a lot of people don't know the difference. If it's been refined, don't eat it!

Athletes from Birth

If you think about it, we are all born athletes. First of all, just coming down the vaginal birth canal is equivalent to doing a marathon! You had to contend with contracting walls and much turbulence just to get here. You may have had to be manipulated, pushed and pulled, as you struggled just to survive the ordeal. Imagine the forces upon your head and neck. And thus begins the training.

Unlike other animals, our human brains take priority over all other development, but nevertheless, we immediately begin the process of developing our muscles in order to get around and get what we want. Just pushing and pulling on a milk-filled breast to get more breast milk is working our jaws and lips, stretching our neck and challenging our arms. In a matter of months, babies begin training for the next level of development, that of turning over, sitting up, crawling, and ultimately, walking on two legs ... and then, parents - well, your life is over! Just kidding! The preferable food that helps us all, at the outset, to develop into these great athletes, is breast milk.

Lars A. Hanson, Professor and Head of the Department of Clinical Immunology at the University of Göteborg, has published more than 500 papers in pediatrics, immunology, and bacteriology. One of his papers, "Breastfeeding Stimulates the Infant Immune System" expresses the importance of human breast milk. Dr. Hanson explains that there are 5 oligosaccharides that are produced by enzymatic attachment of additional residues to lactose. He notes that concentrations of some of these oligosaccharides in human breast milk are as high as those of lactoferrin or secretory IgA. But he also notes that other animal milk contains only trace amounts.

So as our infant athletes have been building their immune systems and developing their bodies, they change into toddlers wherein their physical activity becomes even more strenuous. But the toddler has now been weaned off the breast and the first kind of food he or she eats is usually purėed fruits, cooked vegetables and grains. All the enzymes in these foods have been destroyed via heat and packaging, yet the toddler is totally dependent upon them for his or her mental and physical development.

It's ever so amazing to us how resilient children are, even though so many are being fed such non-nutritious substances. As they try to stand up and fall down, they laugh, giggle, and go for it again. After the toddler has been weaned, however, there is no breast milk with its five saccharides available to help the child develop. Our foods are so incredibly deficient in a number of nutrients. Yet the child, against all odds, continues to grow. We survive because the body will convert glucose and galactose, (the two sugars we do get in our diet), through a large number of enzymatic steps, into the deficient ones. But this process has up to twenty steps in some cases, and it is energy-demanding and error-prone. A famous athlete was once put into a room with a toddler and told to mimic every thing the toddler did. It wasn't long before that athlete was begging to get out of the room. Our children are great athletes, but as they grow up, today's latest entertainment fare robs them of their excellence. They wind up in front of a computer, TV set, Game Boy or Sony Playstation and suddenly, their growing little bodies tend to become obese, their muscles atrophy, their mental focus is erratic, their attention span short, and their desire to go out and play diminishes to the point of lethargy.

If you were one of the lucky kids, your parents entered you into football, Little League, gymnastics, martial arts, basketball, or any fitness program that forced your body to adapt to physical stress. Suddenly, your muscles, ligaments, and tendons had to step up to the plate again, only this time, falling down hurts a little bit more. From aerobic (with oxygen) cardiovascular endurance training to anaerobic (without oxygen) strength resistance training, the muscle fibers were working hard to adapt to the physical stress. The muscle is made up of a group of muscle fibers that are known as the fasciculus, myofibril, myofilaments, myosin, and actin, and oftentimes, these working fibers fail under the stress by truncating, pulling, tearing, or ripping from their attachments. A sports injury is sustained.

Athletic Injury

So when an athlete injures a ligament, tendon or muscle, how does the tissue know what it needs to do to repair the damage and seal itself off again? How does it regulate the inflammation cascade? When an athlete eats, how does his or her digestive tract know which food components to grab hold of and send into the blood stream immediately in order to help heal the damaged area? Well, the immune system is coded to perform many complex involuntary functions. At the site of injury there is a spillage of protein that causes the macrophages to go to the site, phagocytose (eat up) the dead cells, and then through cell-to-cell communication, call in the fibroblasts to rebuild and repair the damage. This is what we call an efficient and specific immune response. It is the coding of the saccharides that completely directs this scenario.

Many athletes who have experienced injured ligaments and tendons are turning to *prolotherapy*. "Prolo" is a shorthand for proliferation because the treatment causes the proliferation (growth formation) of new ligament tissue in areas where it has become weak. The treatment consists of a dextrose (sugar water) solution that is injected into the ligament or tendon where it attaches to the bone. This causes a localized inflammation in these weak areas. This then increases the blood supply and flow of nutrients (including glyconutrients for formation of glycoproteins) the tissue is stimulated to repair itself. Like an elastic band that loses its elasticity, by eliciting an immune response, the body can bring integrity (elasticity) back into the ligament or tendon, especially when the patient is supporting the healing process with all the proper nutrients, including glyconutritionals.

Let's also not forget about the small but chronic injuries that can hinder us from enjoying a certain quality of life. Repetitive strain injuries like that seen in *carpal tunnel* syndrome can become extremely painful. That ligamentous injury occurs when the median nerve, which runs from the forearm into the hand through a tunnel, becomes pressed or squeezed at the wrist. The result may be pain, tingling, weakness or numbness in the hand and wrist, and radiating up the arm. Another common injury suffered by tennis players is lateral epicondylitis, or *tennis elbow*. Golfers also have a similar injury, this time on the inside of the elbow, called *medial epicondylitis*. They can develop this strain from their repetitive swing. To any avid golfer, anything that impedes his or her game is a virtual prison sentence. Martial artists often experience a hip flexor inflammation from repetitive kicking, and a baseball pitcher's greatest fear would be *tendonitis* in the elbow from repetitive throwing. Here the injury occurs not necessarily during the sporting event itself, but rather while practicing the skill in order to become better at the game. Other common injuries due to repetition, which often occur in the upper body, can be from swimming, javelin, discus, shot put, high jumping, or in fact, any kind of sport. Anyone engaging in of these activities could benefit from aggressive supplementation, and of course, glyconutritionals.

We have a tendency to not look upon muscle as an important source of protein for the immune system. However, there is a direct relationship between muscle mass and immune function. The better your muscle mass, the better the reservoir of proteins for the immune system to use in times of need. Muscle wasting is considered the curse of the elderly, infirm and the injured. Where there is muscle inactivity due to illness or incapacitation, i.e., brace, cast or confinement to bed, the muscle will tend to atrophy. This is known as *sarcopenia*. Sarco- meaning flesh or muscle and -penia meaning loss or deficiency. If an athlete has his leg in a cast, the inactive muscles will begin to atrophy or experience what we call "localized sarcopenia." Once a body part is confined, it will experience a wasting away, deterioration, or diminution. When this localized area begins to heal, all the nutrients that this athlete takes in will not only have to support the body, but additional support is then needed for that affected part, just to bring it up to speed. But if the cells can't recognize the additional requirements for food and water, how will all this nutritional help get to where it's needed? Once again, it's the saccharides that are speaking in the sweet language of cell-to-cell communication and directing the healing process.

As our teenage athletes move into bodybuilding, extreme sports, competitive martial arts, and more advanced training, it is a given that the body's chances or risk of injuries increase. With vigorous training or over-training, much of the available protein is being used for muscle recuperation and repair, and therefore much less is left over for the immune system. That is why it would be wise to use carbohydrate/protein supplements, such as a glyconutritional complex with an amino acid, broad-spectrum formula to support the breakdown and repair. Every serious athlete needs to become aware of this. Steroid use is a poor alternative for *repairing* injury, even in the short term.

Competition

What is common among those who are "pushing the envelope" for competition, is the athlete's inability to repair and recover fast enough to keep up with the training schedule and due date of the event to come. As the body is begging, borrowing, and stealing enzymes and proteins, not to mention screaming for saccharides, the immune system can't keep up enough to protect it from exogenous bacteria or invading viruses. It is not uncommon for a prime athlete, ready to make his or her mark in the sports world, to come down with an upper respiratory infection known as URI. This simple illness could prevent a gold medal from ever reaching the hands of a deserving Olympic athlete. It is dreaded and feared by all who are into fitness and sports competition.

Under stress, the athlete will exponentially increase his or her needs for all nutritional supplements, especially glyconutritionals. The higher the stress, the greater the need. From a professional basketball player making $20 million a year to the Formula 1 driver who must stay supremely focused for 90 minutes while driving at incredible speeds, the demand for cell-to-cell communication is great! As for the Formula 1 driver, even though his body is physically under tremendous G-Force stress, he will not incur a physical injury unless he crashes. However, his brain is dictating and demanding more from him than any other part of his body. The fact is, your brain uses more glucose in 20 minutes of intense thinking than your body does in one hour of lifting weights. Glucose is a monosaccharide sugar found in the blood that serves as the major energy source of the body. No Formula 1 driver ever wants to be caught short on this monosaccharide.

From anaeorbic bodybuilding to aeorbic gymnastics, it's not always the training or practice itself that is the most nutrient-demanding, but rather the repair and recuperation that takes place afterwards. The main objective for all athletes is to stay in an anabolic state. You want to keep building up. Without the proper nutritional supplements, the risk of experiencing a downward spiral into a catabolic state is inevitable. You want to avoid tearing down. By getting the proper amount of rest, eating healthy, taking supplements, especially including an adjunct of glyconutritionals to satiate the demands upon the body, an athlete has a fighting chance. He or she will help to prevent a possible URI, and where injuries may be experienced, to heal more rapidly by giving the immune system the tools it needs to do its job.

We believe that a child who sits on his or her butt all day today, will eventually turn into an adult who sits on their butt all day tomorrow. Therefore, we must educate our children. We have to set an example or they could be facing the doctor at an early age to be told to do something to bring down their weight, or their cholesterol/lipid levels, that increase their cardiovascular risk and appear to be robbing their health. Just like a kickboxer breaking capillaries because of the enormous cardiovascular demand on his or her body while entering the ring for round thirteen, so it is with the inexperienced middle-aged, out-of-condition individual who has to shovel his driveway or step on a treadmill for the first time, only to feel their heart pounding dangerously hard to keep up.

As we breathe 17,000 times per day and inhale an average of 16,000 quarts of air for our body's 60,000 miles of blood vessels, we rid ourselves of waste and carbon dioxide. The health of our arterial walls (endothelium) and the epithelial cells that line the cavities of the heart and blood vessels are in constant need of protection. Epithelial cells are separated from the underlying tissue by a basement membrane. The basement membrane is a thin sheet of collagen and glycoproteins that is produced by the epithelial cells themselves and by underlying connective tissue cells, specifically fibroblasts. These membranes are constantly being put to the test every time we experience a physical activity. Incorporating glyconutritionals into our fitness regime would only make sense if we are to support the very membranes that line our blood vessels and heart.

Hormones

Another very important component in the overall health of an athlete is his or her hormones. There are many hormones in the human body and only a few are responsible for sexual reproduction. The greatest misconception here is the notion that only women have a problem with hormones. Quite the contrary. Hormones comprise one of the body's greatest communication networks. A hormone molecule, released by one of about a dozen glands, travels through the blood stream until it reaches a cell with a receptor site that it fits. Every cell has a phospholipid membrane that houses cell-surface binding glycoproteins. This "Biological Braille" communicates which molecules are needed for hormonal balance, along with other cellular wants and desires such as the demand for food, water, protection, apoptosis (cell suicide), etc. Then, like a key in a lock, the molecule attaches itself to the receptor site and sends a signal to the inside of the cell. This signal may tell the cell to produce a certain protein or to multiply. Glycoproteins are key to receiving the message at the cell surface, transmitting the message to the inside of the cell and then implementing the same message there.

Hormones are involved in just about every biological process one can think of including immune function, reproduction, even controlling other hormones. They can work at astonishingly small concentrations (in parts per billion or trillion) which is one reason that small doses of endocrine disrupters are so dangerous, i.e., rbgh, dioxin, diethylstilbestrol (used illegally until 1988), dimetridazole, ipronidazole, and carbodox. These are known human carcinogens used every day in the livestock industry. Even their names sound toxic and poisonous to the body!

Hormones control a vast number of processes necessary for the body to function correctly. They control cellular protein synthesis, enzymic activity, and transportation of nutrients through the cell wall. Without them, we wouldn't be able to reproduce, think, grow, digest, breakdown glucose with insulin, build muscle, repair damage, or get through a fitness routine. If your hormones are out of whack, you're setting yourself up for major maladies, and often, the inability to grow muscle or lose fat. Once again, it's the glycoproteins that are in charge of communication with all the hormones.

We know that if we become hormonally deficient, the state of our wellness is at risk. This hormonal imbalance may lead to estrogen loss or too much estrogen, osteopenia, osteporosis, heart disease or cancer. Another important essential saccharide function is to help retain bone density and muscle mass. The body undergoes wear and tear as we go about our daily routines, or train for our sports or fitness goals. *Cells and tissues need to be replaced, regenerated, remodeled, and renewed continually*. As we exercise, our bodies are developing new blood vessels while increasing muscle mass. However, if we overtrain or become extreme in our training, then the body's fat stores are depleted to severely low levels. In female athletes this can lead to exercise associated amenorrhea (EAA). Studies have found that these young amenorrheic athletes had about twenty-five percent less spinal bone mass than their non-athletic peers, equivalent to those of 50 year-old women. As a result, amenorrheic athletes tend to have more sport-related fractures than menstruating athletes. Essential saccharides play important roles in these processes to help retain muscle mass and bone density while under extreme physical stress.

Conclusion

Clearly, glyconutritionals play an important role in the complex puzzle we call the human body. This role becomes more defined as we slowly learn what secrets nature has in store for us. For now, good nutritional foods, supplementation, and exercise can synergistically work together in order to bring *optimal wellness* to each and every human being, especially those involved in extra physical activity. As far as we are concerned, glyconutrients are a must, not only for amateur or professional athletes, but also for anyone who uses their body to move!

About the Authors
Frank Bredice, DC and Spice Williams-Crosby, BSc, MFS, CFT

Dr. Frank Bredice, obtained a B.S. in Biology at Southern Connecticut State University in 1972, while at the same time becoming a five-time All American Hammer Thrower. After receiving his Masters in Biochemistry, he switched focus and attained the Dean's list at the LA College of Chiropractic, from where he received his doctor of chiropractic degree. He is also a Diplomat in Applied Kinesiology. From 1988-92, Frank was a staff member of the U.S. Olympic Medical Team. He is a member of the American Sports Medicine Council.

Spice Williams-Crosby, BSc, MFS, CFT is an accomplished actress, stuntwoman, world's first vegan bodybuilder, and a nutritional author. She holds a Masters in Fitness Science and a Bachelors in Holistic Nutrition, both with highest honors. She has a Black Belt in Arjukanpo and has been a Certified Fitness Trainer for over 20 years.

Editors Note:

We'll leave the gym or playing field in the next chapter and go directly to the dentist's chair - not for dental work or even cosmetic appliances, but for some good advice on preventative dentistry, a novel application of glyconutrients ...

Chapter 14

Glyconutrients and Dental Health

Dr. Kelly Butler

I will soon enter my third decade of studying dentistry. As long as I am practicing, I will be discovering new things. Dentistry is rapidly and constantly changing, with exciting new advances in technology and science. Of all the new advances in science, the one that most intrigues me is glyconutritionals. As a health professional, I believe that because of glyconutritionals, I have entered into the realm of one of the most important medical breakthroughs in my lifetime. I can't help but be excited about the impact we are seeing on people using glyconutrients. I look forward to what future research in glycobiology will reveal to us.

When you think of improving your health with glyconutritionals, or any other nutritional supplement, you might not immediately think of your oral health. Even as a dentist, I can relate to this attitude or point of view. During a period of time when I was facing personal health challenges, I must admit that my oral health was not the first item on my agenda. But it had to be on the agenda, sooner or later.

As a dentist, I know that good oral health is truly inseparable from optimal overall health. In this chapter, I hope to share with you the importance of glyconutrition from this oral perspective. In other chapters of this book, there is a wealth of detailed information on disease states and the specific action of glyconutritionals. Much of this could be directly applied to issues of oral health. However, I am not looking to simply repeat this information. I would like to share a few of the implications of this information for restoring and maintaining oral health.

All Sugars are Not Equal

Before going any further, as a dentist, I would like to make a comment regarding the 'sugar' terminology, just in case you missed it elsewhere in this book.

Needless to say, for the typical dentist, 'sugar' is a bad word. Sugar means cavities! That's a mantra in my profession. All the evidence confirms that a major consequence of increasing 'sugar' in the diet is an increased incidence of dental caries and other dental diseases.

There's no doubt about that.

Today, the average American consumes about 120+ lbs of sugar per year. That's about half-a-cup-a-day. It comes hidden in soft drinks, fast and convenience foods, prepared foods in the supermarket and in fact, it is almost ubiquitous. We add sugar for taste to so many things that we consume. It is an epidemic in our generation that leads to serious health implications - decreased nutrition, glucose intolerance and mismanagement, and perhaps worst of all, increased obesity.

But language is an unfortunate thing sometimes. The widespread use of white sugar (sucrose) makes the term 'sugar' connote all the unfortunate 'negative' images. We immediately think of concepts like 'sweet', 'fat', 'gluttonous', 'pop', 'junk food', etc. But if we do that indiscriminately, we will miss a fantastic opportunity.

Prevention is a cornerstone of responsible dental care.

Sugar is actually a general term for a class of molecules, known chemically as 'saccharides'. They have a common molecular base structure and yet their properties vary widely. The eight vital sugars that we refer to as glyconutrients have little to do with the typical white table sugar that should be referred to specifically as 'sucrose'. This common crystalline product, usually from sugar cane or beet source, is actually a disaccharide, formed from the combination of glucose and fructose.

Glyconutritionals contain the eight vital sugars that are found to combine with proteins and lipids to form glycoproteins and glycolipids respectively, which we now know have widespread critical function in every living cell. That's the difference. These are vital, necessary, healthy 'sugars' that promote optimal health and wellbeing at the cellular level. That's what glycobiology is all about. Looking beyond the surface, dentists will certainly appreciate this difference.

The Importance of Oral Health

Healthy teeth and oral tissues are necessary for a few extremely important reasons. The most obvious function is in **chewing**. The joy of eating is greatly reduced when teeth are either missing or damaged. But more serious than this are the effects when malnutrition results. Seniors are especially susceptible to the nutritional effects of poor dental health.[1,2] Among the frail elderly, poor oral health is an important contributing factor to involuntary weight loss, which is linked to both increased morbidity and mortality.[3]

A healthy mouth reduces the chances of experiencing pain in our teeth, gums and other oral structures. It is well known that dental **pain** can quickly become an all-consuming issue that demands immediate attention. While practicing in Anchorage, Alaska, for example, I treated a woman who had traveled for six hours to reach me, after spending 24 hours in pain. I relieved the pain and pressure caused by an infection and she immediately fell asleep in my dental chair. For this weary vacationer, the pain of an abscessed tooth was affecting nearly every aspect of her life.

As a dental student, I spent a great deal of time studying the anatomy and physiology of the head and neck region. We became very familiar with the materials and procedures used to deal with the dental problems we would face. We also studied the art of dentistry. In other words, we learned to appreciate the dynamics of a beautiful **smile** and how to preserve and restore it.

While still a student, I was impressed by the profound emotional impact that an improved appearance could have on a person. Nothing brought this home more than the time I put orthodontic braces on a 70 year old woman to straighten her lower teeth. She had been unhappy about those teeth throughout her entire life, and her joy at the final outcome was both infectious and touching.

Teeth themselves can be beautiful. When those healthy teeth are within well-formed, healthy bone and tissue, they support the form of the face. Together, these structures create a beautiful healthy smile. Time after time I have been blessed to watch the personality transformation that takes place in a person who feels comfortable smiling after spending a very long time hiding their teeth. It is a clear illustration that our emotional health and well-being can be greatly impacted by our dental health.

Being instrumental in relieving pain is one of the great rewards of dentistry. Helping people create beautiful smiles also provides much fulfillment. More important, however, is my passion to help educate and support my patients in the prevention of painful experiences and in the maintenance of overall health and beauty. Prevention is a cornerstone of responsible dental care. Glyconutrients have become a powerful resource in my professional arsenal, as I work to alleviate discomfort and help patients reach their goals for beautiful, healthy smiles.

Oral Health & Physical Health

A past Secretary of Health and Human Services, Donna Shulala, in her introduction to the 2000 report on oral health from the Surgeon

General's office put it this way:

> *"The terms oral health and general health should not be interpreted as separate entities. Oral health is integral to general health; this report provides important reminders that oral health means more than healthy teeth and that you cannot be healthy without oral health."*

When most people think of dentistry, they tend to think almost exclusively of teeth. However, oral health goes far beyond teeth, which do not exist or thrive in a vaccum. As with any other portion of the body, it involves many complex structures and systems. Nerves, bone, muscle, connective tissue, blood vessels, glands and skin are all interwoven to form the jaws, gum tissues, tongue, cheeks, palate, sinuses and throat. All these systems and more contribute to the overall form, function and health of the mouth, which in turn contribute to the overall health of the body. And just as importantly, the overall health of the body greatly impacts oral health.

A patient's overall health can enhance or interfere with the dentist's ability to improve their dental health and their smile. At times, I have to suspend treatment until I can consult with the patient's primary care provider. If the patient must necessarily wait for their blood pressure to be controlled, or their blood sugar to be controlled, or for recovery from surgery, the dental problem is often worsened by the delay. Despite the patient's desire to have healthy teeth and gums, the treatment is too often complicated or dictated by their physical health.

You might have to work much harder than others to maintain good health simply because of what your parents passed on to you genetically. Consequently, it would be very important to do all you can to support the natural power of your body to heal itself. The good news is that you can have a tremendous impact on your oral health by the healthy behaviors and choices that you make.

What you choose to put into your body has a huge impact on achieving and maintaining good oral health. Just as with overall wellness, the importance of good nutrition cannot be over-emphasized. Like all systems of the body, your oral systems require that you provide a wide variety of nutrients in sufficient quantities. And just like the rest of your body, the health of your mouth is affected by whatever healthy and unhealthy things you consistently put in it.

The environment of the mouth is unique. The mucosal lining is thinner and more permeable than the outer skin. Oral tissue is very susceptible to the things it comes in contact with, making careful cleaning so very important. Good personal oral hygiene habits at home, in combination with occasional professional cleaning, are foundational to maintaining health. Without this, the bacteria in the mouth will multiply, creating sticky plaque that is toxic to the tissues and can cause both tooth decay and infections in gum tissue and bone.

Even with all our sophisticated dental technology, our daily lifestyle choices are central to maintaining healthy teeth and gums, avoiding pain and keeping a pleasant smile. However, I learned a long time ago that we cannot expect most people to be perfect when it comes to making healthy choices. My husband is a good example of the challenge. Living with me, he hears about the problems of oral disease constantly, and he has experienced them for himself. He gets almost daily advice about oral hygiene. And yet, perfect compliance is not forthcoming. Knowledge is not always power, only the wise application of that knowledge. It is clear that only action produces results. Because we live in an imperfect world, we must make good use of the tools that are available to us to optimize our efforts.

An Additional Choice

We each have a choice to avoid toxic substances, to practice good personal hygiene and to fortify our bodies with proper nutrition to sustain health. We now know that glyconutritionals are foundational to proper nutrition and to all functions of the body.

The evidence you have already seen in this book is overwhelming. And there is more to come. We therefore have another important choice for people that can empower them to better maintain dental health. Whether a person is nearly perfect or has a hard time taking care of their teeth, glyconutritionals can help.

Tooth Decay

It is a well known fact that diet has a great deal to do with how healthy you are. What is not so commonly known is that the mouth is often one of the first places where systemic imbalances may be noticed. Because nutrition affects all the body systems, a change in diet naturally can be seen in oral health. A dramatic example of this was observed in the Australian Aborigines, thanks to the work of Dr. Weston Price.[4] He noted that while these primitive, isolated people were eating their native natural diet, they enjoyed beautiful healthy teeth, in spite of the fact that they wouldn't know what to do with a toothbrush if they had one. However, when introduced to a modern diet containing white flour and sugar, jams and canned food, they soon developed rampant tooth decay. Why would this be? It may not be as simple as it looks.

While many factors are involved in the complex process of tooth decay, in general terms it happens when a susceptible tooth is exposed to bacteria and fermentable carbohydrates. The bacteria happily feed on the sugars, while in the meantime creating plaque. The process results in a sticky goo that sits on the teeth. Being acidic, the goo dissolves the crystalline structure of tooth enamel. So, simply stated, the more 'sugar', the more plaque and acid, the more tooth decay.

However, this does not represent the whole picture. By looking a little deeper we can find a connection between nutrition and susceptibility to decay. Some very interesting studies indicate that systemic nutrition may actually affect the amount of plaque that is formed. One such study compared blood levels of vitamin C and the frequency of brushing per day.[5] They found that regardless of whether teeth were brushed once, twice or three times a day, the people with higher levels of vitamin C had cleaner teeth than the ones with lower levels of vitamin C. Another study reported a reduction of plaque, calculus and stain when vitamin C was daily given for three months to mentally challenged boys.[6] Still other studies report significant reduction in plaque scores when multivitamins and minerals were supplemented.[7,8]

The role of nutrition helps to explain why some people can get away with brushing once a day, while others still have problems when they brush three times a day. We know that glyconutritionals are at the foundation of how vitamins and minerals help the body to be healthier. Therefore the intercellular communication enabled by glyconutritionals should only increase the impact of nutrition on plaque.

Saliva is another factor that influences susceptibility and is a key player in the body's own defense system against decay. There are many important components of saliva which include buffering agents to help neutralize the acid from plaque; minerals to help rebuild the damaged crystalline structure of enamel, and antibacterial agents to help keep bacterial levels in check.

Important *enzymes* are also found in saliva. Research has shown that people with lower levels of ptyalin, a digestive enzyme in saliva, frequently have more decay than those with higher levels of this enzyme. Proper nutrition is essential for the body to make enough saliva and to ensure that the necessary components are included. Tragically for the Australian aborigines, their increase in sugar consumption was accompanied by a decrease in nutrition. But they were not alone, as this is generally the case, and North Americans have been victims of the same trend. This is always disastrous for dental health.

The American Dietetic Association's position paper on the role of diet and nutrition in oral health states: "Diet and nutrition have a direct influence on the progression of tooth decay, a preventable oral infectious disease."[9] The evidence that good nutrition is a major factor in reducing our susceptibility to decay is continuing to grow. Every single function of the human body, including the use of nutrients themselves, is dependent on intercellular communication. Without this cell talk, for example, the body is not able to absorb the vitamin C when ingested, let alone know what to do with it once it is absorbed. The salivary glands would not know when to produce saliva, how much saliva to produce, or when to produce more ptyalin. All this depends on having sufficient amounts of glyconutrients. While there is much research to be done to understand the role of nutrition and the essential role of glyconutritionals on dental decay, it is clear that their contribution is just as important as brushing and flossing.

Periodontal Disease

Periodontal disease, also known as gum disease, is a serious infection that if left untreated, can lead to the loss of teeth. It is, in fact, the most common cause of tooth loss in adults. Periodontal literally means "around the tooth," which is where bacteria hang out if they are not properly cleaned off. Bacteria quickly multiply and create **plaque**, which is toxic to gum tissue, causing infection and inflammation. Inflammation of gum tissue is called gingivitis, where the tissues appear red, swollen and bleed easily.

In the treatment of gingivitis, the current primary clinical focus is the removal of plaque, thereby preventing the initial cause of the inflammation. Patient education in effective brushing and flossing, as well as regular professional cleaning, are the most commonly used approaches. While these methods are very important, we find that many people are still susceptible to gum disease. In a perfect world, we would be able to eliminate all plaque at all times, and prevent infection. Unfortunately, we don't live in a perfect world.

Over time, when plaque is in contact with gum tissue, the **inflammation** causes a pocket to develop between the gums and the teeth. The pocket fills with even more plaque and tartar. In this pocket, the toxins trigger a chronic inflammation in both the gum tissue and underlying bone. The inflammatory response of the immune system is a huge factor in exacerbating periodontal disease. The body essentially turns on itself, and in so doing, **destroys the tissue and bone** that supports the teeth. However, if the immune system is depressed, the body cannot effectively defend itself from the invading forces. If the immune system is confused, the inflammatory process goes into overdrive and speeds up the destruction of bone and connective tissue.

For me, the prevention of tissue and bone destruction due to the immune response is an exciting oral health application for glyconutrients. You can read more about the immune system modulation provided by glyconutrients in other chapters. Suffice it to say here, that the immune system is a grateful beneficiary of glyconutritional action. Empowered by glyconutrients, the immune system can more appropriately respond to the challenge of plaque generated toxins and better resist periodontal disease. Once again, poor nutrition and a lack of glyconutrients can often be implicated in compromising the body's immune system. Because periodontal disease is fundamentally a serious infection leading to tissue and bone destruction, the immune system is critically involved. Optimal nutrition and the foundational role of glyconutrients are crucial to enable the body to prevent, control and recover from this disease.

While plaque and inflammation are the major players, there are other conditions that increase our risk of developing periodontal disease. These risk factors include tobacco use, genetics, stress, medication and physical disease. I am excited by the fact that glyconutritionals can play a role in modulating the effects of these other factors.

Let's look at diabetes as an example. It is well documented that people with diabetes are more likely to have periodontal disease than those without diabetes. The disparity is due in part to the fact that diabetes lowers the function of the immune system. Conversely, periodontal disease can increase the severity of diabetes. On this two-way street, periodontal infection can make it more difficult for diabetics to control their blood sugar levels, making the diabetes more severe. A study was conducted on a group of diabetics who supplemented their diet with a nutritional program including glyconutrients.[10] After supplementation, 97% of the participants reported overall improvement in health and improved sense of well-being. More controlled diabetes correlates with more controllable periodontal disease.

The diabetes example raises the issue of the interplay between oral disease and overall health. Periodontal disease is linked to heart disease and stroke, respiratory diseases and preterm low birth weight. By reducing periodontal disease, we reduce the risk for these diseases as well. Once again, we are back to the circle of health. By improving oral health, we improve overall health and vice versa. Sound nutrition, including the vital sugars of glyconutritionals, gives me a way to address the holistic nature of my patients' health.

So what do we find in practice? In a preliminary study, all participants, whether they had mild, moderate or severe periodontal disease, reported significant improvement after nutritional supplementation which included glyconutrients.[11] Clinically, they showed less plaque, less inflammation, substantially decreased pocket depth and less bleeding. In addition, we find that patients using glyconutritionals have exceptional healing after such periodontal procedures as grafting and implants. The body truly functions in amazing, integrated ways when intercellular communication takes place as it was designed.

Oral Cancer

You will find information on cancer and glyconutritionals in other chapters in this book. I just want to briefly mention oral cancer because, for me, it is particularly devastating. Earlier I spoke of the fact that oral health is both about good functioning of the teeth and the entire oral environment, and maintaining a pleasing physical appearance. Oral cancer can be particularly devastating in both these areas. No matter how much of this disease condition I see, it still moves me when I see someone who has lost part of their jaw as a result of surgery to remove a tumor. Such surgery can drastically alter a person's appearance.

And function can be just as severely altered. I feel for those who have lost the sense of taste due to surgery or radiation, or whose salivary glands have been destroyed. And some people will have significant loss in their chewing ability due to the removal of a tumor. Without this ability, it is very difficult to maintain adequate nutritional intake, and life is far less enjoyable.

By improving oral health, we improve overall health and vice versa.

It is nearly impossible to recognize when oral cancer has been completely avoided through the use of glyconutritionals. However, I believe someday we will have numerous stories of individuals with precancerous lesions in their mouth who never needed radical surgery because they empowered their natural defenses with glyconutrients. What a contrast between the crude impact of surgery after the fact, and the precision of the body's own ability to destroy cancer cells before they wreak havoc.

Herpes (Coldsores)

Obviously, the impact of herpes on the lips or in the mouth, does not compare to that of oral cancer. However, for many patients, herpes is a big concern. One common complaint of my patients is that of ***herpes labialis***, commonly known as fever blisters or cold sores. These painful lesions are usually 1-2 single or multiple nodules found on the border of the lip or inside the mouth on gum tissue that is covering bone. The blisters first appear as fluid-filled vesicles which then give rise to the encrusted lesions. Usually, they last anywhere from up to 7-10 days. While these lesions are not life threatening, they are a sign that the body's systems are not in balance.

Patients who suffer, sometimes for many years from the intermittent nuisance, will often report that they are usually under stress for one reason or another at the time of breakout, leading to a significant suppression of their immune system. They may or may not also report the presence of a body fever which itself could indicate something is happening to the immune system. The herpes simplex virus (HSV-1) resides in the nerves surrounding the mouth and are kept in check by the active immune defense of the healthy body. When that defense is inadequate, the virus finds expression in the common symptoms. No wonder then that some people are much more predisposed to these lesions than others, at least in frequency and severity. But it is believed that up to 90% of the population in general are carriers of HSV-1, while more than half have some degree of susceptibility to the lesion recurrence.

Another kind of painful oral ulcers found in the mouth is ***recurrent aphthous stomatitis***, commonly known as canker sores or just aphthous ulcers. In fact, this is the most common disease of the oral mucosa, with a prevalence of 5-25% in adults. (Oral candidiasis is probably more common in small children). These relatively larger lesions (up to 5mm) are quite painful and tend to be irritated more by acidic or salty foods. They also hang around a bit longer than 'cold sores.' They tend to appear in similar fashion (stress, nutrition or immune deficiency) and also sometimes with hormonal changes in women. There is an associated familial component but the true cause of the disease is still unknown.

Partial ***symptomatic relief*** is usually provided with saline mouthwashes, topical analgesics, and in severe cases, topical corticosterioids. Yet patients are continually asking for new and better ways to prevent or cure these types of lesions. The usual request is for a simple quick-fix. Understandably, they want some pill to prevent these annoyances and if they ever occur, they look for a method of instant recovery.

But that's not the way the story goes. Building from the inside out, always takes time.

Here again we see the two sides of dentistry. Herpes is not only painful but also impacts appearance. For some reason, the site of a sore on someone's lip is not esthetically pleasing. In my experience and that of other professionals, patients who are on glyconutritionals excitedly report much fewer outbreaks.[12] In addition, if they do occur, they are much smaller, less painful and last only a few days. We see similar results with canker sores.[13]

Ray N. Kinley, DDS has advanced some preliminary ideas regarding possible mechanisms by which glyconutritionals and other supplements could impact the immune defense in cases like these [12,13], but a full understanding of exactly how these things work will have to await much more research. But we need not wait for those answers, the benefits are available now!

And talk about emotional impact - these **patients are overjoyed**. My reward is seeing their joy, and knowing that while glyconutrients are helping to manage their outbreaks, all the other cells in their bodies are also communicating better, improving areas they may even have no awareness of.

Medications

Over the counter medications are formulated to impact symptoms, with little regard to dental health. Companies that prepare these formulations seem to buy the statement that a "spoonful of sugar helps the medicine go down". Anything that I can do to help patients avoid sugary medication is a benefit. Glyconutritionals help to modulate the immune system and interfere with many cold viruses. Therefore, especially in children, there is less need for typical cold syrup medications that coat the teeth with the sugar that bacteria love.

Medications, whether over the counter or by prescription, can reduce salivary flow and may also hinder the ability to ingest, digest and absorb an adequate diet. As previously discussed, saliva plays an important role in dental health. These medications can seriously compromise oral health by leaving the mouth dry. Glyconutritionals can have an indirect effect on available saliva by reducing the need for medication that tends to dry mouth.

Dental Specific Research

A story on a new treatment for breast cancer will always get more headlines than a technique for reducing plaque. The truth is people often don't view dental health with the same importance as physical health. And let's face it, if I have a choice between losing a kidney and losing a tooth, I am choosing to protect the kidney. This means less research funding is available for oral health. However, there is much to learn about glyconutrients and oral health. It is with the understanding that oral health and overall health are inseparable that I look forward to more research in this area.

Conclusion

My personal health has dramatically improved from enhanced nutrition based on glyconutritionals. I can honestly say that I feel my life has been given back to me. The joy that I feel grows daily as I see family, friends and patients experience the amazing benefits of these nutrients. The fact that this benefit results from something that is part of the wonder of nature and the human body, makes me even more thankful to have found it. My life has been truly blessed. My hope is that you too will enjoy a partnership with your dental professionals to use the blessing and power of glyconutrients in your pursuit of wellness. The dental future looks bright indeed!

About the Author
Kelly Butler, DDS

Dr. Kelly Butler, graduated at the top of her class from Loma Linda University School of Dentistry. She was recognized for both her academic and clinical skills with several awards: from the Academy of Periodontology, Pierre Fauchard Academy, Southern California Academy of Oral Pathology, American College of Dentists, Southern California, among others. Dr. Butler, her husband and young daughter live near Seattle.

Editors Note:

The images of youth are not preserved with fine dentition and contagious smiles alone, but every organ system is at risk of premature aging. Let's bite the bullet next and face the inevitable prospect of the passing years, to learn what glyconutrients might do to delay or alleviate the inevitable ...

Chapter 15

Glyconutrients and Aging

Dr. Linda Hansen

W***ho's really 'Old'?*** As I wrote that question, immediately my brain began to search through a mental list of patients whom I consider old...Yes, there is the 83 year old with osteoporosis, marked kyphosis (dowager's hump) and loss of several inches in height as a result of the collapsing vertebrae in her spine. When she first came to me, she was taking drugs to increase bone density, heavy duty pain medications, and NSAIDs (non-steroidal anti inflammatory drugs) to try to help her sleep at night and function during the day. Approximately two months later, after taking glyconutrients, she came in the office to tell me that she was off all her medication and was sleeping through the night without pain. She was even able to work in her garden for 30-45 minutes before needing to rest. I can still picture her at that point, putting her hands on her hips and declaring "But after all, I am 83 years old!"

Then there is the 93 year-old woman who is doing pretty well, in spite of a recent fall that fractured her hip...She was quickly back on her feet after having taken glyconutrients before, during and after her hospitalization.

Just imagine ... 83!....93! That's old. Really Old. Yet these patients testify to the benefits they have received from glyconutrients even at such advanced age.

But it's all relative.

Preparing dinner this evening, I was suddenly struck with the realization that I too, am among the elderly! How could I forget that when my children (and grandchildren) are constantly reminding me of the reality. They really think I'm old - relative to them, of course! Not only that, but my practice consists of 85% or more persons over the age of 50. There are a lot of "baby boomers" whom I have treated in recent years. But to put it simply, I don't think of them as "older"! After all, quality of life is what makes the difference! Being able to feel strong, to be mentally alert, and to be useful citizens of society, does not have to be lost simply because of one's chronological age.

So when do we become "older"? The American Association of Retired Persons (AARP) sends you a card around 50 years of age. They are sending you a message. Perhaps the change happens at 55, when you qualify for a "senior discount" at some restaurants. Traditionally, it is age 65 when one is eligible for "Medicare". But many persons remain vigorous at that age and far beyond. In contrast, some people may be ready for retirement at 40 because they are early victims of chronic disease or are just weak and worn out. They are no longer able to be active and energetic. Still, others may be vibrant and useful, well into their 80's and beyond.

The question remains: Can we influence the aging process? More appropriately, here: can we postpone aging using glyconutrients? Is it possible to live an active and productive life, more or less until death?

It would appear so. There are several areas of the world where people live to be over 100. Some are still active and appear to be in reasonably good health. These people tend to have several environmental and lifestyle (including good nutrition) factors in common.

Coping with Oxidative Stress

It has been shown that a combination of glyconutrients, with certain antioxidants and phytonutrients from fresh fruits and vegetables, help to protect our bodies by reducing free radicals.[1] Free radicals are caused by oxidative stress. Oxidative stress in the body may be compared to what happens to your garden tools when you leave them outside in the weather for any period of time. They gradually rust from exposure to oxygen. Similarly, the same oxygen that is indispensable to life can form highly reactive molecular intermediates inside the cells of the body during the course of normal metabolism. These oxygen species are lethal if not effectively neutralized or quenched. They create more unstable free radicals. Chemically speaking, free radicals are unstable compounds that are lacking an electron. To attempt to become stabilized, the free radical may pull an electron from a different molecule in the cell, with resulting damage to the cell. This can create a cascade effect, with progressively weaker free radicals being created.

In the final analysis, damaged cells are what cause aging!

We must have adequate antioxidants to maintain healthy bodies. These important molecules are present in unprocessed natural foods.

That makes these nutrients exceedingly critical. Yes, they are protective, defensive, anti-aging weapons. Why? Because damaged cells are what cause aging! Not only that, but according to Dr. Les Packer in his book, The Anti-Oxidant Miracle, "73% of all premature death is the result of oxidative stress from free radicals."[2]

It is imperative that we consume adequate amounts of the necessary anti-oxidants in our diet. Glyconutrients have been shown to raise glutathione levels when they are taken orally. Glutathione is the most powerful antioxidant produced by your body. Glyconutrients not only raise the glutathione levels, but also help to maintain them against free radical destruction.[1] It is nearly impossible to get enough anti-oxidants in our modern, industrialized diets.

Energy

In chiropractic care, we seek to correct the flow of energy in the body by manual adjustment of the spine and/or extremities, or utilizing therapeutic modalities such as ultrasound, cold laser, electric stimulation, vibration, percussion, massage, ice, and heat. Einstein showed that mass and energy are but different manifestations of the same thing.[3] Necessary nutritional support for the individual patient is just another means of optimizing the flow of energy necessary for proper bodily function. Unfortunately, it has become clear that our foods have been increasingly adulterated, and we must supplement those missing elements in order to achieve the healthiest body possible. Everyone needs basic building blocks in the form of proteins, fats, carbohydrates, minerals and vitamins. Looking at these energetically, they are but molecules with spinning and vibrating atomic particles necessary for the body to function at its best. But lacking the right ones will definitely spell malfunction!

Glyconutrients have made a tremendous change in my practice. Since I have done much nutritional counseling over the years with my patients, using whole food nutritional supplements, and realizing that these were necessary sugars, I wondered what I might do to further encourage or even inspire my patients to get more of these in their diets. About three weeks after first learning of them, a nurse practitioner came into the office for a treatment. When I stopped to explain the glyconutrient deficiency step, she stared at me and said, "Do you know that there is a supplement that has all eight of those sugars in it?" I replied that I did not, but I knew then that they were vital to health in the same way that we need essential vitamins, minerals, amino acids and fatty acids...all necessary to give our bodies the building materials to achieve optimal health. Glyconutrients are not meant to cure anything, but our bodies are awesome energetic creations that are programmed to respond and function in health, if we supply what is necessary for repair, regeneration, communication, detoxification and energy.

Challenges

So what are the problems that concern the aging population the most? The simplest tasks can become all-important. Just being able to retain a driver's license or maneuvering to catch public transportation, negotiating stairs, shopping for necessities, fixing meals, maintaining proper hygiene, avoiding communicable diseases, preventing falls; in brief, just being independent!

Let us look at some of the ways that glyconutrients may help us maintain quality of life and enthusiasm.

Visual Decline

The most common changes that occur, as we grow older, involves the eyes. Even those people fortunate enough not to require glasses earlier, find that between the ages of 40 and 50 they begin to have some difficulty focusing objects closer than about two feet. Many find that they need increasing light to be able to distinguish detail. These conditions may be the result of deterioration of the muscles of accommodation, the lens of the eye, or the cells of the retina at the back of the eyeball. From all that you have read earlier in this book, you would suspect that supplying the body with the necessary glyconutrients may help to maintain the cellular health of the eye and delay visual problems indefinitely. You will not be disappointed.

Consider what happened to one of my patients - a 69 year-old female, who came to me with macular degeneration, having been told by her ophthalmologist that she would be legally blind within two years. This lady also suffered from diabetes and mild depression. After starting the glyconutrients, she noticed almost immediately, an increase in energy, and her depression began to subside. She also credits the use of glyconutritionals during the past year for the curtailment of the macular degeneration. Plus, an age-related hearing loss has improved in the past two years, and her blood sugar levels have stabilized. Pangs of joint pain in her knees, hips and hands have lessened too. She has remarked that she often hears those who have known her over the years declare that they can't believe the positive changes they see in her attitude, energy and complexion. She frequently hears how good she looks these days!

That's not an isolated case.

Joint Pain

Arthritic pain plagues many of the aging population. Whether the cartilage was destroyed by physical abuse in sports or because of poor alignment (osteoarthritis), or whether it was consumed by inflammation due to auto-immune disorders (rheumatoid arthritis), the morning stiffness and joint tenderness can become quite debilitating as you get older. The good news is that glyconutrients are found to act as foundational elements in the formation of proteoglycans in the joint cartilage. This relatively new intervention has made natural *glucosamine* almost a standard therapy in arthritis management today. We now know that supplementation with the essential sugars can result not only in repair of the cartilage, decreased pain and increased mobility, but it may also help retard further arthritic development.[4,5,6,7]

V. is a 56 year old female who had a lengthy history of rheumatoid arthritis. It caused such acute pain in her hips and feet, that it was extremely difficult for her to perform activities of daily living. Imagine her excitement when she sent an e-mail which stated that after three weeks on the glyconutrients she was able to shop at the mall for three hours without pain. Eight weeks later, she went camping with her family and was able to hike the hills without suffering ill effects.

S., age 59, has been taking glyconutrients since July of 2000. She carries approximately one hundred pounds in excess of her optimal weight. As a result she was unable to step up the height of a curb without knee pain, and she had to curtail her beloved golf game. Her x-rays showed bone-on-bone in her knees. In other words, she had destroyed her cartilage pads and was left with nothing to cushion the weight. She had taken prescription NSAIDs (non-steroidal anti-inflammatory drugs) for about ten years, but they were no longer relieving her physical disabilities. About the time of those x-rays, she began to take minimal amounts of glyconutrients. Shortly thereafter, she added phytosterols to her regimen because of her menopausal symptoms (hot flashes), and increased her glyconutrient intake significantly.

Today this patient, who lives to golf, can now play 18 holes or more without pain. Last summer her medical doctor, who specializes in physical therapy, told her that her x-rays showed marked improvement. And now, she no longer suffers with hot flashes!

What is it that allows for these dramatic turn-arounds? It appears that there are significant changes in the process known as glycosylation, not only in rheumatoid arthritis, but also with a number of other rheumatic diseases. The term glycosylation means that 'sugars' (hence, *glyco*) are attached. In cases of rheumatoid arthritis, at least the protective Immunoglobulin G does not have the correct glycosylation, and painful debilitating inflammation can be the result. In some instances that have been reported, it seems that supplying the essential nutrients may bring remission from these symptoms.[5,8]

Muscle Loss

Another age-related problem is weakened muscles. It's called sarcopenia. Muscle breakdown from lack of exercise, malnutrition and individual genetic factors within the body, account for much of the muscle/fat imbalance seen in the elderly. This tends to increase anxiety and propagates fear of falling, thereby decreasing the willingness to exercise or try to change or slow the muscle wasting. Further deterioration of joints and loss of bone density often become serious in the elderly. This can result in pathological fractures from minimal trauma.

The typical American diet that most elderly persons consume does not include the required five servings of fresh fruits and vegetables a day. They tend to consume white flour which is missing the nutrients found in the hulls polished off the grain; add to that white refined sugar which has had the nutrients in the cane or beet removed, and excess fats, many of which have been converted into trans fatty acids through refinement and leading to free radical damage. The general population suffers gross lack of necessary nutrients to maintain health. Common vitamin deficiencies seen in the elderly are Vitamins B12, B6, C and E, folate, niacin, iron and zinc. These micronutrient deficiencies can mimic the damaging effects done to the DNA from radiation![9,10] In fact, all the *micro*nutrients are essential for optimal *macro*nutrient metabolism so that both of these classes are necessary in the diet.[11]

The term *macro*nutrients refers to proteins, carbohydrates and fats. A person cannot build or maintain adequate muscle tissue without essential amino acids to build proteins. Many of the elderly are not only lacking in the necessary sugars, but they are also deficient in proteins and essential fatty acids. Sometimes, because of difficulty chewing due to teeth missing and gums deteriorating, decreased digestive juices, lack of finances, limited mobility to acquire proper foods, and yes, a myriad of other reasons, there may be a significant lack of macronutrients as well as micronutrients Providing missing micronutrients together with necessary sugars to aid macronutrient metabolism as we age, will result in improved health and increased life span.[11]

D., age 53, suffered with scleroderma and severe joint pain for over five years. She had been taking an average of five or more medications on a regular basis to try to find relief. Patients with scleroderma commonly exhibit thickened, leather-like skin, and connective tissue that over time becomes hard and rigid. When told of the possibilities of supplying her body with nutrients that might be crucial in helping her tissues heal, D. began to take glyconutrients. After four weeks of supplementation with the glyconutrients, she said that she no longer had joint pain. That was just the start.

Still another patient, R. a retired schoolteacher, came to me covered from head to toe with a blotchy rash. The itching alone was intolerable. She was a sight to behold when she presented at the office, having bathed her body with a mysterious pink lotion to try to soothe the irritation before coming in. Glyconutrients, phytosterols, phytonutrients and essential fatty acids were recommended; the glyconutrients and phytosterols to be applied topically as well as taken internally. She experienced immediate relief from the itching as applications of these were made topically. However, it took several months before the rash totally disappeared.

We must realize that aging simply requires more effort to maintain a healthy and fit body. Inactivity for lengthy periods of time will result in more rapid muscle deterioration and bone loss. The old slogan "*Use it or lose it*!" becomes especially pertinent in our senior years. Numerous things become really necessary. One cannot have optimal health without proper nutrition and glyconutrients represent one of the most vital classes!

Cardiovascular Problems

Studies have shown that optimal levels of certain minerals may reduce some risk factors and in turn, the incidence of atherosclerotic heart disease.[12] But once again we realize that the body must have all the essentials, including glyconutrients for cellular communication, to have these positive changes occur successfully.

M. was a tall, pleasant looking gentleman with gray hair, in his 70s. He came with his wife for the first visit because he had great difficulty communicating verbally after suffering a stroke. When asked questions, he would often look at his wife with pleading eyes for her to produce the words of response that he could not bring forth. His frustration was very evident. Now, months later, M. comes into the office regularly to pick up glyconutrients which he has faithfully taken since his initial visit. He displays a delightful sense of humor as he transacts his business with office personnel. Only those who knew him prior to the stroke would ever know that he had suffered ill effects from it. Today, he enjoys a full life and rides his bicycle approximately eight miles several days a week over steep terrain near his home.

Another stroke victim, J., prior to his first visit with me, had been hospitalized to have both knees replaced with prostheses. But while in surgery, J. suffered a stroke that left him with an inability to walk or talk, having affected the left side of his body. Prior to surgery, this 65 year-old worked full time in construction, exercised regularly at the gym, and was considered quite fit.

When he first came for treatment about 4 weeks after surgery, his wife and his daughter assisted him and he was using a walker. At that time the patient was non-communicative, with little use of his left side. It was with considerable difficulty that any treatment was given to him initially, but after several months on the glyconutrients, and a regular exercise program, he has recovered remarkably. Recently he was able to return to the department of motor vehicles and pass the tests to again be able to drive his car. His speech continues to improve and he and his wife are once more working out regularly at the gym and enjoying their retirement!

Body Fat

Another common result of aging is an increase in body fat. Some people may maintain their weight yet find that body composition has changed greatly. Body fat increases, but at the same time, there is a loss of muscle mass and strength.

Others find a gradual gain in weight. This seems to correlate with the decline in hormone production. Besides the hormonal changes that occur with the inevitable shut down of a woman's ovaries at menopause, or decreased testosterone production from the testes of the male in andropause, other hormones play a part in weight gain. Atrophy of the reproductive organs and the resulting changes in our bodies can be very depressing, if we are not aware of any means for changing the picture. The skin and mucous membranes throughout our bodies tend to become drier. Loss of collagen tissue adds to developing wrinkles. Some may suffer from dry eyes, sinus problems, incontinence, and/or pain, inhibiting intimate sexual relations.

Diabetes becomes more prevalent with increasing insulin resistance. That triggers the body to store the excess blood sugar as fat, instead of utilizing it as energy. The beta cells of the pancreas may be pumping insulin out into the blood stream, but lacking the essential glyconutrients on the surface of the cells. The communication of the cells may not be sufficient to allow the pancreatic hormones to do their job. Insulin resistance can often develop because of excess cortisol levels, which result from stressful lifestyles placing too much load on the adrenal glands.

Decreased hormone production and imbalances aggravated by nutritional deficiencies can result in a myriad of negative symptoms. Giving the body plant-based glyconutrients, together with phytonutrients from vine-ripened, tree-ripened fruits and vegetables, and plant-sourced phytosterols along with a source of essential fatty acids, can result in dramatic positive changes.

Malnutrition in the elderly

Many people do not realize that they are malnourished. At age 30, I had two healthy sons, having given birth to them when I was 24 and 26 years of age. After the second pregnancy, my lower front teeth shifted quite dramatically so that I had rather large spaces in front. Wishing to correct the problem, I consulted an orthodontist who told me that I would lose my front teeth within five years, and that there was no value in straightening them. The gum recession and periodontal disease had progressed too far.

First, depression set in! After all, I was only 30 years of age. Then I became angry and finally I decided to try to learn just what was missing nutritionally from my body that had caused such deterioration. Thus began my quest for nutritional knowledge. My nutritional supplementation has added a dimension of health 35 years later, such that most persons incorrectly guess my age as being much younger. Incidentally, I still have my own teeth!

Malnutrition in the elderly may be the consequence of missing teeth and ill-fitting dentures; depression and loss of elasticity of the walls of the stomach thereby decreasing appetite; inability to absorb nutrients from the intestines; dependence, isolation and even limited incomes that prevent the elderly from acquiring the basic foods to eat. These factors and more contribute to the often manifest anemia. Insufficient iron results in inadequate oxygen being delivered to the tissues. It can be the result of abnormal (and dangerous) bleeding, or lack of certain vitamins and minerals, the most common being vitamin B12, folic acid and iron.

The usual symptoms of anemia are seen as fatigue, weakness and pale appearance. In older people, anemia may contribute as well to confusion, depression, listlessness, and agitation. They may be unsteady or have difficulty walking, not just from aging, but also from inadequate oxygen and other nutrients. Some elderly folks may develop anemia so slowly that they do not notice these symptoms until they experience physical stress. If the anemia is great enough, some may experience shortness of breath, lightheadedness or even chest pain. These symptoms manifest more quickly if blood is being lost rapidly. And then, one must always be suspicious of what doctors call 'anemia of chronic disease.' Your physician can easily order blood work, if you suspect anemia is your problem.

The story of 92 year-old M. is worthy of mention here. She began having major health problems at age 82. She had been diagnosed with marked osteoporosis and degenerative disc disease at age 62. As a result, she walks with a bent-over posture. At age 82, she was taking prescriptions drugs for acid reflux resulting from a hiatal hernia; synthetic hormone replacement for hot flashes; potassium to alleviate cramping; a diuretic for swelling in her legs and feet; two blood pressure medications, and a medication that was meant to alleviate dizziness.

A few months later, M. began to hemorrage and was hospitalized for six days with a diagnosis of diverticulosis. While there, she was transfused with six units of blood. Her daughter brought her home and began giving her significant doses of glyconutrients, after reading the possible side effects of the drugs her mother had been taking. They seemed to match her major symptoms. After a few months, the daughter gradually reduced the glyconutrients to minimal dosage. Then about nine months after she had been hospitalized for hemorrhaging, blood was again seen in her stools. Again, M. was given large doses of glyconutrients and within twenty-four hours the bleeding had stopped. After six weeks of this, she was again reduced gradually to minimal dosage of the glyconutrients.

M.'s physician tests her blood every three months now. Her cholesterol, triglycerides, and blood sugar levels are within normal ranges which is an added plus, since there is diabetes present on both sides of her family tree. Today she has no dizzy spells, no more problems with acid reflux or hiatal hernia or hot flashes, and her legs no longer swell. The only medication she is still taking is to regulate blood pressure. She is very alert, loves to work crossword puzzles and seems in much better health than ten years ago.

J., age 58, has a long-standing history of ulcerative colitis. She has had numerous colonoscopies over the years, and she has had to take many pharmaceuticals to prevent diarrhea, bloody stools, and bowel cramping. Hearing about the possible healing aspects of glyconutrients for her bowels, she began to supplement with generous amounts. When she recently went to her physician to get the results of her most recent colonoscopy, the doctor was astounded, because almost two thirds of her colon appeared to be healed, and the other third was much improved. He told her, "This just doesn't happen!" and advised her to keep on doing whatever she was doing.

A healthy gastrointestinal tract becomes increasingly important for the assimilation of needed nutrients. Balance in intestinal flora (beneficial organisms) will improve the way foods are digested and used to repair and regenerate tissues, but of great importance is supplying the right nutrients, including the glyconutrients necessary for cellular communication. It is not just what you eat, but what you digest, absorb and assimilate that counts.

Decreased Immune Response

Aging means a less effective immune system. Malnutrition is prevalent in the elderly and as a result they are prone to invasion of infectious agents in their bodies. Proper nutrition is a deterrent to infection. "Malnutrition enhances the propensity to and heightens the intensity of infections, by weakening the various host defense mechanisms."[13] Immune response is enhanced with the glyconutrient supplementation.

Allergies are very common. My practice is located in the central valley of California, where products used in agriculture and the petroleum industry affect many of my patients with serious allergic reactions. Certain times of the year, cotton is sprayed for defoliation and the almond orchards are shaken during harvest, releasing fuzzy particles from their outer shell. Dust, herbicides, pesticides, pollens and petrochemicals sometimes result in some serious health problems.

One of my male patients, age 58, has lived in this valley since 1980, but did not begin to suffer allergy problems until 2001. At that time he just thought he was suffering from a bad cold that was accompanied by usual complications such as a streptococcal throat infection. He normally would expect to contract at least one such infection each winter, but when he went to his medical doctor in 2001, expecting to be prescribed the usual antibiotics, he was told that he suffered from allergies! He couldn't believe it at first, but the symptoms didn't go away. For over two years he used numerous antihistamine prescription drugs, including nasal cortisone spray...anything that was available...to try to alleviate the runny nose and cough. In the fall of 2003 he learned about glyconutrients and began taking large doses. After about four months of faithfully taking the glyconutrients each day, his symptoms totally cleared. Today he has no allergies, no runny nose or cough. He has no negative symptoms at all!

Yet another patient has a history of yearly trips to the hospital emergency room during seasonal bouts with allergies. H. had for 6 or 7 years suffered difficulty breathing that required the use of many different inhalers, decongestants and sometimes injections of epinephrine to open up his airway. At 60 years of age, his energy level was low and he also suffered from sleep apnea. Six years later he is allergy free, has high energy, takes no medications and no longer has sleep apnea. He attributes freedom from his former debilitation to glyconutrients.

Filling the Gap

The glyconutrients are basic nutrition for everyone, but even more so for the older person. As we age, cell regeneration slows and there are fewer cells in the stomach that produce hydrochloric acid and enzymes for the breakdown of foods for absorption. Many enzymes are glycoproteins and without necessary sugars, these enzymes cannot be made. Cell processes throughout the body slow down to some degree. Many older patients complain of some form of indigestion; acid reflux, hiatal hernia, burping, bloating, burning, abdominal cramping and flatulence. Supplementation with the essential vitamins, minerals, glyconutrients, fatty acids and possibly amino acids becomes necessary, if one expects to maintain or restore health.

> ***I****t is not just what you eat, but what you* ***digest****,* ***absorb*** *and* ***assimilate*** *that counts!*

One of the major problems I see when a new patient comes to my practice is related to their inability to assimilate the foods that they are eating. If they supplement, they may be guessing as to their needs and do not realize that there are dangers of synthetic supplementation. Selection of supplements should be done carefully. It has been shown that many of the nutrients purchased over the counter are synthetic extractions without a whole food matrix. Often the body is unable to recognize and/or assimilate these, and they may actually put an additional load on the organs of elimination.[14] Again, because the kidneys tends to get smaller as a person ages, elimination of waste through the urine is less, which means a greater toxic load on the entire body. Supplementation for the elderly can be very beneficial since that can aid the enzymatic breakdown of foods so that they may be absorbed, and then improve the elimination of waste products.[15] In particular, fiber-rich foods, supplements and lots of water go a long way to favor good bowel regularity.

The foods that we consume are lacking in many of the needed nutrients because they have been grown on soils depleted of minerals and beneficial organisms. They have been green harvested which means they are lacking essential phytochemicals that are only present when the fruit or vegetable is fully mature. They may be stored in warehouses for lengthy periods of time. **From the time fruits and vegetables are picked, they immediately begin to utilize the anti-oxidants present in them to stay alive.**

Processing of our foods allows them to remain on the shelf for weeks, months or sometimes years. Many are so processed, preserved, irradiated, and/or overheated, that any semblance of live food is gone, and contrary to advertising and perception, so-called fortification does not replenish what has been stripped from them! Dr. Roger Williams uses an illustration of fortification of grain flours that is classic. When grains are "polished," removing valuable B vitamins, and then synthetic vitamins are added back, he says it is like a robber holding you up for hundreds of dollars, and you in turn asking the robber to please give you five dollars so you can get a taxi! In addition to that, foods are often contaminated with herbicides, pesticides and other toxic substances.[16]

A Makeover

Changing your health profile will take time. Don't be surprised if you feel worse before you feel better. Cleaning out metabolic wastes...toxic substances, parasites, candida debris...things that may have been present in the body for years, can cause a person to experience negative symptoms. To change the health picture, one needs to be consistent in the manner in which the nutrient building blocks are supplied. Everyone has different needs. We have different genes, emotional makeup, environments, stressors, lifestyles and problems in our bodies, some that we may not even be aware of. But the body must first correct underlying issues before dealing with symptoms that we wish to see changed.

Cells age and die off at differing rates. It may take days or weeks, or perhaps months or even years to correct symptoms after improved health takes place on the cellular and molecular level. Homeostasis (balanced function) is a goal, but how long it takes to achieve that is a major challenge - more so for some people than for others

No matter how long it takes to give the body what it needs to heal itself, we must not shun responsibility for our health. That responsibility requires intelligent choices in lifestyles as well as choices of foods consumed. Loading the body with carbonated drinks; artificial sweeteners and flavorings; food dyes; hydrogenated and partially hydrogenated oils and trans fatty acids; preservatives, MSG and other taste enhancing additives, homogenized, pasteurized, fortified dairy products; meats that contain hormones or pesticides or herbicides; grains that have had their nutrients stripped in processing and more, -- all these can play a huge part in our health or lack thereof. One should not expect to maintain good health with supplementation, yet eat artificial junk food, imbalanced meals, and lead a sedentary lifestyle.

Fortunately for us, the restorative powers of the body are truly remarkable. Considering that besides the many conditions in the body we deal with as we age, there are numerous biological stressors that may affect us significantly. These include negative thoughts, electromagnetic pollution, negative drug effects, radiation exposure, physical stress/exhaustion, environmental pollutants, "super bugs", social isolation, psychological pressures, allergies and nutritional deficiencies. Some, or all of these, may impact our lives at one point or another.

Conclusion

Research has only scratched the surface in the understanding of the functions of these vital and necessary sugars. The study of Glycomics is an emerging field of research, the vastness of which is difficult to grasp, because of the myriad ways in which the sugars may function at the cellular level. There may be billions of combinations of them attached to bits of protein (as glycoproteins) or fats (as glycolipids) in the matrix of the cells of our bodies.[17]

Relying largely on pharmaceuticals to relieve the symptoms of common ailments associated with aging is not the answer for optimal health. We must seek to supply necessary components to eliminate the cause of our infirmities. Health *begins* at the cellular level. Health and vitality are also *maintained* at the cellular level. Let's also remember that we are spiritual beings having souls living in awesome bodies. Therefore, we must also aggressively seek to maintain health and active lifestyles with positive attitudes, regular exercise, mental stimulation, a well balanced diet and wise nutritional supplementation. With such applications, may the generation known as Baby Boomers change the definition of what it means to be "old"!

About the Author
Linda Ann Hansen, MTASCP, DC

Dr. Hansen earned her doctor of chiropractic degree from Los Angeles College of Chiropractic (now Southern California University of Health Sciences). She holds a BS in Medical Technology from the University of Puget Sound in Tacoma, Washington, and a BS in Human Biology from Los Angeles College of Chiropractic. She completed her internship in Medical Technology at Tacoma General Hospital in Tacoma, Washington and is registered with the American Society of Clinical Pathologists as a Medical Technologist. She currently practices as a DC in Bakersfield, California.

Editors Note:

Sooner or later, everyone succumbs to the inevitable, and it's left to the pathologist to find out why. After years of such practice, one can look back to learn some lessons of life that can help those who yet remain. In the next chapter, a pathologist shares that perspective ...

Chapter 16

A Pathologist Looks Back

Dr. Norman Peckham

All that will get you, is expensive urine" That was the response I got from an ear, nose and throat (E.N.T.) doctor when I asked him about taking vitamin supplements. We were sitting around the house after a fine dinner. I had had a series of upper respiratory infections and was experiencing a typical stuffy nose. Our topic of discussion was sweets and refined sugar as inhibitors of white cell function and promoters of infections. My E.N.T. colleague advised me to, "just eat a variety of foods, drink plenty of water and get adequate rest," and he promised that once I did that, all would be well. It was when I asked about supplementation with Vitamin C, that I got the "expensive urine" comment.

A bit surprised, the statement stopped me for a while, as I contemplated the implications of his words. I had heard that reference before, but never had it put so directly to my face, and especially from a colleague who I would think, ought to know better.

Or, should he?

A Belief System

There is a whole belief system behind such a statement that deserves some exploration. It's more than just a bias. It is symptomatic of a professional culture, a clinician's paradigm. What was it that made him come back with such a comment? How does that belief system impact his ability to see new information concerning nutrition? How could I help him see that supplementation is becoming ever more important for a popular culture that is willing to exchange good nutrition for expediency?

I have heard it said, "If glyconutritionals are so great, why haven't I heard of them before?" As a physician, I want to let you know that there are good reasons why you are not learning about glyconutritionals from mainstream medicine. In exploring the development of the belief system behind the "expensive urine" comment of my colleague, I hope to help you understand the position of most physicians.

Medical Schools Promote Business As Usual

Let's start with the role of his medical education. As both of us went to the same medical school, I have some knowledge of his education. Our education represents the curriculum of essentially every medical school, at least at the time we went through the system. We received only a few limited hours of formal instruction in the field of nutrition. Because it has been some time since I went to medical school, you might expect that things have changed. However, just a few days ago, I asked the person responsible for the curriculum of the current class at a nearby medical school how much nutrition training medical students receive. Five hours was the answer. That compares to 60 hours of lecture time for pharmacology, the study of drugs. It is easy to see that a medical student could get the impression that pharmacology is more important than nutrition in the work of a physician. This is further reinforced in practice, with all the new drug information provided by the pharmaceutical companies.

There is a course in biochemistry, the study of how the chemical machinery of the body works. Here students study how food is converted into energy to be used by the various body organs to perform their individual functions. It is in this course that they learn of vitamins, minerals, co-factors and the many enzymes needed to make it all happen. Here is where they learn that sugars and carbohydrates are converted to glucose which is used for energy production. In this course however, the information is not tied to disease states. Therefore, there is no structure to discuss the role of nutrients to maintain optimal health.

Pathology is yet another course. This is the one where students learn of the many diseases that plague us. As an interesting aside, it happens every year that as the students study the symptoms and signs of diseases, they find some correlation with their own case and become convinced they have the disease under study, only to repeat the process when the next disease is examined. So it is, that in this course they learn of the deficiency diseases like scurvy(lack of vitamin C) and beri-beri (lack of vitamin B). But again there is no information on the quantity of nutrients necessary for optimum health.

And by the way, even that is a 'red-herring'. We are all told that the federal government (US Department of Agriculture) has determined recommended dietary allowances (RDAs) for many nutrients. But the meaning of such recommendations in terms of health and wellness is hardly explored. Optimum health is a foreign concept in that nutrition-deficiency disease paradigm. By government standards, most of us are just 'healthy statistics.' After all, if we don't see cases of scurvy around today, for example, what is the need for vitamin C supplementation? If we don't have patients with beri-beri, why increase B-complex intake? What would result if thinking professionals would approach nutrition from an optimum health standpoint. Something tells me, we've got that all backwards. Optimum body function, not lack of disease symptoms, should be our studied goal. But that's in a different paradigm altogether. For now, we will continue examining physician education.

Learning the Art of Conversation Control

The courses above are usually taken in the first and second years of medical school. They are given in typical lecture format. In the third and fourth years of medical school, the style of education changes from classroom lecture to clinical exposure. Students rotate between clinical services such as medicine, surgery, psychiatry etc. The students now work with patients. Each student must take a history and do a physical examination. The findings along with recommendations are presented at rounds to the attending physician and other residents and students. Having been involved in this process as both a student and as an attending physician, I know how much pressure students feel to do well with their presentations. Often it appears that the duty of the attending is to grill the student's knowledge of the case and the disease to the point of embarrassment. Students become skilled at elaborate explanations of what they know, hoping that there will be less time for the intense questions. Sometimes intelligent guesses are presented with an air of authority.

A clinical presentation is as much about skillful communication as it is about information and knowledge. With enough oral skill, sometimes a student can make up for lack of knowledge. In so doing, the student avoids embarrassing themselves in front of the attending physician and classmates.

> ***O**ptimum body function, not lack of disease symptoms, should be our studied goal.*

Unfortunately, this skill is retained and is sometimes used when a patient asks a question about a topic with which the physician is less familiar. Doctors can be known to bluff and sometimes appear confident about things that are not well understood. It is a practiced art. Medical school is not the only place where physicians are expected to be right. Patients expect answers to questions and physicians feel an obligation to give good answers. Those answers tend to be consistent in the mainstream, but as soon as you digress from the classic diagnosis and treatment, anything is possible.

Doctors' Information Overload

The drive to provide useful expert opinions can result in the physician being "down on anything that he/she is not up on". Physicians are able to maintain an air of authority, even with a lack of knowledge. Much worse is the fact that the physician may not recognize that there is a true lack of knowledge. Introduce 'ego' and 'pride' and the situation then becomes serious. In fact, often , in the doctor-patient relationship, there is a tension between maintaining the position of authority and exposing a lack of specific knowledge. The patient who wants to know, comes to the doctor who is supposed to know. But the boundaries cannot be unlimited when discussing issues outside the physician's formal specialized knowledge and skill, and in matters of general inquiry and personal lifestyle values, there is a level intellectual playing field. The patient, not the physician, may have more and better information on the topic. *Doctors can't be expected to know everything and should not be always given a blank check or prescription pad.*

Yet, physicians did not go to school for so many years, with the intent of being put in the position of "I don't know what I don't know". It is just a result of the system of education and the volume of new information. I remember when I started medical school being told, "Half of what we are going to teach you is wrong. The problem is that we don't know which half it is." We were taught to rely on the established sources of information to keep us properly informed.

Although every physician intends to do their best for patients, after graduation physicians get busy. Time is totally consumed in keeping their hospital and office practices running smoothly. They work hard to keep up with the mass of new information and knowledge in their area of practice. The established sources of information become even more important to manage the overload of new medical advances.

One could go on to describe the typical doctor's sources of information; for that in itself is revealing. Doctors spend most of their time with, and are most inclined to listen to, other doctors. We read announcements, updates, magazines, etc that tend to be dominated by the pharmaceutical industry, almost exclusively. They are essentially our key suppliers. The implications are obvious.

Even knowledge in accepted sources, but not in our specific field or area of interest, may be totally missed and frankly, never come to consciousness. It is humanly impossible to keep up to date with even a small percentage of the huge amount of research and the developments in every field of medicine. The National Library of Medicine has some 12 million articles from 4000 Journals online, and that is just from the mid 1960's. Unable to read everything, your doctor may have major gaps in knowledge of areas that are not directly associated with his/her type of practice.

That's just the way it is.

Hard to Change

Another major issue comes to play when you ask your physician a specific question or request a special treatment. The government and society demand that your physician treat you according to the "standard of practice" in your area. The standard of practice is the current practice used by the majority of physicians in the area. For example, treatments common in the more urban areas of the country may not be available in a rural area. Your physician has to be continually watchful that he/she does nothing that could be interpreted as experimental or unusual to a patient. This is especially constraining in the current litigious climate where almost everyone is inclined, if not eager, to bring a lawsuit forward - whether it be frivolous, unsubstantiated or malicious.

Your physician can do things to themselves that they would not choose to do to a patient because of the "standard of practice." Get outside the standard of practice and a physician is at risk of being punished with large court judgments. Staying within the standard of practice is called "defensive medicine". I know a physician who is very willing to take supplements for himself, but will not recommend them to his patients. Other physicians have refused medically accepted treatments for themselves (such as radical surgery) yet will recommend the same surgery to patients because such treatment is within the standard of practice.

One of the primary methods physicians use to ensure that they are not outside the standard of practice is to generally use only treatment methods that have passed the statistical standards of randomized, controled, double-blind studies. Because physicians are trained in the use of drugs, they automatically use the thought processes that apply to drugs. A drug is a molecule that is made to affect one and only one enzyme or other factor that can modify a single body function. An example is the function of pain. The sensation of pain is the result of many biochemical reactions. Ultimately a nerve ending is triggered and the pain message is transmitted to the brain. Pain medications are designed to block only one of the body's chemical reactions in the pain process or the nerve pathway transmitting it. The series of studies required by the FDA is designed to evaluate this one effect. If there are other effects or benefits discovered by the study, they are considered confounding elements and are considered to weaken the value of the study.

Because the FDA uses this "single effect" method of thinking, a physician runs into intellectual conflict should he/she decide to recommend products that claim to benefit many organ systems. The FDA has set up an elaborate process of animal and human testing and trials that use the "single effect" thought process, to assure that the desired result is indeed received and that the side effects are minimal. As a matter of fact, it was illegal for a physician to tell patients about the clinical benefits of a nutritional product prior to 1994. Fortunately, the passage of the DSHEA law changed all that. **But most physicians still use the pre 1994 thinking. Prior to giving you a prescription, your physician will want to be sure that the material has passed the proper clinical trials. It is the trials that define the benefit to a patient. Material that has not gone through the trials will be met with significant suspicion.**

The body is a whole and not a collection of parts.

Two serious problems are present with these clinical trials. First as stated above, these FDA approved studies are designed to study only one benefit. So a drug that goes through the process is only approved for one benefit or disease. It will require another complete set of studies prior to approving another disease or benefit. Secondly, a multifaceted impact can easily be lost in clinical trials.

Before we change the subject, it may be useful just to note that despite all the emphasis on randomized, double-blind, placebo-controlled clinical trials today, the fact remains that many, many of the interventions used by doctors today have never been subject to those rigorous RCT standards ever. They have become common practice, initially by trial and error, then by anecdote and case reports, then by collaborative exchanges and finally by common practice.

Take the use of aspirin, for example. It has been for many years, that anyone could buy aspirin over-the-counter. That was long before any RCTs had demonstrated its wide-ranging effects of analgesia, anti-inflamatory, anticoagulation etc, etc. That was also long before statistics were reported on the thousands of annual deaths due to the inappropriate use of the same 'wonder drug'. If aspirin were to be first introduced to doctors and to the market today, could you imagine what the

FDA would demand and how it would be used? Enough said.

The Approval System

Nutritional products are essentially food. If you were to starve yourself, how many functions or body processes would you expect to be affected? Ultimately, all would be impacted. Conversely, if you begin to feed a starving body, you can expect that all of the body organs and processes will be improved. Unfortunately the total body impact of nutritional products, does not fit into the established way of evaluating effectiveness of treatment. **The model of**

"Single Diagnosis → Single Drug → Single Cure"

is *NOT* the single solution. The body is a whole and not a collection of parts. So how does one determine the real benefit of a food?

Another problem is that the FDA has no way to evaluate a food product, and as such, there can be no FDA approval. What's more, you can't patent food; therefore companies are not willing to spend the millions for evaluation studies (even if a method existed) without the potential of significant profit. So, your physician is not likely to get the FDA approval that he/she is used to requiring. The result in practice is: no FDA ruling means no cover or protection, and that means no likelihood of a strong recommendation from the person in that white coat.

Then there is the problem of the Recommended Daily Allowance or RDA that we mentioned earlier. Scurvy has been recognized as a problem for as long as 1500 years before Christ. The British Navy lost 10,000 men to the disease. In 1747 a British physician discovered that two men with scurvy were cured by eating oranges and limes each day. He didn't know it, but he had just supplied the nutrient that allowed the body to make the "glue" that keeps the cells of the vascular system tightly together and prevents the hemorrhage of scurvy.

Later in the 1940's the National Academy of Science (NAS) set forth the RDA for several nutrients. The amount was just enough to prevent the symptoms of the disease plus just a bit more. There was no attempt to discover the amount for optimum health and vitality. But this approach has become ingrained in the thinking of society. Every few years the NAS and FDA revise the numbers.

There is no cheap good way to determine scientifically the amount of nutrients to take for optimum health. So the regulating agencies use the following logic. It is assumed that the American people are generally in good health; therefore we can set limits based on the amount of these nutrients that Americans eat. The fact that cancer, heart disease, immune system problems, diabetes and a host of other chronic diseases beset us, is generally ignored. The fact that we spend more on health care than any other nation and remain near the bottom in fitness seems to pass by them. So, if your physician wants to recommend a program of supplementation, he/she will have to stick his/her neck out and move away from the standard of practice and he/she will usually be very reluctant to do that.

It is easy to see that training, social and legal pressures, with a good dose of ignorance, may all predispose your doctor to subscribe to the "expensive urine" idea. But it may be that there is a significant cost to patients and the public for such an attitude.

Yes, there is a price to pay. As a pathologist, I think I am witnessing it every day. Let me explain.

Looking Back

I am a pathologist. The doctors in my specialty are trained as specialists in the multitude of disease processes and their consequences. We make early diagnosis from tissue specimens by careful histological examination under the microscope. That is our bread-and-butter. Surgeons, dermatologists, some radiologists and others, prepare the indicated biopsy specimens and send them to us in the laboratory. We make rigorous analysis of all the data to come to specific diagnosis which can have major consequences in terms of clinical management.

That is our work in life.

When all else fails, we are obliged to examine our patients in death - the classic post-mortem examination. That is often a revealing experience. We follow a near standard procedure, sometimes as mere routine to uncover the obvious. But at other times, the findings are quite surprising, and occasionally, embarrassing to my professional colleagues. It is not uncommon to discover missed diagnoses. But then, 20/20 hindsight is always so much better, and the Monday-morning quarterbacks never deserve any trophies.

What's always disturbing and at times depressing to many pathologists like me, however, is to see the dire consequences of neglect, abuse, violence or iatrogenicity (doctors errors). The sight of a cancerous lung of a chronic life-time smoker; or a cirrhotic liver in an alcoholic; or a spleen ruptured by a drunken driver's folly; or atherosclerotic vessels around a heart or a brain, or a small kidney destroyed by drugs; etc., etc., -- none of these observations can ever be taken for granted. Each one is the story of a life - another human being like me.

The foremost question in the pathologists' mind is pathogenesis. Where did this come from? What was the underlying cause? How did it get to this? But soon follows the obvious next question. Could this have been avoided? Was this inevitable? Did someone make a mistake? The patient, the doctor, the society? But then, in the end, all roads lead back to the deceased individual. How did they choose to live? What were their priorities in life? Not in a moral or judgmental sense, but in a practical one. If half the causes of death in adults are consequences of lifestyle choices, including nutrition - it is not unreasonable or illogical to question one's diet and the possible role of supplementation.

I wish you could have been there.

It was time to do the **autopsy**. The patient had finally succumbed to the tumor that started in his large bowel. It was an aggressive adenocarcinoma. He had had surgery to remove the tumor six years before, which was followed with chemotherapy and radiation. While he was having the chemotherapy, he had stated that the treatment was worse than the disease. The poisons that comprise chemotherapy made him so terribly nauseated and weak. It was one of those times when first he was afraid he would die of the treatment, then came to the place where he was afraid that he might not. He would just begin to recover, then they would start the next cycle of injections. About a year ago he was told that the tumor had returned. Now it was in the liver. That was about the time he just gave up the fight. For the last three months he had been too weak to do much but sit around the house or just lie in bed.

Now, as he lay on the autopsy table, his abdomen was greatly distended and you could feel that it was full of fluid. His skin was yellow with jaundice. We made the incision from his breast bone to his pubic bone and opened up the chest and abdominal cavities. There it was, all over everything, a condition we call carcinomatosis. The liver was about twice the normal size. The surface was lobulated with circular masses of yellowish tan nodules from ¼ inch to 4 inches in diameter. When we cut the liver in half the entire cut surface had similar masses. The liver was 80% replaced with tumor. The tissue that connects the bowels to the back of the abdomen was filled with similar masses as was the abdominal wall. These masses had leaked about three quarts of yellowish fluid into the abdominal cavity. We found tumor nodules in the adrenals, lungs and bone marrow. His body just couldn't support that volume of energy-demanding tumor.

Earlier, liver cells had broken away from the original tumor, floated through the blood stream only to set up "house keeping" in these other organs. One has to wonder how things might have been different if he had had the opportunity to flood his system with the sugars that assist in cell-to-cell communication and cell-to-cell adhesion. Maybe his immune system could have covered the tumor cells with these sugars and used up all the attachment sites thereby preventing the tumor cells from setting up "house keeping" in other organs. Maybe the sugars could have made his body's killer cells more efficient and destroyed the tumor cells in the first place. What if his doctor had just known?

Just maybe, things could have been different.

Maybe his case could have been more like the case of a relative of mine. She was diagnosed with lymphoma, a malignancy of lymph nodes. Devastated by the diagnosis and feeling confused she called her son. His wife had recently renewed her life with dietary supplementation. Between the two of them they convinced his mom to supplement her diet with vitamins, minerals, hormone precursors and several monosaccharides. She went to a major cancer treatment center and was told that they thought they had an excellent chance of putting her tumor in remission.

Now that is not a cure, but it is a lot better than active disease. She began her chemotherapy expecting to lose her hair and have days and weeks of nausea and weakness. To her surprise she did not lose her hair, was not nauseated and she only had one day of fatigue and that was on a day when she took her grandchildren to the park for the day. That would make anyone tired! She had the usual rounds of chemotherapy given to anyone with her diagnosis. There were others in her "group" who did lose their hair and had all of the other side effects of the chemotherapy.

At the end of the treatments she had some additional laboratory studies done to check on the treatment progress. The physicians told her that because she had done so well and showed such a good response, they now felt they could affect a cure if she continued treatment with a course of radiation therapy. Thinking that a cure sounded like a good idea, she underwent the radiation and appeared to have the desired result.

She was then given another oncologist closer to her home for the rest of her continuing care. Because radiation therapy continues to have effects on the body after the treatments are finished, she was to have an expensive ($4,000) shot to boost her hemoglobin. The new oncologist began to ask her question after question about her previous disease and treatment. Finally, the patient said to the physician that perhaps she could get the medical record as all of the information was in there. The doctor said. "I have your record; I just can't believe what I am seeing. No one with your diagnosis has done this well. We need to study you." Then the oncologist said that she could not give the shot as the most recent laboratory studies showed she did not need it and no insurance company would cover it.

What did the supplementation do? I don't know for sure, but her body seems to have been able to protect her from the toxicity of the chemotherapy and radiation treatments while not interfering with the desired action of the therapy. That's called **a positive adjuvant effect**. It is the best of both worlds! Were the sugars able to do for her what they were not able to do for the other cancer patient because his physician did not know? Who knows?

Before I describe another case scenario, a word of explanation is in order

We know that platelets are a vital part of the complicated system that controls the balance between blood clot formation and destruction. Both of these processes are going on within our bodies at all times. Clots are formed, clots are destroyed. Platelets attach to a protein called fibrinogen. As the clotting process goes forward, fibrinogen is broken down into fibrin which is the tough stuff of a blood clot. It's important to note here that specific sugars are a part of this reaction. Needless to say, having normal platelet function is vital.

It was a Saturday morning when he awoke with a pain in the middle of his chest. It felt like a heavy aching weight on the center of his breast bone. He had heard about heart attacks and chest pain so he asked his wife to take him to the emergency room. She drove, and by the time they got to the ER the pain was gone. They started an I.V., drew blood for a panel of blood tests and did an EKG. After a few hours, all the tests came back as normal. The doctor looked at him and said "because of your age and symptom of chest pain, I am going to have to keep you here for 24 hours of observation."

The next day the physicians said "it must have just been heartburn because we can't find any evidence of a heart attack." That was good news. In preparation for discharge from the hospital they turned off the medication in the I.V. Within a few minutes the pain was back and the heart monitor was going crazy. One look at that picture and they restarted the I.V. medication and scheduled an angiogram for the next day. That showed a 90% blockage at two places in one of the coronary arteries. They then proceeded to place two wire stents at the site of the obstructions to keep the blood flowing.

A specialist who had done years of research on platelet function said "You shouldn't have had this episode, your laboratory lipids are normal. Maybe it is a platelet problem." He did some platelet function studies in his laboratory and came to the conclusion that the platelets were too "sticky". He recommended taking some fish oils which reportedly have a beneficial effect on platelet function.

Once a year, for the next 5 years, he would check the platelet function and always the platelets were too sticky. He added flaxseed oil, later primrose oil. The patient experimented with anything else he could find. No change was made in the platelets.

About six months prior to the next test he began to take a variety of glyconutrients just for good measure. At the next test, his platelets were normal! What a relief. Perhaps the platelets now had the proper complement of sugars on their surface and were able to normalize their behavior. Again, who knows? The patient doesn't care, as long as they behave right.

Conclusions

As I sit in my office looking at the tissue cells from patients with tumors of all kinds, infectious diseases of various causes, and autoimmune disorders of all varieties; I can't help but wonder and hope that they have had the good fortune to have a doctor or friend who has introduced them to this new science of glyconutrition.

We are in a rather unique time, a time in which there is an abundance of basic science information on the topics of glycoproteins and glycolipids. There are thousands of personal cases that have benefited from advanced good nutrition. The problem is that all this information has not yet reached the main stream medical community in a form that makes it "official" for them. I believe that physicians will respond when they get the "OK" from their information resources. Maybe the educated public can influence the process by asking questions of physicians and presenting literature to stimulate their paradigm until they too become believers.

Until that time, as for me and my house, we will rejoice in the benefits of "expensive urine"- if that's what it takes.

About the Author,
Norman Peckham, MD

Dr. Norman Peckham, graduated from Loma Linda University Medical School in 1962. After a residency in Pathology he spent two years in the US Public Health Service in Baltimore, MD. He spent several years as Medical Director of United Medical Laboratories in Portland, OR. He and his family enjoyed three years as pathologist for a Tanzanian Government Hospital on the southern slopes of Mt. Kilimonjaro in Africa. On returning from Africa he joined the pathology staff at Loma Linda Univesity Medical Center in Southern California in 1979. For the past 10 years he has served as Chief of Pathology and Laboratory Medicine Service in the Loma Linda Veterans Administration Medical Center in Loma Linda, CA.

Editors Note:

Fundamentally, the body always heals itself at the most basic level. As such, healing is a truly natural phenomenon - even when supported by medical intervention. Naturopaths emphasize this holistic approach and find special appeal from the value of glyconutrients. Here's one to tell us more ...

Chapter 17

Natural Healing and Glyconutrients

Dr. Marcia Smith

A 3-year study conducted at Johns Hopkins University concluded that 3 out of 4 Americans will die of a chronic disease.[1] With new diseases being named on a regular basis, there is growing concern about what is really happening. In fact, a recent Harris Poll noted that concerns about our health is one of the key factors keeping us awake at night.

The emergence of many chronic diseases occurred only after the beginning of the 20th century. Before the last century most people died of infectious diseases (from viruses or bacteria). That was essentially a "war without". The fact is that our natural habitat is also populated by microorganisms with an agenda totally different from ours. They seek to survive just like we do. But unfortunately they choose to do so at our expense. "Life breeds life," so these microbes find their most natural support by infecting other living systems, like humans and animals. They have a field day but unfortunately for us, if left untreated, they destroy our life in the process. For centuries, if not millennia, they were our biggest enemy.

Today, in the industrialized nations, most people are not dying from the "war without;" they are dying from chronic diseases, i.e. the “war within.” The leading causes of death are primarily heart disease and stroke, followed closely by cancer. You could add to this, the many years of suffering with complications of hypertension, diabetes and arthritis, just to mention three of the leading chronic conditions.

The question we should be asking is "Where are these diseases coming from? We know that the widespread occurrence of these diseases has little or nothing to do with infection by microorganisms per se. They are not contracted illnesses like influenza, small pox or polio. There is no obvious "war without" in these cases.

What then are the causes? Why are these chronic diseases so prevalent now?

These questions are not generally being asked but the answers are essential for real movement toward true wellness and away from our current health crisis. But before we begin to address those questions, we need to explore the emergence of modern medicine.

Modern Medicine

Before the 20th century, medical treatments were generally herbal (naturalistic) or homeopathic (energetic). They were limited in scope and effectiveness but both of these approaches worked with nature. At the beginning of the 20th century, there was the emergence of a more chemically based and less natural medicine in the United States. This approach was solidified with the publication of the Flexner Report in 1910 which ushered in a new medical education in the United States that focused on the use of synthetic chemicals instead of natural substances. There was such a strong bias in this report for a more chemically-based medicine, that most of the existing Naturopathic Colleges quickly disappeared. The Flexner Report only applied to medical education *in the United States*. In other parts of the world, including Europe, natural medicine (herbs and homeopathy) continued to be used with success and complemented the emergence of chemically-based pharmaceuticals.

It is interesting to note that the United States, which veered away from natural approaches toward the more chemical-based medicine, recently earned a ranking of only 37th place by the World Health Organization in terms of overall health. This ranking was in spite of the fact that the United States is ranked in 1st place in the world with regard to healthcare expenditures. Obviously, something is terribly wrong with this picture. We spend the money on health, but we don't see the proportional return in health!

These observations, combined with the statistics on chronic disease, are so dramatic that you would think that there would be a shock wave in the medical system and a huge coordinated effort to find the underlying causes. I don't see evidence of either. It appears to be "business as usual" in the medical world, treating the symptoms of disease and hoping for the best.

There can be no doubt that medical doctors do a commendable job in helping the acutely ill. A day in any emergency room, intensive care unit or even a delivery suite or operating theatre, would impress any observer of the "magical power" of modern medicine. You would witness the heroics of surgeons who stop bleeding in the brain, remove bullets from internal organs, reconnect a severed limb, deliver a baby by C-Section from a comatose mother, resuscitate a massive heart attack victim, or stabilize a child with status asthmaticus gasping for the breath of life, etc. Such combinations of surgical skill, life saving medicines and life-supporting therapies would impress the most die-hard skeptics of the remarkable success of modern medicine. It could easily be the latest "wonder of the modern world".

All this was romanticized on TV by *Doctor Kildare* and *Marcus Welby, MD* in the last generation and dramatized in this generation by the heroes on *ER* which popularized this type of medicine for all the nation to see. People are fascinated by it and they buy into that particular view of sickness in the world. But that paradigm is the unusual, the rare event, and most people are silently and inadvertently killing themselves in ways that doctors are totally impotent to affect.

Epidemiologists at Harvard have estimated that if one were to quantify the relative factors that advance the length of life and quality of health we enjoy, the ratio would be:

The "Health Care" system	10%
Genetics	20%
Environmental Factors	20%
Lifestyle issues	50%

These statistics make a clear case. Medicine is most effective at the bottom of the cliff where humanity tumbles, often prematurely and unnecessarily. The hope for modern man (and woman) is that we change our focus, away from the valley below with all its drama and excitement, to the guard-rails that are on the top of the same cliff, work towards strengthening those protective barriers.

It is time that even doctors re-evaluate how they think about health, i.e., what is the true nature of disease and what is the real meaning of health? That's what you and I and the general public need to know.

The current medical paradigm is clearly not working. The system of mainstream, chemically-based medicine in the United States holds a lot of power over its citizens ... including doctors and their associates. We are in a sort of national hypnotic trance about disease and illness. We are led to believe that the cure for all disease is just around the corner, as soon as new drugs and/or procedures are discovered. This paradigm presupposes the possibility of finding a single cause for each disease and that the discovery of the cause will lead to a single drug or class of drugs that will cure each disease.

The ongoing, multibillion dollar, *War on Cancer* (declared by President Nixon), still not won after 30 years, and the many *Races for the Cure* all maintain the illusion that it is only money and time that keep us from the cure.

The current medical paradigm prevents individuals from truly understanding the state of their health. Doctors are treating disease labels and far too often, are not assisting patients in building their health. Since chronic diseases often have no cures, doctors simply manage the symptoms as best they can. I have had many clients tell me that they were healthy, despite multiple diagnoses and a long list of prescribed medications. Their definition of health was the absence of symptoms (because their drugs kept their symptoms under control) and after all, they were not missing work. There is an economic cost to health, but health is not an economic value. It is an intrinsic value, right up there with "life, liberty and the pursuit of happiness."

Even when a cure is claimed, this usually does not equate to restoring health - only to an absence from the disease-label. With regard to cancer, for example, you are technically considered cured if you are cancer-free five years after diagnosis. Not only may the cure (the treatment) have left you ravished, but, if the cancer recurs more than five years after diagnosis, you are still counted as one of those who was cured. Does that really make sense?

Defining Disease

Just the very term disease should cause us to pause and think. DIS-EASE implies that some natural state of ease has been disrupted in the body or mind. It is a consequence of dissonance in the whole person. What should otherwise be a healthy, vibrant, stable and integrated organism has become a disorganized, vulnerable, symptomatic and deficient caricature. Disease begins with the whole body as a focus and then blurs the margins as individual parts come into view.

But that's not the popular way to think. We have been hypnotized by the establishment - the medical profession, the pharmaceutical industry and the media acting in concert - to foster the use of diagnostic labels for pharmaceutical solutions. The establishment has therefore perpetuated several popular myths. Let's take a closer look.

Myth #1 The Power to Name Implies the Power to Cure.

Here lies the crux of modern medicine's hypnotic trance. Western medicine generally translates a symptom or complex of symptoms into a disease name. Some diseases are referred to by the organ involved, like the general term heart disease. Other disease names are derived from the translation of symptoms into Latin or Greek. The disease lupus (more precisely, systemic lupus erythematosis, SLE) is a good example of the translation process. The lupus patient typically has a 'butterfly' rash on the face that simulates the mask-like pattern on the face of a wolf. *Lupus* is the Latin name for "wolf," thus the name lupus for the disease. Another very good example is the disease diabetes. One of the symptoms of the disease is the presence of sugar in the urine. The complete name for diabetes is diabetes mellitus. The translation of those words means passing honey. *Diabetes* is the Greek word for passing; *mellitus* is the Latin word for honey. The symptom of passing sugar is translated into Latin and Greek.

> ***H****ealth is not an economic value. It is an* ***intrinsic value****, right up there with "life, liberty and the pursuit of happiness."*

Many times in medicine, a so-called "disease" is really defined clinically by a group of associated symptoms which collectively is called a syndrome. Many syndromes are labeled by the name of the clinician who first described his/her observations of such in a patient. Syndromes and diseases are often used interchangeably, especially by the lay public.

In any case, the classic medical model involves taking a good patient history, doing a careful clinical examination, then ordering specific laboratory and diagnostic tests where necessary. This model is designed to proclaim a diagnosis.

The patient is usually relieved to have a diagnosis. They make the assumption that the doctor fully understands what is going on with them. The diagnosis validates the patient and their complaints. The problem is that having a disease name often creates an artificial reality or illusion that there is a cure, and if not now, there will be one someday. The process of translation described above does not, in fact, contribute to a cure. All it really does is create a kind of communication shorthand - a name and code number that allows doctors to communicate among themselves and to obtain insurance reimbursement. It also enables controlled studies to be designed and carried out so that drugs, specific to the name of the condition, can be hopefully developed and evaluated. Unfortunately though, it also fosters a recipe-book approach to treatment - that is, one drug or class of drugs for each separately-named disease. A current example of this, is the very popular statin drugs for cholesterol management and the associated heart disease risk.

Myth #2 Disease is Universal not Individual

Robert Aronowitz, MD, Associate Professor at Robert Wood Johnson Medical School discusses the disease definition issue in his insightful book Making Sense of Illness.[2] In that book he makes the distinction between specific disease and individual sickness. Dr. Aronowitz defines specific disease as essentially a mental construct created by a committee of doctors and scientists; individual sickness, he says, is the unique experience of the individual and may not always fit into a convenient definition. Dr. Aronowitz describes in detail the definition and naming process involved with specific disease. The essence of this process is clear in his quote from Dr. Charles Rosenberg, Professor of History and Sociology of Science at the University of Pennsylvania. "In our culture a disease does not exist as a social phenomenon until we agree it does." In other words, a disease doesn't actually exist until we say it does! The decision to declare that a specific disease exists, gives the doctors an insurance billing code.

Chronic Fatigue Syndrome is an excellent example of how a condition did not become real until a group of doctors agreed that it did. For many years prior to the naming of the specific disease, there were thousands of individuals experiencing symptoms of chronic fatigue. Dr. Aronowitz would classify those symptoms as their individual sickness. Those who were suffering were very frustrated because their doctors often didn't believe in the reality of what they were feeling. Many were told that the symptoms were psychosomatic. Finally, there were so many people suffering with the same or similar symptoms that a formal process was initiated to define and name the group of symptoms as a legally recognized specific disease. The codification of the illness really did nothing to solve the problem, it merely provided a kind of legitimacy! However, many chronic fatigue sufferers felt frustrated with the disease name that was chosen since it was only the description of their symptoms. Perhaps they would have felt comforted if the symptoms had been translated into Latin or Greek.

Chronic fatigue syndrome is now widespread. Few doctors are looking for the real cause or asking the important question, "Why now?" Yet, those who have finally been diagnosed somehow feel a sense of relief (they are entranced by the fact that their symptoms finally have a name), and they can now receive insurance reimbursement for any treatment prescribed by their doctor. Their doctor is now taking them seriously and will now acknowledge their sickness; the symptoms are no longer just in their heads. And with the diagnosis, the patient assumes there will be a cure. Unfortunately, that supposition is an illusion, part of the hypnotic trance. There is no cure in sight, and from my experience, it is unlikely that a cure will come from mainstream science and medicine alone.

I trust these examples will clarify Dr. Aronowitz's distinction between specific disease (the legal definition) e.g. lupus, diabetes or chronic fatigue syndrome, and individual sickness (the individual's specific set of symptoms). Hopefully you are now clearer about how the naming process and the creation of a billing code contributes to the hypnotic trance. As long as the medical system is centered around disease names and codes, and not individuals, there will be little progress in dealing with chronic disease. Remember most disease names are descriptions of symptoms, not causes! It is time to break the Disease Code!

Myth #3 Healing is Medical, not Personal

While the hypnotic trance surrounding disease lingers in our culture, you have a choice to make. You can continue to subscribe solely to the symptom-treatment approach and the one disease, one class of drug theory, or you can embrace a new health consciousness - a newly emerging natural health paradigm - a complementary approach which includes medications where absolutely needed. The natural health paradigm teaches that symptoms are, in fact, the very language of your body alerting you to poor health!

You can be thankful that those symptoms are alerting you to a problem in your body's regulatory mechanisms. The symptom-suppression approach of modern medicine is actually turning off your body's warning signals. It is similar to taping over the warning light in your car and continuing to drive, or grabbing a mop (instead of turning off the faucet) when your sink is overflowing onto the floor! Getting you to a symptom-free state only through the use of drugs does not address the real causative issues and does not provide you with true health. In fact, artificially eliminating symptoms often drives the problems deeper and provides you with a false sense of security. Your symptoms, with or without a disease name, are only the tip of the iceberg.

Let's illustrate to make sure this point is abundantly clear, for it is pivotal.

Consider the symptom of pain. Pain is a natural response to danger inside the body. Sometimes the more serious the danger, the more severe the pain. Why is abdominal pain sometimes localized in the right lower quadrant, or the right upper quadrant or the flanks on either side and the lower back? And why is increasing headache or chest pain (angina) so important? Because appendicitis, gall stones, kidney stones, cerebral hemorrhage and heart attacks can kill, and sometimes in short order. Pain is the symptom. It is the body's alarm system. To lack sensitivity to pain is to be vulnerable to all kinds of insults and injury. Analgesics (pain-killers) are very widely used medicines, but just imagine what real problems are masked by turning off that alarm.

What we just observed for pain may be said of so many common symptoms that become complaints, driving patients to doctors' offices to demand attention and relief. Think of vomiting, diarrhea, fever, etc. Relieving the symptom is usually the easy part in medicine. And far too often, it stops there.

But real healing requires numerous lifestyle changes that can move you towards optimal health and away from chronic disease. You will therefore need to deal with imbalances in your body's regulatory mechanisms, compromised due to the 20th century modernization process itself. It is a long-term process!

Myth #4 Modernization always Leads to Health

Nobody can deny the remarkable benefits to health the world over from the introduction of good public health infrastructure development: the provision of clean water; regular universal hand-washing; the development of some good agricultural practices; the preservation of food in transport, storage and distribution; the invention of vaccines against epidemic diseases; the design of safe roads, traffic control and safer automobiles; mandatory health and safety practices in the workplace, etc. These and many more advances that we take for granted every day, have made the world a far healthier place than it would otherwise be.

Symptoms are, in fact, a natural response, alerting you to danger inside the body.

But modernization has not always led to improvements in the health of society or of individuals in particular. The very term chronic disease implies that the underlying problem is not acute or sudden or simple. It is something that accumulates over time. It derives from a set of multi-factoral conditions "known and unknown" and tends to exacerbate over many years, causing much suffering and morbidity.

Donald O. Rudin, MD, longtime Director of the Department of Molecular Biology at the Pennsylvania Psychiatric Institute, has created a very succinct term to describe the chronic diseases of the 20th century. The name he chose is not a description or translation of symptoms;

it is a description of cause: The Modernization Disease Syndrome. A syndrome is a complex of disease manifestations grouped under an umbrella and treated as a whole. Dr. Rudin argues that underlying this syndrome are imbalances in the regulatory mechanisms of the body resulting from "changes in lifestyle factors involving exercise, stress, smoking, drugs, pollutants, and especially a multiplicity of interacting dietary modifications which have not...been evaluated for their collective effect."

In short, the modernization process has been an uncontrolled experiment with disastrous ramifications for our health. Dr. Rudin puts it this way: "*The real costs - economic and human - of the modernization disease epidemic exceed that of any World War.*" He puts special focus on the repair of nutrient deficiencies - making it clear that we will not solve our current healthcare crisis until we do the following:

- Take our focus away from treating separate disease entities and dealing with diagnostic codes;
- Understand the effects of the modernization process; *and*
- Focus our creativity on finding practical solutions to reverse the effects of that modernization process.

The Iceberg of Chronic Illness is a conceptual representation of what I have addressed here. The tip of the iceberg is *individual sickness* whether or not it has been translated into a *specific disease*. Biological stressors, most of which were delineated in Dr. Rudin's quotation above, are the causes which may be considered to be below the water line. They constitute a much greater part of the iceberg. Biological stressors produce dysfunction in multiple systems, precipitating a complex of symptoms. As an individual resolves these biological stressors, the whole iceberg (including the tip) will naturally begin to shrink. Sometimes the tip will shrink to the point where disease disappears, i.e., the individual loses his or her disease label. Individuals who are already on medications to treat the tip of the iceberg by alleviating the symptoms, will usually need to continue their medications during the process. They should reduce them only under the guidance of a professional, while working actively to shrink the iceberg and to strengthen their multiple systems by restoring the biochemical integrity of the body.

Many doctors and health consultants educated in the emerging natural health paradigm are using symptoms (individual sickness) as clues to the imbalances below the water line. They understand that biological stressors are, in fact, the cause of chronic conditions. These stressors are often intertwined, each person having a unique combination of many biological stressors along with their own unique genetic predispositions.

These health consultants suggest various lifestyle and dietary changes that are known to address the Modernization Disease Syndrome. They are speaking out against the negative behaviors that so many indulge in today. Just think of the impact of smoking, alcohol abuse, and misuse of both prescription and non-prescription drugs. Each of these factors could form an iceberg of chronic illness by itself.

But on the positive side, there's something more important still.

Myth #5 Drugs do More than Foods

This is the ultimate deceit of the hypnotic trance we referred to earlier. In the world of acute sickness, of course drugs are almost indispensable. They are fast-acting and dramatic in their relief of symptoms. They save many lives in emergency and they relieve pain and other unwanted symptoms when you need them most. But that is not the important health factor.

Food provides all the building blocks to repair and replenish body tissues and organs. Food provides all the essential nutrients for efficient metabolism in every cell in the body. Food fuels the entire system, allowing us to do everything from thinking and dreaming, to running and playing. Food protects us from all the environmental stressors and threats on the outside, and all the malfunctions and mutations on the inside. Food perpetuates life and heals its wounds from every single moment to the next. There is nothing more important, save universal oxygen and water.

Wise health practitioners understand that deficiencies in key nutrients can cause imbalances in at least four major regulatory systems: 1) The immune system; 2) The endocrine system; 3) The gastrointestinal system; and 4) The cellular communication system. It is worth emphasizing further that a dietary deficiency cannot be corrected with drugs or anything else other than the missing nutrients. All the body's building blocks are derived from foods - food nutrients only - never from drugs!

Dietary deficiencies can produce negative effects that manifest in ways that go way beyond the typical understanding of nutrient deficiency. There will inevitably be an interaction of all the external factors with the individual's genetics. Your genes are your book of life. Most people believe that their book of life is doomed to be read only one way. They have no idea that there is a new avenue of scientific exploration which is called by a new name, in a new health vocabulary for the 21st century.

Nutritional Genomics

It is clear that it is the interaction between the individual genetics and the environment that creates the outcome of disease or health.[3] Perhaps the most important inputs from the environment are air, water and food - especially food, as the source of essential nutrients. There is an emerging scientific discipline referred to as *nutrigenomics* or *nutritional genomics*. The science of nutrigenomics is the study of how naturally occurring chemicals in foods alter molecular expression of genetic information in each individual.[4]

There are numerous researchers in this field and a department at the University of California at Davis has been dedicated to this research. There is also research in Nutrigenomic Modulation occurring at the University of Colorado. In 2002, the University sent out a press release with some of the following quotes. "Food molecules enter our body and modulate our genes ... One's diet can be more powerful than drugs ... Antioxidants are gene modulators that turn on and off appropriate genes." They concluded by stating that "If we had diets more enriched with the right plant foods, we would likely live longer, and more importantly, maintain a higher quality of life as we age."

With the understanding of the power of food molecules to even modulate genetic expression, it becomes crucial that we consume all the necessary nutrients to ensure optimal metabolic function. Research on the composition of food has spanned a century, starting with the discovery of many classes of nutrients necessary for optimal function: essential vitamins and minerals, essential amino acids, and essential fatty acids. At the end of the 20th century a new frontier in nutrition opened up with the discovery that certain sugars in plants were necessary for optimal cell communication. This book is intended to document the power of these "sugar" nutrients in health and healing - hence, its title: The Healing **Power** *of* [8]**SugarS®**. Nutrients are so important that they can actually have an effect on genetic expression. Glyconutrients are now proven to be vital and necessary in both health and disease. And so I urge you to add this new class of missing nutrients to your program of optimal health.

Conclusion

In summary, if you suffer from a chronic health problem, the cause is not something that just happened to you, either by accident or by genetics alone. Instead it is something that emerged from you...from an interaction between your unique genetic predisposition and your lifestyle. **Chronic disease is not due to a pharmaceutical drug defi-**

ciency. Coronary heart disease is not caused by a lack of statin drugs. Infectious disease does not come from a lack of antibiotics. However, most of the chronic and infectious diseases can be traced, clearly in part, to a lack of optimal nutrition. The choice is yours. Every time you take a bite of food or a dietary supplement you are telling your book of life how it is to be read. My wish for you is that you will pick the nutrients that will cause your book of life to be read with joy and good health.

Strive to become the best that you can be!

About the Author
Marcia Smith, PhD., ND

Dr. Marcia Smith is a Naturopath who discovered alternative health for herself over 30 years ago when she reversed her long-term nearsightedness with the help of Dr. R. Gottlieb, the developmental optometrist, and later assisted him. She trained for three years with Dr. Dwight McKee, a well-known holistic physician and cofounder of Integral Health Services in New England. She subsequently earned a PhD in Holistic Nutrition from the American Holistic College of Nutrition and a Doctor of Naturopathy degree from the Clayton College of Natural Health. She is the mother of four.

Editors Note:

Any health care professional who comes to appreciate the true nature of healing will be frustrated in one sense but relieved in another. In the next chapter a physician lifts the veil and shares how this awakening and the introduction to glyconutrients changed his medical practice ... it's an eye-opener. He now expects healing and you will too.

Chapter 18

How Glyconutrients Changed my Medical Practice

Dr. Bruce Hyde

We are fearfully and wonderfully made! By design, we are made not only to be healthy, but also to be able to recover health.

We often take it for granted but just think of how many ways and almost on a daily basis, life is maintained by critical immune defense and restored by spontaneous repair. This is naturally an indispensable characteristic of life. It distinguishes the animate from the inanimate and it seems the more sophisticated and complex the design, the more efficient is this life process, as we go from simple cellular organisms to plants, to animals and finally to man, the crown jewel of creation.

Let's take a simple example to illustrate the point further. Imagine you received a cut on your finger in the kitchen. In fact, suppose it was a more extensive laceration with severe bleeding, requiring a couple stitches at the local clinic. Could you imagine the doctor's response with a pressure bandage to control bleeding, a local anesthetic to control pain, a few sutures to close the wound and a tetanus shot to prevent infection. The doctor made four major interventions to:

- Stop bleeding
- Close the wound
- Control pain
- Prevent infection

In all likelihood, the wound healed in a week or two, almost without a trace of the injury and the patient is delighted. But now, let's revisit the same incident to observe that each of the four intervention steps were superseded by natural phenomena that most patients would hardly recognize. The common response is to thank the doctor for a job well done. But surprise, surprise! The real healing that took place had little to do with the medical intervention, when compared to the body's natural response. Let's take a second look.

True Healing

How did the bleeding stop? Applied pressure created stasis so that the blood could spontaneously coagulate by a long and complicated cascade process of protein biochemistry and oxidation. If the patient had low platelets for example, clotting times and bleeding times could be much longer and continuous hemorrhaging could be disastrous. Many deficiency states could make this a major problem (coagulopathy). Without clotting factors and vitamin K, how could you even stop recurrent bleeding?

How did the doctor control pain? Injecting a small amount of topical or local anesthetic was enough to reversibly affect nerve conduction so the sutures could be put in without the patient jumping off the table. But when that anesthetic wore off, how could nerve conduction be restored? What if you continued to feel no pain? Just try to imagine the consequences to your health if you could feel no pain. This all-important natural alarm mechanism would become dysfunctional and the necessary warning signs would fail to alert you to many a major threat or physical insult. So the question remains: what's more important, the anesthetic to dull your pain or your nerve recovery when it wears off?

Take it the next step. The doctor put in sutures to close the wound. Sutures hold the skin in apposition so that the severed layers can touch. But *what constitutes the wound closure*? The cells of the epidermis, the dermis and underlying soft tissues including capillaries and nerve endings all regenerate and form a bridge. They do such a clean reconstructive job, tailored to that local tissue environment, that in a few weeks there is not only new skin integrity but in most cases, hardly a sign of previous injury. That is the amazing capacity of nature to heal and usually, to heal without even a trace!

Finally, the doctor used tetanus prophylaxis, just as a precaution against possible infection. But *what's the real protection* against the host of infective microorganisms? That's the body's own immune system. No more and no less. The body ultimately defends itself. It uses a wide variety of cells acting in concert to identify, isolate, attack and destroy any enemy that dares to pose a threat.

Take the complete incident as a whole. You get a laceration in the kitchen, you go to the local clinic, the attending doctor fixes the problem. But does he? He may get the credit for sure, but it's really your body that heals. **Medical intervention is at best, the secondary event.** The primary response is always the body rising to whatever challenge, and adapting to heal itself. This is true of almost any type of disease condition. **The body itself is its own greatest asset in maintenance, defense and repair.**

The surgeon in the operating room must remember this, both before, during and after whatever surgical procedure is carried out. Similarly, this applies for the internist doing routine 'rounds' in the hospital. As he or she follows each patient, noting whatever progress is being made - there must be constant recognition of the patient response to whatever management protocols are devised. The family physician in the office must be always aware of the patient's responsibility to make wise lifestyle choices to avoid the many premature degenerate conditions. So much so, that it matters far less what happens in the ten or twenty minute office visit and much more what happens between visits. That's where the body will maintain itself and that's when effective healing will take place - almost spontaneously, when it comes right down to it.

*If we take proper care of our cells, our cells will **then** take proper care of our bodies.*

Wellness by Design

Wellness is by Intelligent Design. That is an opportunity but not without responsibility. To put it simply, if we take proper care of our cells, our cells will then take proper care of our bodies.

I write this now and it seems so obvious. How else could one imagine health and wellness to take place. But I remember clearly when this all dawned upon me. The year was 1988. I was at that time, two years into a three year family medicine residency. Suddenly, I realized that none of my patients were really getting well. I was caring for chronic patients with chronic conditions. I was treating symptoms and not addressing the root causes for those many diseases. As a result, the unresolved root causes only resulted in ever more persistent signs and symptoms, requiring even more and more medications.

I came to a different understanding of the nature of disease. In real terms, disease was not the real problem. Disease was the indicator trying to send a message. Put it this way - disease is actually your body's natural way of helping you know that there are root issues that must be properly addressed before it will stop "complaining." Therefore, instead of a disease-care plan, we need a health-care plan! We need a way to enable the cells of the body and therefore the body as a whole, to find the resources and the environment they need to function optimally to maintain health and to heal and repair when necessary.

During my work with the USAF as an emergency medicine physician, I would often encounter individuals experiencing acute signs and symptoms of gastroenteritis, for example, with nausea, vomiting, and diarrhea. They had their own agenda. "Doctor, please help me feel better." I would tell them that there were two treatment options. The first option would keep the problem. I could give them anti-nausea pills and motility drugs to quickly "relieve" these undesirable circumstances, but at the same time, cause them to "keep" the root problem longer and actually delay recovery. The second option got rid of the problem. I would let them know that these unpleasant responses were actually the very processes necessary to get rid of the root problem. It was better to support the elimination effort by simple care, which would include bowel rest, adequate hydration and cleansing support. Those who chose the first option lost more work time and usually their recovery would take several days. Those who chose the second option usually went back to work the next day with recovered bowel health.

The problems pertaining to treating symptoms instead of root causes are manifested by the persistence of the corresponding disease. The removal of the symptomatic care can only intensify the signs and symptoms. Let's take another example. If you have hypertension and you abruptly stop your high blood pressure medication, you expect that your blood pressure will surge higher. Or again, if you have diabetes and you abruptly stop your diabetes medication, you expect that your blood sugar will rise higher. So therefore, we need the medications! Or do we? The medications are restraining a process that's otherwise out of control. It is not changing the process per se, which is still fundamentally there. As long as the 'problem' remains, then the need for more medication will also remain.

But medications should be best used temporarily, while seeking better options that get to the root of the problem. I tell people to think of the medications as you would think about a cast on your leg and crutches under your arms. The sooner the fracture heals (addressing the root problem), then the sooner that the cast and crutches (supportive symptomatic care) are not needed.

Treating Patients, Not Numbers

I was taught in medical school not to treat numbers, but instead, to treat patients! That is still a good mantra. The question should always be 'how is the patient doing ?' The patient's condition is the problem. The patient's real need is the focus. The patient's health is the goal.

I am in the business of helping people get well, not stay sick. Therefore, I expect healing! Progressive disease is not an acceptable option. Palliative care for chronic conditions is not good medicine today. There is another way. Proactive cellular support, with adequate nutrition and appropriate supplementation, and complete lifestyle overhaul, are indispensable to ideal contemporary health-care.

And how do we evaluate progress? Laboratory tests and diagnosis are sometimes so deceiving. Just because numbers look better does not mean that you are better. Good numbers obtained the proper way will usually parallel optimum health, while the converse equates with progressive disease. As an example, the statin drugs will make cholesterol numbers look better (lower). They will also lower the C-reactive protein number. These results are actually accomplished by blocking or hindering the normal biochemical pathway for cholesterol synthesis. My response is that you should never interfere with the normal cellular functions of the body in order to "improve" your health! That always comes with a price.

But lifestyle intervention with proper cellular care, that involves detoxification and nutritional supplementation, can result in the same numbers without interfering with normal functions. That program might even enhance normal functions. On the other hand, I can give you more and more statin drugs and lower your cholesterol even below a necessary level. The current guidelines recommend that your LDL-cholesterol should be below 70 if you have elevated coronary artery disease risk. It used to be less than 100. I could give you enough medication to make the LDL 0. Is that even better? Of course not! By proper care, health is maintained by modulating the numbers in a healthy range, neither too high or too low.

An Alternative Program

For more than 15 years, I have helped people get well by teaching them how to take care of their bodies through proper lifestyle, physiotherapy and nutritional supplementation. All these establish the basis for predictable health recovery. Proper lifestyle is the foundation of life, health and healing. Physiotherapy enhances the normal physiologic functions and assists the detoxification effort that removes any cellular toxic burden. Nutritional supplementation provides the necessary nutritional cellular support that is inadequately provided by the diet, or because of the disease process, the necessary support that is inadequately provided for by the cells (body). Stated another way, there are two basic nutrients. Those you eat, and those that your body makes. If either or both are lacking, then the nutritional supplementation bridges the gap.

It is still humbling to observe that even the best of interventions do not heal. Certainly, medicines do not heal. Physicians do not heal. Lifestyle does not heal. Therapy does not heal. Nutritional supplements do not heal. These modalities of care only, at best, support the healing process. Healing only occurs at the cellular level. The cells do the healing! It is called **wellness by intelligent design**. Every cell has intelligent, purposeful and health giving functions when properly supported. With proper cellular care, expect healing! That's what the Great Designer intended. Every physician and every person suffering with health problems should share that hope for healing. Actually, the Great Designer is also the Great Physician.

In my work, health recovery is expected, and tremendous health recovery has been observed for many diseases, including diabetes and its complications, coronary artery disease, asthma, allergies, arthritis, hypertension, obesity, and so many more. These results occurred in response to improved lifestyle habits and from the benefits of physiotherapies that enhance health by improving circulation, immune function and physiologic detoxification. Not everyone, however, responded as well as others. In particular, those with autoimmune diseases and cancer were predictably not consistently helped. In these latter cases, we've seen a few "miracles", but usually a lot of disappointment.

Believing that healing is to be expected based on "better promises", I am never content with failure. I expect healing recovery from all diseases. That is the standard. That is the goal. Lack of success does not mean that the principles of care are inadequate or that the "promises" are faulty, but instead, we are challenged in understanding how to cooperate with both, so that the expected recovery becomes reality.

The Glyconutrient Difference

This is where glyconutrients make the difference. The rapidly emerging science of glyconutrition establishes at the cellular level, the vital nutrients required for proper cell-to-cell communication. This cellular communication is accomplished through a wide range of specific glycoproteins synthesized by the cells and based upon the genetic code. Since every cell has the same genetic code, all cells "speak" the same language. When all the cells communicate effectvely and purposefully, then health is maintained and health recovery is expected. Efficient cell-to-cell communication within the immune system is the natural function that keeps us all healthy, even with our many varied lifestyles.

By contrast, when chronic progressive disease enters the picture, one can assume correctly that the cells do not have complete, coordinated and purposeful function. Until that function is restored, health recovery is not possible and diseases only progress. When we focus on treating the symptoms of disease (managed care), we should not wonder why, if no one is really getting better. Diabetics remain diabetics, hypertensives remain hypertensives, arthritics remain arthritics. The sick remain sick.

Simply aiming to re-establish the proper cell-to-cell communication by supplementing with these vital glyconutrients restores that lost function and health recovery can then be expected. Impaired cell-to-cell communication can be the direct result of genetic alterations (inherited or acquired) or a result of impaired cellular synthesis of these necessary glyconutrients. We have found that supplementing with glyconutrients has resulted in significant help for individuals with a wide range of diseases. The nutrients obviously do not diagnose or treat any disease directly, but rather can help restore the cellular functions that enable the spontaneous recovery of impaired functions. In a real sense, that is cooperation with nature.

Results, Results!

So many books could have been written about the many dramatic health recoveries that I have personally witnessed in individuals supplementing with glyconutrients. From my point of view, results are everything and the results I have observed in my practice are clear and convincing. Here I will present just a few cases.

J. is a 13 year old boy with Down's Syndrome. He had obvious impaired cognitive abilities and physical variations from the expected norm. His verbal skills were limited to one word responses, his artistic skills were very simple, and he had significant difficulty with learning. Physically, his mouth was too small for his tongue that protruded from his mouth; he lacked proper coordination that affected his posture and gait; he had a chronic folliculitis that nothing seemed to help. Within weeks after taking the glyconutrients, his verbal skills dramatically improved. He now spoke in sentences comprised of many words, and his drawings became very detailed and elaborate. "Something" seemed to suddenly link his brain with his tongue and hands. After several months, his skin started to clear up and over time, resolved in a manner never before realized. After a year, his tongue, posture, and gait issues are also "normalizing". The body is somehow healing itself, even when detailed explanation is not immediately obvious.

D. is a 64 year old man with end-stage diabetes. Diabetes is a disease that impairs both large and small blood vessels. The consequence of the large vessel disease is atherosclerosis that can result in strokes and heart attacks. D. has already had a stroke and a heart attack. Neurologically he continued to have impaired speech, facial asymmetry and poor gait. After the heart attack, he developed congestive heart failure. The consequences of the small vessel disease parallel end-organ complications that affect the nerves, the eyes and the kidneys. D. had no feeling below his knees. He was having laser therapy on his eyes. When he presented to me, he was experiencing rapidly advancing kidney failure. His creatinine level was 4.9, which represents about 1/5 of normal kidney function. Despite taking more than 20 drugs, his health was only getting worse.

Upon instituting lifestyle changes (diet/exercise), undergoing physiotherapies, and utilizing glyconutrition, D. began to demonstrate dramatic health recovery. His exercise capability was previously severely limited. He started by walking 30 seconds three times a day. Two of four diuretics were held. The statin drug was stopped. By the third day, the use of insulin was stopped. From that time forward, his blood sugar control was better without insulin and *with* diet change and limited exercise, than before with insulin but *without* proper diet and without exercise. By the end of 2 weeks, D. was walking a total of 30 minutes a day in divided sessions, he had lost over 20 pounds which was mostly weight from retained water (better eliminated by lifestyle changes than by diuretics), and his creatinine was at 3.7 (better than ¼ of normal kidney function). Every two weeks he went to the lab for blood work. His creatinine went from 3.7 to 3.5, then 3.3 to 2.7, then 2.3 to 1.7, then 1.2 to 1.3, and finally to 0.9 after a total of 4 months. A creatinine of 0.9! Normal kidney function! For someone who had been in progressive renal failure over a 3 year period! D. had faithfully followed the care plan that he was given and after 4 months, he was walking 30 minutes four times each day. He lost more than 60 pounds, and he was taking only 4 medications. A changed life!

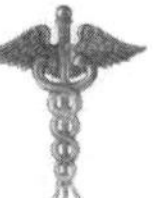

N. is a 45 year old female physician diagnosed with liver cancer. She had been given 3-6 months to live. She chose to come to our wellness center where the emphasis is upon improving lifestyle habits, providing physiotherapy, and specialized nutritional supplementation including glyconutrients. By observation, she appeared to be pregnant. The mass in the liver was the size of a large grapefruit. After two weeks of care, she returned home to continue the care she learned. After 2 months she consented to surgery. Upon removing the mass, it was discovered that the composition of the mass was predominantly dead cells.

Now, almost 4 years later, she continues to be in vibrant health without recurrence of her liver cancer. With regard to this case, as glyconutrients help to restore the cell-to-cell communication with the immune system, that system is very capable of finding and destroying cancer cells. This is the understood basis for the success in this case, and for so many other cases involving people with cancer.

M. was 23 years old when she was diagnosed with lupus. Her case was quite severe and soon she was requiring very strong immuno suppressants, including both steroids and chemotherapy medications. Her condition was so bad that at one point, she was expected to die. Her pharmaceutical care was altered from one extremely toxic chemotherapy protocol to one that was less toxic, and she survived. She was told that her disease condition would never improve, that she would need these medications for the rest of her life, and that she would never be able to have a baby. The disease severely affected her kidney with a very high grade of inflammation that caused excessive protein loss. On inspection, her urine had a frothy, foamy appearance as a result.

Five years later, upon learning about glyconutrition, her uncle provided her with these nutritients so that she could benefit from what he believed might offer better hope for a better life. M. was determined to continue with the care that she was already receiving. She was afraid to do anything different. After having possession of the nutrients for over 4 months, and after repeated urging from her uncle to "try just a little", she finally consented. For the first 3 days she experienced flu-like symptoms, and also on the third day she noticed that her urine was clear and not foamy for the first time that she could remember. That got her attention. However, she was not excited about taking "that stuff" and soon quit taking it. But then she soon noticed the return of the foamy urine. So she resumed taking the glyconutrients and her urine cleared again. She persisted in taking the glyconutrients this time, at ever higher and higher serving sizes, and in time she was taken off her chemotherapy medications. In the last year she not only got pregnant, and had an uncomplicated pregnancy, but recently gave birth to a healthy baby boy! Her quality of life is excellent, practically normal! Now she has hope for life and purpose.

H. is a truck driver, but for the 9 months before he came to me for help, he had unrelenting bloody, mucous stools. Imagine trying to drive truck at the same time. His diagnosis was chronic ulcerative colitis. He also had the diagnosis of chronic myelogenous leukemia. Nothing that he tried had really helped. Finally, he heard about the real meaning of hope and came for care. Right from the start, he was introduced to glyconutrients, but at a low serving amount. He was also receiving physiotherapy and made lifestyle modification. After 8 days of a planned 2-week course of care, he came to me saying that he was not responding at all to any of the care. He was committed to cooperating with the recommended care, but was wondering if anything else should be done so that he might soon get some relief and come to believe that this was the right course of care for him. In response, the next change was to increase the glyconutrients to a high serving amount while the rest of the care continued, but unchanged. Two days later, H. said that something was changing in his bowel function. Three weeks later his bowel function was so normal for him that he began to wean his serving size and by the end of another three weeks he was taking the same amount he started taking at the beginning. For one year at that lower serving amount, he never had another flare-up of colitis. Also at the end of that year, his doctor told him that his leukemia was almost not detectable. Where before, every white blood cell (with leukemia) looked like a cancer cell, now only 1 in every 1000 cells appeared abnormal! Health and vitality for him were at an all time high! In fact, he recently told me that every day he feels a little better. We are not supposed to wear out, every day feeling a little worse! We were made to have life, and have life more abundantly!

W. is from California. He has lymphoma that is found in numerous locations throughout his body. He is followed at a major university medical center in California. He is a man of great faith and prayed that God would be in charge of his cancer and that God would lead him to the right people for the right care. His wife plays the harp and she shares her talent everywhere. In fact, together they travel a circuit around the US, giving concerts in churches and prisons. As she plays, she also gives their testimony that includes the challenge they face with his cancer. A few years ago, I saw a notice in the paper regarding their concert that would be in Battle Creek, Michigan where I live. As a family we went and upon hearing their testimony, I felt compelled to give W. my card which had a message penned in, stating that I work extensively with cancer patients using natural remedies with wonderful results, and that I would be happy to talk with him, should he so desire.

That same evening he called and the next day he met with me and another doctor at the health center. I have now incorporated the glyconutrition technology in my patient care for over 7 years, but the year that I first met with W. we were inadvertently not using these nutrients. He was started on a plan and one year later he came back through Battle Creek. When we met again together, he was quite excited because his cancer was not worse, but neither was it better. I told him that was not good enough. I told him that we needed to add glyconutrients. He was still 5 weeks from home and I urged him to take enough of the nutrients with him to be able to take an aggressive amount during that period, before being able to receive additional nutrients at home. He was willing to take only enough glyconutrients for one week at the serving size I recommended. Still I urged him to take more, but he kindly took enough for one week. I expected to see him one year later, but instead he was at our door one week later. He wanted more glyconutrients. He stated that in one week his large lymphoid masses in his groin were already noticeably smaller.

Healing only occurs at the cellular level, where intelligent and purposeful functions need to be properly supported.

He was excited and committed. By 6 months his doctors were surprised and grateful that the disease was not progressive as expected. But he had not yet received any conventional treatment with chemotherapy or radiation. About 7 months later, he was told that his spleen was twice normal size. Also the CT scan revealed 30-40% increase in lymphatic tumor mass throughout the chest, abdomen and pelvis. At this point he consented to immune enhancing treatment, but no chemotherapy. Prior to that therapy, W. intensified the glyconutrition support to extremely high amounts for 10 days, followed by lower-end high amounts continually thereafter. For the past 7 months he has continued to be very diligent with the care plan that I recommended to him.

Two weeks ago the repeated CT scan revealed drastic reduction in the tumor mass, and for the first time the word "partial remission" was being used. The doctor said, "the results that we are now seeing are exceeding any expectation that we could have had for you". Furthermore, the comment on the most recent labs are not just normal, but "perfect". All his labs are normal and his spleen is back to normal size. They further said, "whatever you are doing to boost your immune function, keep it up." The next recommended care plan is to return in 6 months for a follow-up checkup. W. gives God all the credit for guiding his journey and the conviction, that he had all along the way, that he needed to build up the body and its defenses as the only logical long-term hope for recovery. His results seem to validate the benefits of a cellular-based health plan, rather than a symptoms-based disease plan.

And on a lighter side, I want to add the case of G. with several health challenges, but the issue to be presented here pertains only to the common and chronic fungal infestation of particularly the nails of the big toes (onchomycosis). His thick and ugly nails resulting from fungus have been a problem for many, many years. But upon instituting the use of glyconutrients, G's nails are no longer thick and ugly. Since this experience, this finding has been observed and reported many other times. This condition is extremely difficult to treat normally. But often we observe benefits in subtle areas where need is not identified but change is noticed upon providing the glyconutrients support. It is all about cells working together to maintain health and also for recovering health. In a nutshell, the principles: **Take proper care of your cells, and your cells will take proper care of you!**

CONCLUSION

Nature is so full of wonder! The best of medical technology today and the sum total of all we've already learned about the human body is but a very small part of the cellular reality. Life itself is still a continuous miracle. By Intelligent Design, each cell performs beyond all expectations and surpasses all the consequences of every intervention we make. The best that doctors can do is to only fulfill the supportive role. The cells are the true superstars!

But the critical step may still lie in our hands, not as experts and specialists, but as simple responsible human beings who must choose to provide the best of nature's resources, in the most supportive environment, for cells to function at their optimal best. We give them the tools and they get the job done. That's why we expect health!

You can too.

About the Author
Bruce Hyde, MD

Dr. Bruce Hyde graduated from Loma Linda University Medical School, CA after an undergraduate major in Biochemistry at Andrews University, MI. He did a family practice residency at Florida Hospital in Orlando and served four years as an emergency physician in the US Air Force. For the past decade he has focused on integrative medicine, first at the Newstart Lifestyle Center in Weimer, CA and then at the Battle Creek Lifestyle Health Center, MI. He has been a short term medical missionary to Nepal, Marshall Islands, Uzbakistan, China, Russia, Belize and Canada. He is now an International Medical Health Consultant.

He and his wife are proud parents of 9 children.

Editors Note:

Now we're at the frontier. We're on the verge of radical change in the way we approach health and disease. We need more research for sure, but what we're finding out already points to a brighter future. The next chapter is but a preview.

Chapter 19

Clinical Trials, Stems Cells and The Future of Glyconutrients

Dr. Gary Anderson

A Friend Recovers

It was November of 1999 when my wife and I learned that a friend, --we will call her Cathy-- had just been scheduled for surgery to remove one of her kidneys the following July. We had known Cathy and her family for several years and had first learned of her serious kidney problems in October 1998 when she began dialysis at a local renal unit. At that time, we had just started on our glyconutrient supplementation program and were feeling pretty good about it. My immediate thought when I first heard about Cathy's kidney problems, was that she probably should be using glyconutrients as well. Perhaps there could be some benefit that she would derive. At least it was worth trying, and at worst, we knew it could do no harm.

We knew the cost of her personally buying the supplements would be an unreasonable burden on her family. Therefore, we offered to provide her with the recommended minimum levels of glyconutrients for the next year if she would agree to take them. She agreed and had been doing so very faithfully for a year when we learned that her doctor had scheduled her for the kidney removal. Throughout 1999, her kidney function had continued to degrade, in spite of the glyconutrients, and was down to 15% of normal. The problem was not low kidney function by itself (that was being supported by dialysis) but the greatest danger she faced was that of possible infection spreading through her body from the dying kidneys.

When we learned of her scheduled surgery and asked if she would be willing to increase her intake, Cathy agreed to take as much glyconutrient as we would personally recommend. I consulted with the experts and we settled on 3 - 4 tablespoons per day. Previous experience had established that intake of up to 10 tablespoons per day was safe, so we felt there was no risk of harm in recommending this level of intake. Independent research had also established that, when the body is under stress, it requires greatly increased amounts of the eight vital monosaccharides.[1]

We were able to make special arrangements for a charity to provide

Cathy with the glyconutrients at no cost to her, under her exceptional circumstances.

She began this aggressive supplementation program in early January of 2000. Her doctor had scheduled her for kidney function tests and visual kidney investigations near the end of each month until her scheduled surgery in July. Amazingly, her tests began to show an immediate and rapid rise in kidney function. After her February examination, the doctor hugged her when she came in for her results and said he saw evidence of new flesh on the visual examination of her kidneys. Her kidneys were healing!

By the end of May, her kidney function was approaching 70%. The doctor had originally said the surgery would be called off if she reached 75% of her normal kidney function by July. Although she became ill in June and did not make it to the desired level by July, her surgery was called off.

It is now almost five years later. Not only did Cathy not have a kidney removed, but she has continued at approximately 75% kidney function and has required no further dialysis since mid 2000. In 2001, she had a complete kidney assessment by renal specialists in Toronto. She was told her kidneys are 100% healthy and the reason she has less than normal function is because she has smaller kidneys. A significant amount of tissue had been removed during surgical intervention when her kidneys were dying and suffering from infections. She was told that this reduced level of function is perfectly adequate for a normal life.

Such personal experience that I witnessed first hand raises several obvious questions, especially for me and I am sure also, for any thoughtful reader.

CLINICAL TRIALS

The Gold Standard

What did the glyconutrients really have to do with Cathy's recovery through this very difficult time? If you ask a typical nephrologist (renal expert) about their opinion on what happened to Cathy, and I have done so, you would get very aggressive, side-stepping expressions of disbelief that a nutritional component alone could have had any significant role in what happened to her. I don't think we should be too surprised at such a reaction. After all, would you really believe a food component could have this effect without something more than this single case report to go on?

So, what would be required to establish that intake of large quantities of glyconutrients, over a period of time, actually can influence the ability of the human body to regenerate dying kidneys? What can we do? What, if any, is the standard approach to this kind of challenging question? The answer is a Randomized Controlled Trial or RCT. It is the gold standard today. Let me take a few paragraphs to explain what I mean by an RCT and show how it would be applied to this or a similar question about the role of glyconutrients in human health and wellness.

By training, I would be referred to as a professional Biostatistician. In our field, we use statistical methods to rationalize observations of living systems and draw conclusions and generalizations of cause and effect. We look for associations and measure the influence of different factors on determining outcomes. The methodology is that of rigorous mathematical science. As a result of my training and career, I have had a considerable amount of experience in the design, organization and conduct of RCTs.

RCT Definition

An RCT is a study in which consenting participants are assigned at random to receive one of two interventions. One of these interventions will be a standard of comparison or control. This control is very often a placebo (a so-called "sugar pill") or no intervention at all. It may also be an existing standard intervention against which the "new" intervention is being measured to determine if it is a more effective alternative. To eliminate biases, both the researchers who are administering the intervention and the study subjects themselves must all remain unaware (blinded) about which intervention is being administered to them. They must remain blinded for the duration of the study. Note that both researchers and subjects are blinded - hence it is a double-blind study. A more comprehensive title we may hear for such a study is a Double Blind, Placebo Controlled, Randomized Clinical Trial - quite a mouthful! You can see why the term RCT is most commonly used.

The greatest potential impact of glyconutrients will be helping people stay well, remain productive every day, and become less dependent on the health care system.

In Cathy's case, the research question to be addressed by an RCT might be stated as follows: "Do glyconutrients, consumed in sufficiently large quantities over a specified period of time, significantly influence the human body in its ability to perform kidney regeneration and repair, beyond that observed when taking a placebo?".

The study would consist of observing two groups of kidney dialysis patients, one group consuming large amounts of glyconutrients and one group taking a placebo. We might well ask, however, why do we need the controls, the randomization and the double blinding. What do these complicated steps do for us that we couldn't do by just measuring the results in two groups after a sufficient period of time?

It is true that there are many less complex and less difficult study designs than an RCT that can be used. All of them, however, are open to questions of confounding, bias and lack of control that make the results obtained less solid. If we want the answer from our study to survive the attacks of the critics, then it needs to stand on the strongest possible research grounds.

To expand on the various study designs that might be considered, and to identify the issues they face when compared with an RCT, is beyond the scope of this chapter. For the interested reader, there are many good books available for further reference on clinical design, execution and analysis. Perhaps one of the most comprehensive and up-to-date is *Design and Analysis of Clinical Trials: Concepts and Methodologies, Second Edition*, by Chow and Liu 2 which was published in mid 2004.

RCT Requirements

The actual job of designing, organizing, conducting and analyzing the resulting data and then publishing the results of a proper RCT is a very complicated and expensive process. It is not something that can be done by just anyone and is best done by a well-trained team of individuals with various backgrounds and disciplines. We would need a significant budget (likely a minimum of $500,000), investigators interested in working on this question and a research organization experienced, qualified and available to conduct a proper RCT.

It would be exciting to conduct such a study, especially if the result established that the consumption of large quantities of glyconutrients dramatically influenced the human body's ability to regenerate dying kidneys. The impact for those suffering from kidney failure would be phenomenal and the potential cost savings to the health care system could be very dramatic. However, such a study just will not likely happen anytime soon for at least three reasons.

First, the question we are asking would be considered so absurd by most researchers that we would find it very difficult to identify specialists willing to be involved in such a study. It is just not conventional wisdom that a nutritional intervention could have this dramatic an impact on human physiology. Finding a source willing to fund such a study would be even more challenging. This study would likely be considered a waste of time, talent and resources.

Secondly, we must ask whether it is even appropriate that we set out to answer disease-treatment specific questions about glyconutrients. Since they are used at such a fundamentally basic and broad level of biochemistry within the body, glyconutrients have the potential to affect the body's ability to deal with every aspect of human health. They are a support for the body to help it achieve and retain wellness. Even if we were to begin considering them as treatments, there are just too many disease conditions to consider. Just reflect on the variety of benefits to patients referred to throughout this book. They span the breadth of clinical conditions that doctors regularly see. We can't test the role of glyconutrients on all of them. It would take too long and would obviously be cost prohibitive.

Thirdly, there is always the challenge to find appropriate patients to consent to such a study. Generally speaking, patients who have mild to moderate conditions are less likely to risk missing out on the perceived benefits of standard therapy - whether it be with established or known drugs or regular surgical procedures. The option to use the 'unproven,' 'unrealistic', 'unimaginable' solution of a 'food product' as a hopeful alternative would usually seem too risky to the patient and even more so, to their attending physician who must give their professional opinion and advice. Hence, the tendency is to get 'informed consent' generally from the very sick patients, for whom standard, orthodox medicine has done its best and for whom the prognosis is grim. In simple terms, the normal pattern is to get the support of patient volunteers when ALL ELSE FAILS. That means, you would get isolated worst-case scenarios and that makes a huge challenge for the practical application of an RCT.

But there is an even bigger hurdle to cross.

Food, Not Drug

A glyconutrient supplement containing all of the necessary monosaccharides, has now been available commercially since 1996. Since it is a food supplement, it did not require the extensive regulatory approval process that a drug or any other product making a disease treatment claim would require. As a result, it became available for human consumption as quickly as its qualification as a safe food supplement could be established.

What if any manufacturer were to make the claim that consumption of large amounts of glyconutrients was a treatment for kidney disease, or for any other type of disease condition? In almost every developed country in the world, glyconutrients and glyconutrient products would then fall under that country's drug regulatory system. Almost certainly that would mean appropriate clinical trials would be required to show safety and effectiveness before glyconutrients could be marketed to anyone. That would also mean many years of research and millions of research dollars before any benefits could be derived from this new technology.

Today, literally hundreds of thousands of people are supplementing their diet with glyconutrients and realizing significant health benefits as a result. Further, since it is a food, which is safe in any reasonable quantity, anyone with a major health challenge can consume as much as they wish, if they feel it might help their body fight their problem, with no constraints other than cost. The drug approval process generally takes a minimum of ten years (often 15 or more years). Therefore, if the availability of glyconutrients had required a disease treatment approval process, no one would have access to them today unless they were taking part in a clinical trial. This would be a most unfortunate situation.

The Better Way

If disease condition studies are not the most appropriate direction, what type of RCTs should we be doing to assess the true value of glyconutrients?

We live in a world where new drugs and the quest for scientific solutions to all our human illnesses receive an ever increasing portion of our attention and resources. For the last 60 years, we have increasingly turned to science to find solutions to our problems of pain and disease. This has allowed us to learn a tremendous amount about how the human body works. There have been wonderful discoveries to help in the alleviation of pain and the treatment of disease. This investment in science has also led to great progress in treatment of trauma and the surgical replacement of body parts.

The development of the pharmaceutical industry, over these same 60 years, has been a direct result of this emphasis on scientific solutions to human health problems. But this development has been both a blessing and a curse. On the one hand, drugs allow us to save lives and control the pain of disease as never before. On the other hand, however, properly prescribed drugs are now the fourth leading cause of death in North America .[3]

The increasing burden of illness and our almost complete dependence upon our health care system to rescue us when we get into trouble with our health, is quickly leading us into a health care system cost crisis. It presently costs approximately $4500 per person each year to provide health care in the US. To put this in context, that would exceed the per capita income of more than 90% of the world's population. It is estimated that it will cost approximately $10,000 per person by 2012.[4] This will result in an increase from the $1.5 trillion US national health expenditure in 2002 to an estimated $3.1 trillion in 2012. This will raise the present 15% of gross domestic product for health care to between 20-25% in the US. The result will be a staggering and ever increasing burden on the economy. For those who live in Canada, the national health expenditure is expected to rise from the present $130 billion spent in 2004 [5] to a whopping $205 billion in 2012 providing a similar burden on our economy.

The total cost of illness includes these direct expenditures plus the indirect social costs, such as loss of productivity on the job, missed school days, etc. It is this total cost of illness that needs to be addressed if we are to gain control of this economic monster.

The greatest potential impact of glyconutrients will be helping people stay well, remain productive every day and become less dependent on the health care system. How much could the total cost of illness be reduced by regular consumption of a comprehensive, glyconutrient based, supplementation program? A major RCT designed to assess the potential of glyconutrients for reducing the burden of illness and to provide cost savings estimates could be completed in two-three years by the right team with adequate funding. I believe that this is the type of RCT that needs to be done and that this is where our future clinical research emphasis should be placed for glyconutrients.

I will expand on this later in this chapter and provide an outline for such an RCT. But before we go further, however, let's look at some of the clinical studies that have been done with glyconutrients to date and gain some sense of why there is good evidence that we could significantly reduce the cost of illness by their widespread consumption.

Why So Few?

As we review the clinical research studies done with glyconutritionals, we will find that there have not been very many RCTs to date. We might well ask, in light of a great number of amazing cases like Cathy's and very positive pilot studies, why haven't more RCTs been done? There are some very good reasons why more definitive clinical research studies have not been done to date.

1. **They were not required for marketing** - No treatment specific claims are made for glyconutrients. Therefore, there is no requirement by the regulators for RCT quality pre-marketing studies.
2. **Proper RCTs are very expensive** - As has been indicated, the cost of a single RCT would likely start at $500,000. A nutritional company is unlikely to fund such studies when it is not required to do so, and especially if they can show sufficient benefit for marketing purposes by much less expensive, albeit less powerful, study designs.
3. **Supplementation with glyconutrients is a new idea** - The idea of supplementation with vitamins, minerals, amino acids, essential oils, etc. has been under investigation for well over half a century. Consequently, there has been much more clinical trial investigative work done in these areas. The complete glyconutrient complex has been available as a supplement for less than ten years and is the result of the work of one company that has patented the idea of supplementation with these monosaccharides.
4. **The case has not yet been made to the major funding agencies** - Billions are being spent annually by government agencies on health research in North America. For example, the National Institutes of Health in the US was given a budget of $28 billion in 2004. [6] In Canada, the Canadian Institutes of Health Research spent $688 million on research in 2004 with approximately $33 million of that spent on clinical trials.[7] The funds are certainly available if an effective case could be made for funding.

RESEARCH REVIEW

What clinical studies have been done?

The most comprehensive compilation of the published studies to date on glyconutrients is found on the site www.glycoscience.org. This award winning site is maintained, to bring together in one place, access to as much of the available scientific information about the nutritional aspects of the necessary monosaccharides as they are able to identify. It is a very comprehensive and useful site. In addition to compiling references and linkages to abstracts, when available, the site provides a great number of actual copies of papers in PDF format and many survey and review papers which summarize available knowledge in this field for both the professional and lay audience. At the time of this writing, 59 studies are referenced. Of those involving human subjects, 21 are individual case reports, 11 are listed as prospective or retrospective studies, 17 are listed as clinical trials and 2 are listed as double-blind, placebo controlled clinical trials.

Case Reports

The case reports are documents describing interesting individual responses to glyconutrient supplementation. These are generally similar to Cathy's situation described at the beginning of this chapter. This book has included dozens of different case reports, made by the contributing doctors to illustrate their specific subject in each case. Case reports have been documented on improvements in a broad spectrum of conditions including cerebral palsy, cancer, muscular dystrophy, diabetes, periodontal diseases and hepatitis C, just to name a few. But case reports are truly the weakest evidence. They are similar to a testimonial in that they represent the experience of a single individual. They are important though, as they do tell us what is possible and what has happened in particular situations. Since they are formally documented, they can be checked out and verified. They are not adequate bases for making universal recommendations or developing public health policy. Case reports do not provide strong evidence of what might be true in others or in the general population under similar circumstances. They provide a good starting point that can trigger and guide further research.

Retrospective and Prospective Studies

The 11 retrospective and prospective studies referenced to date, provide a somewhat stronger level of evidence. In a retrospective study, a group of individuals with a particular condition or outcome are investigated to see what they did in the past (retrospectively) in an effort to assess what impacted their condition or outcome. The retrospective studies done so far with glyconutrients have largely selected a group of individuals with a particular condition such as diabetes or lupus and then looked back at their glyconutrient intake and asked for their self-reported changes in symptoms and quality of life. In a prospective study, in turn, we identify a group of individuals with a condition of interest (such as diabetes or lupus) and then follow them forward through time and observe outcomes.

For both retrospective and prospective studies, the strength of the results are significantly increased if the study individuals are matched with individuals who are as similar as possible to those we are studying and who also have the same condition or disease, but who are not exposed to the intervention (did not consume glyconutrient supplements). If we see significant improvements in the glyconutrient group over what we see in the matching group, our conclusions are much stronger than if we are only reporting on improvements seen in the glyconutrient group by itself. All of the retrospective and prospective studies referenced to date show very positive results and are of great interest in providing evidence of the benefits of glyconutritionals in many disease conditions.

Clinical trials

There are 17 papers and poster sessions referenced to date that report on the results of 12 clinical trial studies. These studies are almost entirely pilot studies which, although the results are all exciting, require more extensive controlled studies before the results could stand up to critical appraisal. If we look at the areas covered by these 12 studies, however, we see a broad spectrum of health issues. They include; alcoholism, ADHD, fibromyalgia and chronic fatigue, failure to thrive, autism, oxidative stress, cancer and Hepatitis C.

Finally, two papers are referenced under the title of "Human Interventional: Double-Blind, Placebo-Controlled Study". These two, relatively simple studies, represent the study design, care and rigor that need to characterize more of the glyconutrient studies in the future.

There are likely a number of RCTs underway or not yet published. For example, C.E. Pippenger and Mary VanderWal have completed a very successful RCT looking at the effects of glyconutrient supplementation on mild and moderate asthmatic children which is yet to be published.[8]

In addition to these very limited RCTs on glyconutrient supplementtion *per se*, we should point out that there have been numerous RCTs done using natural products that are known to be significant sources of glyconutrients. In particular, you may recall the dozens of research papers referenced by Dr. Mondoa in his chapter on Cancer (Ch.10). Researchers, particularly in Asia, have observed many dramatic benefits of naturally occuring mushrooms (including shiitake, maitake and oyster, for example) as well as extracts (like polysaccharide P and K, aloe vera and sarcodan, for example) in both laboratory animals and humans. This body of scientific data is yet to gain prominence in the western literature and is still far removed from the typical doctor's radar screen.

Before concluding this brief overview of existing clinical studies conducted so far on glyconutritients, I would like to comment on a major series of studies on glyconutrients done by the Health and Medical Research Foundation.[9] That foundation, based in San Antonio, Texas, is directed by Dr. Gilbert R. Kaats. Through the foundation, Dr. Kaats has conducted a great amount of research for the cosmetic, nutraceutical and pharmaceutical industries. His research has been directed primarily at weight loss, cholesterol control, bone density and osteoporosis, and has spanned more than 20 years. Although Dr. Kaats' work has involved many other technologies, his studies with glyconutrients provide some of the most interesting clinical research to date.

The work of Dr. Kaats, is especially interesting because it centers around weight management and related issues identified with improving overall wellness. Also, his studies are well designed and although he hasn't published a proper RCT, the published work available does involve placebo control and relatively large numbers. His work convincingly shows that taking glyconutrient supplements benefit body composition, bone density and cholesterol levels.

One very interesting finding, which is indicative of the work he and his group is doing, was published in the Journal of the American Nutraceutical Association in 1999. [10] This 60 day study convincingly demonstrated that consuming glyconutrients as an adjunct to an exercise program helped the body modulate cholesterol toward normal levels. The comparison exercise group receiving the placebo showed no significant changes in cholesterol levels. If verified in other studies, this would be a very desirable, wellness promoting event.

Dr. Kaats' group routinely collects total-body DEXA scans of bone density and soft-tissue composition at conferences and other locations around North America.[11] His foundation presently has a database of some 15,000 individuals who have had one or more scans over the last 10 years. About half of these measurements are on individuals who have been on glyconutrient supplements and have provided information on their usage at the time of each scan. More information on Dr. Kaats ongoing work with glyconutrients can be obtained by contacting the foundation directly. [9]

Reducing Health Care Costs

Based on the studies which have been done and the experience of thousands of users over the last several years, it seems clear to me that widespread regular consumption of glyconutrient supplements would lead to a significant reduction in the total costs of illness within our society. It is not enough, however, just to make a statement to this effect. As I have said, we must do the necessary research to establish whether or not this is indeed true. In this section, I will outline briefly a study intended to address this issue. My challenge is that we need to do whatever is necessary to bring about the completion of at least one major RCT of this type as soon as possible. A positive outcome may be enough to start the ball rolling towards realizing the real benefits that glyconutritient supplementation holds for our nation and potentially for all the people of the world.

The research question that such an RCT needs to address can be stated rather simply as follows: "In the general population, does regular glyconutrient supplementation significantly reduce the costs of illness when compared with use of a placebo supplement?" This is but a suggestion. The actual research question would be given careful consideration by the research team that ultimately comes together to do the RCT.

The term "cost of illness" rather than "health care costs" is being used because the study needs to look at more than just the reductions in the number of doctor visits, diagnostic tests, hospital stays, prescription and over the counter drug usage. It needs to make a real effort to assess cost savings due to increased wellness. For example, the study needs to measure the impact of an increase in productive days when work gets done. That would include measuring days at school, days at work, days when housework gets done, days without colds or other infections, etc. between the two groups. In other words, the study needs to get cost measurements that can be projected into cost savings and productivity gains for the population as a whole.

The study should be done in a suitably representative sample of the general population. Practically speaking, however, it may need to be done in a more controlled environment such as within the work force of a large industrial company. It is often more practical to gain cooperation, obtain the required measurements and control study costs in a more readily defined and accessible population.

To carry out such a study, a study team of interested researchers needs to first come together to refine the study question, design the study and seek funding. A study of this nature also requires the enlistment of a properly equipped and experienced research organization to conduct the study once the funding is received.

The costs of the study would be determined, based on the complexity of the design, by the study research team prior to submitting the study for funding. My experience tells me any reasonable study, capable of addressing this question, would require a minimum of $750,000 but would more likely cost a few million dollars to do in the US or Canada. Maybe this sounds like a lot of money. It is trivial, however, in light of the huge and presently rising health care costs.

STEM CELLS

The Truth about Stem Cells

Let's move to an entirely different subject for this next section. At the time of writing this chapter, we have been hearing a lot in the popular media about stem cells. During the 2004 Presidential election in the US, the press and many high profile individuals led us to believe that the research into potential benefits of stem cells is all about *embryonic* stem cells. After you read this section, I think it will be obvious to you that embryonic stem cells are not the whole story at all. In fact, embryonic stem cell research may turn out to be totally unnecessary.

In an effort to try to put this subject into proper perspective, we need to define what stem cells are and then provide a brief overview of the present state of research in this exciting area. It turns out that glyconutrients do seem to play a very significant role in your body's use of stem cells. This may well be the most exciting news you will receive about glyconutrients in this entire book and I feel privileged to have been allowed to be the one to discuss it with you here.

First of all, let's look at what stem cells are. A good **definition** comes from a very informative stem cell information web site maintained by the NIH.[12] They define stem cells this way: "*Stem cells have the remarkable potential to develop into many different cell types in the body. Serving as a sort of repair system for the body, they can theoretically divide without limit to replenish other cells as long as the person or animal is still alive. When a stem cell divides, each new cell has the potential to either remain a stem cell or become another type of cell with a more specialized function, such as a muscle cell, a red blood cell, or a brain cell*".

Stem cells, then, are a foundational component of our body's amazing ability to heal, repair and regenerate itself. The beginnings of a comprehension of the full implication of stem cells and their everyday role in our body is a very recent phenomenon in science. Although bone marrow transplants have been carried out for over 40 years, only recently was it understood that it was stem cells (called hematopoietic stem cells, or HSCs) that were responsible for the success of this procedure. It was not until 1998, when a group led by Dr. James Thomson at the University of Wisconsin developed a novel technique that allowed scientists to begin to isolate and grow stem cells from human tissue and fluids that the science of stem cells began to expand and flourish.

Embryonic vs Adult

There are two current sources of stem cells. Embryonic stem cells originate from fertilized human embryos that are less than a week old. At that point, each of the cells in this miniature ball of cells has the potential to develop into any of the 220 different types of cells that are known to make up our body. In contrast, adult stem cells are taken from living tissue or body fluids after birth. The source of adult stem cells can be the umbilical cord at birth, an infant, a child or any one of you or me. The realization that many types of adult stem cells are present in our body all our life is a very recent discovery and an area of increasingly active ongoing research.

There is a great scientific (and political) controversy centering on the question of whether or not adult stem cells actually have the potential to regenerate all the different types of tissue cells in our body. Clearly, embryonic stem cells do have this innate potential since that is exactly what they do as they develop from an embryo to a fetus in the human mother. Everything about embryonic stem cells yielding successful treatments, however, is only conjecture at the time of this writing, since there is none. Also, research with embryonic stem cells is plagued with many problems including moral and ethical issues, immune system rejection and tumor creating tendencies, to name but a few. None of these problems is an issue with adult stem cells since they are taken directly from the tissue of the patient themselves.

As research progresses, it is becoming more and more evident that there are adult stem cells that do indeed have the potential to develop into almost, if not all, tissue types in our body. In July, 2002, Dr. Catherine M. Verfaillei and her team at the University of Minnesota reported discovering multipotent adult progenitor cells (MAPC) that appear to do just that.[13] As a result, research and resulting treatments are moving forward rapidly using adult stem cells. To see an up-to-date list of the treatment areas where adult stem cells are being successfully used as treatments and to find specific references to the actual work, anyone can visit the DoNoHarm web site.[14] As of mid January 2005, this site lists 56 current adult stem cell treatments in the following disease conditions; Crohn's disease, rheumatoid arthritis, systemic lupus, stroke, corneal regeneration, heart damage, Parkinson's, spinal cord injury, 20 types of cancer and many more. As I said above, in contrast, **there are no successful treatments using embryonic stem cells at this time.**

A review paper written in July of 2003 by David A. Prentice, Ph.D., a senior fellow for the life sciences for the Family Research Council,15 illustrates very directly the rapid expansion of stem cell research since 1998. This paper provides a review of the published literature, up to that time, regarding the identification of adult stem cells in various body tissues and the present understanding of the mechanisms for their observed differentiation into both their own tissue type and into types other than their tissue of origin. He cites 192 references for this paper with all but four published since 1998. Almost 40% of the 192 papers were published in the first half of 2003 alone.

A further illustration of the **rapid growth in the area** of adult stem cell treatments is illustrated by an announcement from Argentina on January 11, 2005.[16] A team of doctors announced that they had transplanted stem cells taken from a diabetic patient's own body into his pancreas. His type I diabetes resulted from the fact that his pancreas had ceased to produce insulin. As a result of the treatment, his pancreas is now producing insulin again and he no longer requires insulin treatment. We are clearly only beginning to see the potential for adult stem cells as successful medical treatments.

The final paragraph in the paper by Dr. Prentice referred to above, provides a very good concluding statement for our introductory discussion of stem cells and I present it here before we move on to the impact of glyconutrient supplementation on adult stem cells: "*In summary, our current knowledge regarding adult stem cells has expanded greatly over what was known just a few short years ago. Results from both animal studies and early human clinical trials indicate that they have significant capabilities for growth, repair, and regeneration of damaged cells and tissues in the body, akin to a built-in repair kit or maintenance crew that only needs activation and stimulation to accomplish repair of damage. The potential of adult stem cells to impact medicine in this respect is enormous.*"[15]

Glyconutrient Support

The last two sentences of the preceding paragraph provide an accurate description of the role that glyconutritients seem to play in the body's stem cell growth, repair and regeneration activities. Recent evidence is indicating very clearly that providing the body with an abundance of glyconutrients through aggressive supplementation of these necessary monosaccharides, supports and tremendously enhances the activation and stimulation of this maintenance crew of which Dr. Prentice speaks. In the example that follows, I think you will see that **glyconutrients may be a primary key to unlocking the human body's enormous potential of healing and regeneration through the support of its own natural use of adult stem cells.**

Dr. Reg McDaniel in a recent paper,[17] presented the results of work done in the late 1980s at the Fisher Institute for Medical Research that clearly shows a tremendous increase in monocytes in peripheral blood sample after seven days of glyconutrient supplementation. Monocyte is a name given to adult stem cells that, although they are not able to differentiate into all cells types, still retain the ability to be converted at least to some other cell types. Keep in mind, of course, that in the 1980's they were not called adult stem cells. At that time, they were just known to be part of the body's healing and repair process. The flow cytometry scattergrams, which show the results of this analysis (Figure 1) are included below by permission. Let me also quote Dr. McDaniel here as he explains what is seen in this analysis:

"What one sees in this slide (Figure 1.) are two assays done on the same research subject a week apart. At the top are two different assays done on the same day on blood before dietary glyconutrients were taken. On the left, one sees all the different types of white cells grouped together with their size or diameter plotted on the horizontal line and the complexity that scatters light on the vertical axis. The pattern on the right top shows the addition of a specific fluorescent antibody that tags to monocyte/macrophages, i.e. RE (reticulo-endothelial) cells, and they are under 150 microns in diameter. These tagged cells are displayed on the vertical axis as a cluster of dots above the majority of white cell types. Each tiny dot represents one fluorescent cell counted. Monocyte/macrophages have many functions. They not only defend the body against infectious agents, but like the military Seabees or engineers in a war zone, these white cells have the capacity to repair and heal damaged cells. They are committed at this stage to the immune and healing system of the body.

Now give attention to the two lower scattergrams of white cells from this same individual after adding the polymannose glyconutrient to the daily diet for one week. Note that a much larger in size, low complexity, new population of cells is in the peripheral blood. By adding the same fluorescent Leu M3 antibody, it can be shown that these cells greater than 150 microns in diameters, as was noted on the peripheral blood smears, are labeled by the same antibody that binds with the monocyte/macrophages that defend, repair and replace damaged tissues. These new populations of cells are stem cells that come from the person's own bone marrow".

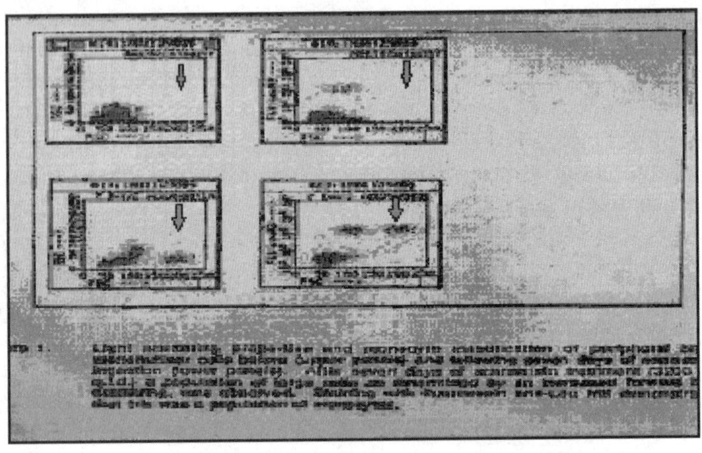

At the conclusion of his syllabus, Dr. McDaniel goes on to say:

"Starting in the fall of 1985 and continuing to the present date, there have been multiple restorations of lost function in the central nervous system, beta cells of

the pancreas, lung, kidney, and heart patients that defy explanation for how such a turn around in health could transpire. Such challenging events have been reported in infants, children, youth and adults that include some that are quite elderly. Previously thought hopeless health situations and irreversible damage have been noted to repeatedly be reversed and corrected. Only recently, the events being recognized by science regarding the capacity of transplanted stem cells to replace damaged or destroyed organ cells could be correlated with laboratory observations made in the late 1980s at the Fisher Institute for Medical Research. A large population of very large cells appeared in the peripheral blood within one week in individuals who added a glyconutrient formulation to their diet. Now it is known that ***these cells are stem cells*** *coming from the individual's own bone marrow*".

As Dr. McDaniel points out, we have seen multiple hundreds of examples of restoration of function in the presence of high intake of glyconutrients that truly have defied explanation. The example of Cathy's kidney regeneration described at the beginning of this chapter is such a case. After a year of taking minimal levels of glyconutrients, no significant improvement in the condition of her kidneys was noted (other than perhaps helping to control infections). It was when the intake of glyconutrients was increased dramatically that her kidneys began to regenerate. What Dr. McDaniel has shown us would indicate that, in the presence of an abundance of the necessary monosaccharides, her body's innate stem cell process (her "maintenance crew") was stimulated and activated to repair the damage.

To have proposed such a solution for what we saw take place with Cathy at the time it happened, would have been termed preposterous and impossible. Today, in light of the progress in knowledge about adult stem cells and taking into consideration what Dr. McDaniel explained above, this now provides a very reasonable explanation. *It may not be certain, but it is reasonable. And that is the basis of research.* A reasonable hypothesis always points the way forward. It stimulates thought and prompts further inquiry. It raises as many questions as it may appear to answer but all good science is initiated by the timely and judicious insight that such questions provoke.

Here, we are provoked by an amazing possibility that the simple addition of essential sugars - glyconutrients , in adequate quantities and under the right clinical conditions - could give rise to the most surprising and beneficial regeneration of live human tissues and organs. The import of that is not yet in our conscious minds - it defies our normal instincts and expectations.

I hope this also provides you, the reader, with a heightened awareness of the importance of supplementing with glyconutrients.

THE FUTURE

What does the future hold for Glyconutrients?

The above discussion on adult stem cells and the role that glyconutrients appear to have in supporting our body's use of them should give us great excitement about the future of glyconutrient supplementation. Let's look briefly at a few of the implications that glyconutrients may hold for the future.

Laugh, then Think

The thought that merely supplementing with eight simple monosaccharides can have such dramatic effect on the body's ability to defend, heal and even regenerate is considered foolishness today by the majority of the medical establishment.

But a quote from the IgNobel Prize website is most pertinent here. The IgNobel Prizes are intended "to celebrate the unusual, honor the imagination - and spur peoples interest in science, medicine and technology." Their editors could not be any more astute than to observe that every prize winner ' has done something that first makes people LAUGH, then makes them THINK.'

It seems that all medical breakthroughs as in much of science too, arise after a number of important phases that include:

Phase 1 • **An idea** or hypothesis that at best seems speculative and pre sumptuous and at worst, seems ridiculous and foolish.

Phase 2 • Later the idea finds some support in **preliminary observation** like Case Reports and noted 'exceptions to the general rule.'

Phase 3 • Then other researchers are attracted to **the possibility** and design experiments that confirm the predictions.

Phase 4 • Reluctantly, the establishment opens up the professional communication channels. New **dialogue** ensues, the evidence grows as everyone wants to investigate or review, and to take a position.

Phase 5 • Finally, the consistency of results establishes a **new paradigm** and the original idea becomes a new mantra or widespread technology.

Keep in mind that it has seemed a bit *unbelievable* to those of us who have been involved with these amazing nutrients long enough to have witnessed these wonderful examples as well. There just didn't seem to be any mechanism that could explain how just consuming lots of glyconutrients could turn on the body's ability to regenerate kidneys, for example. Then at just about the dawn of the new millennium, all of these adult stem cell discoveries began. After all, the thought that we had within us adult stem cells that were as capable as the MAPC cells Dr. Verfaillei discovered in 2002 was considered impossible until that discovery. Now that the power of adult stem cells is readily accepted, we appear to have one of the mechanisms identified for how glyconutrients may be assisting in the healing and regenerative process. We are obliged to then ask: What steps need to be taken to get the medical community to accept the role glyconutrients are able to play in activating and stimulating our body's adult stem cell forces?

I have just finished watching a video recording of Dr. Verfaillei as she spoke before the NIH on Feb. 11, '04 about her work with MAPC adult stem cells and the progress made since the announcement of her team's discovery in 2002 (http://stemcells.nih.gov/info/media/verfaillie.asp). One of the limitations she stressed is the difficulty in finding a sufficient quantity of the MAPC stem cells in a donor. These cells are extremely rare. This same problem exists for bone marrow transplants and will be true for all stem cell therapies as this science moves rapidly into actual treatments. Whatever the particular stem cell required for a treatment, there will be great interest in finding ways to increase the number of stem cells in the patient's bone marrow, blood or tissue available to be harvested and used in the treatment.

As we saw on the flow cytometry scattergrams in Figure 1, a large cloud of stem cells are seen after one week on glyconutrients that were not there in the earlier analysis. Dr. McDaniel believes that high intake of glyconutrients for just a few days increases the stem cell count by several hundred fold. If this increase applies to all types of adult stem cells, then incorporation of glyconutrients would be of great value to any adult stem cell therapeutic program. **We need to find ways to link up with adult stem cell programs presently underway.** We need to cooperate with them and conduct the clinical trials necessary to establish whether or not they are able to obtain better yields of adult stem cells by incorporating glyconutrients. This could serve to reproduce the results of Dr McDaniel's analysis described above and provide validity for glyconutrients in a field that is generating tremendous excitement at the present time.

This is but one example of how glyconutrients have the potential to greatly complement medicine in the future.

A Health Economic Crisis

Earlier in this chapter, I discussed the rising costs of health care in the US and Canada. This is not a problem limited to North America. All the economies of the world will be pulled into the vortex of the health care economic black hole within a few short years without some solution being found. I maintain that **the only solution that can possibly work is to help people stay well and therefore out of the health care system**. I challenge the reader to identify anything that has the potential to do exactly that better than glyconutrients.

If studies are completed that establish the cost savings and enhanced productivity that could be achieved through glyconutrient supplementation, I believe we would see programs put in place to encourage widespread use. When we look at the impact that improved wellness can have in pulling us back from the brink of the imminent health care disaster, it becomes very clear that the future role of glyconutrients will be very significant indeed!

A Pandemic Orphan Crisis

Our world is in the midst of an AIDS epidemic that is robbing millions of children of their parents. In Sub-Saharan Africa alone, the UN estimates that the number of children orphaned by HIV/AIDS will reach 25 million by 2010. Many of these children have HIV/AIDS themselves. As we all know, this disease weakens these children's immune system and sets them up for poor health, illness and high mortality. This situation is not restricted to Africa. It appears that the disease is spreading rapidly in China, India and Russia, and that each of these countries may have 12 million cases of the disease by 2010. As a result, a whole generation of children is being affected.

Interestingly, glyconutrients have the potential to make a significant difference in this worldwide dilemma. One of the results of sufficient glyconutrient supplementation is a much enhanced immune function. Providing these children with glyconutrients might give them tremendously improved resistance to disease and a chance to survive until a cure for this disease can be found. Not only that, but the child gains a quality of life that could approach that of children without the disease. A great challenge to us, as we consider the future of glyconutrients, is how can we get these supplements to the HIV/AIDS orphans of the world?

Fortunately, an avenue for doing just this already exists and is ideally positioned to rise to this challenge. The mission of MannaRelief is expressed in the motto: "Bringing Health and Hope to the Children of the World". As a non-profit, non-government organization, MannaRelief presently supplies glyconutrient supplements to orphanages and medically fragile children in over 30 countries. The nutrients are made available through the generosity of sponsors and through charitable gifts. MannaRelief provides an avenue to truly help the children of this world with health and will play a very significant role in the future of glyconutrients.

As a reader, you might be pleased to learn that a portion of the sale price of each copy of The Healing **Power** *of* ^{8}**SugarS** is being contributed directly to MannaRelief to further their mission. To that extent, you have made a modest contribution.

Conclusion

Finally, I must emphasize that I firmly believe that the greatest benefit of glyconutrients will come from their widespread use, at maintenance levels, to promote greater wellness for everyone. However, it is very exciting to witness the impact of glyconutrients on the human body's ability to heal when there is a health crisis.

All the evidence to date confirms that we are experiencing a break-through whose time has ome. Glyconutrients will indeed be one of the top emerging technologies that will change the world. May that begin with you.

About the Author:

Gary D. Anderson, Ph.D.

Dr. Anderson completed a Ph.D. in Biostatistics at the University of Washington in 1969 and joined the Department of Clinical Epidemiology, Faculty of Medicine at McMaster University in Hamilton, Ontario that same year. In 1984, he founded Innovus Inc., a company that has become a world leader in clinical, health economics and outcomes research. He was President up to 1996. Since his retirement in 1998, Dr. Anderson has devoted much of his attention to studying human nutrition and health. He now conducts regular seminars on nutrition for health, wellness and anti-aging. He and Marilyn have five children and presently thirteen grandchildren.

References

Chapter 1, The Discovery of Glyconutrients

1. "Carbohydrates and Glycobiology," *Science*, March 2001; Vol. 291, No. 5512, pp. 2263-2502.
2. C. Wang; R. T. Pivik; R. A. Dykman; "Effects of a Glyconutritional Supplement on Brain Potentials Associated with Language Processing," Glycoscience and Nutrition, April 20, 2002.
3. C. Wang; R. T. Pivik; R. A. Dykman; "Effects of a Glyconutritional Supplement on Resting Brain Activity," Glycoscience and Nutrition April 20, 2002.
4. www.glycoscience.org. Copyright 2000. All rights reserved.
5. Acta Anatomica, the International Journal of Anatomy, Embryology and Cell Biology, 1998, Vol. 161, pp. 1-4.
6. R. K. Murray, "Glycoproteins," Harper's Biochemistry,24th edit.,R. K. Murray, D. K. Granner, P. A. Mayes and V.W. Rodwell (Appleton and Lange,1996), pp. 648-666.
7. T. Gardiner, "Biological Activity of Eight Known Dietary Monosaccharides Required for Glycoprotein Synthesis and Cellular Recognition Processes: Summary," GlycoScience and Nutrition, 2000, Vol. 1, No. 13, pp. 1-7.
8. Bill H. McAnalley, Ph.D., and Eileen Vennum, R.A.C., "Introduction to Glyconutritonals," GlycoScience and Nutrition, January 1, 2000, Vol. 1, No. 1.
9. B. D. Campbell, D. L. Busbee, H. R. McDaniel, "Enhancement of Immune Function in Rodents Using a Proprietary Complex Mixture of Glyconutritionals." Proceedings of the Fish. Inst. for Med Res, 1997, Vol. 1, No. 1, pp. 34-37.
10. M. J. Montvale, "Medical Economics," 2001 Physicians' Desk Reference for Nonprescription Drugs and Dietary Supplements, pp. 508, 819, 820.

Chapter 3, Structure and Function of Glyconutrients

1. D. Lefkowitz, "Glyconutritionals: Implications in Inflammation," www.glycoscience.org Copyright 2000. All rights reserved.
2. J. Ramberg. "Can You Tell Me About the Peer Review Process for Articles" *ibid*, 2000-2004 All rights reserved.
3. R. Murray, "Glycoproteins: Crucial Molecules for Health." *ibid*, Copyright

2000-2004 All rights reserved.
4. R. K. Murray, "Glycoproteins," Harper's Biochemistry,24th edit.,R. K. Murray, D. K. Granner, P. A. Mayes and V.W. Rodwell (Appleton and Lange,1996), pp. 648-666.
5. R. Murray, J. Ramburg. "Glyconutritionals: Implications in Cystic Fibrosis." Glycoscience and Nutrition, Aug 1, 2004, Vol 5 No. 4.
6. R. Fleming., T. Monte, Stop Inflammation Now!, Copyright 2004. Published by G.P. Putnam's Sons, a member of Penguin Group USA.

Chapter 4, Glyconutrients and the Immune System

1. R. K. Murray, "Glycoproteins," Harper's Biochemistry,24th edit.,R. K. Murray, D. K. Granner, P. A. Mayes and V.W. Rodwell (Appleton and Lange,1996), pp. 648-666.
2. Ishihara Y, et al., "The role of neutrophils as cytotoxic cells in lung metastasis: Suppression of tumor cell metastasis by a biological response modifier (PSK)." *In Vivo* 12(2): 175-182, 1998.
3. Mondoa E, Kitei M, Sugars that Heal, The Ballantine Publishing Group, 2001, 53-54
4. Adachi et al., "Host-mediated antitumor activity," Chem Pharm Bull, 1987; 35(1): 262-270.
5. Adachi K, Nanba H, Kuroda H, Kuroda H, "Potentiation of host mediated antitumor activity in mice by Beta-glucan obtained from Grifola frondosa (Maitake)." Chem Pharm Bull, 1987; 35(1): 262-270
6. Liu C, Lu S, Ji MR, "Effects of Cordyceps sinensis (CS) on *in vitro* natural killer cells." Chung Kuo Chung His I Chieh Ho Tsa Chih 1992, 12(5): 267-269,
7. Kossi J, et al., "Effects of hexose sugars: glucose, fructose, galactose and mannose on wound healing in the rat," Eur Surg Res. 1999: 31(1): 74-82
8. Kelly GS, Larch arabinogalactan: clinical relevance of a novel immune-enhancing polysaccharide. Altern.Med.Rev. 1999: 42(2), 96-103
9. Takata I, et al., "L-fucose, D-mannose, L-galactose, and their BSA conjugates stimulate macrophages migration." J.Leukoc.Biol. 1987; 41(3), 248-256
10. Dwek RA, Lellouch AC, Wormald MR, "Glycobiology: the function of sugar in the IgG molecule." J.Anat. 1995:187 (Pt 2): 279-292
11. Sathyamoorthy N, et al., "Evidence that specific high mannose structures directly regulate multiple cellular activities," Mol Cell Biochem. 1991; 102(2): 139-147

12. Tizard IR, et al. "The biological activities of mannans and related complex carbohydrates. Mol.Biother. 1989; 1(6): 290-296.
13. Flowers HM, "Chemistry and biochemistry of D- and L-fucose." Adv.Carbohydr.Chem.Biochem. 1981; 39:279-345
14. Adachi Y, et al. "Enhancement of cytokine production by macrophages stimulated with (1.3-)-beta- D-glucan, grifolan (GRN), isolated from Grifola frondosa." Biol Pharm Bull, 1994; 17(12): 1554-1560
15. Campbell B, Busbee D, McDaniel H. "Enhancement of immune function in rodents using a proprietary complex mixture of glyconutritionals." Proc Fisher Inst. Med Res. 1997; 1(1): 34-37
16. Tomassini J, Maxon T, Colonno R, "Biochemical characterization of glycoproteins required for rhinovirus attachment." J Biol Chem 1989; 264(3): 1656-1662
17. Saavedra J, et al., "Gastrointestinal function in infants consuming a weaning food supplemented with oligofructose, a prebiotic. J Pediatr Gastroenterol Nutr" 1999; 29(4): 95A
18. Saavedra J, et al., "Effects of long-term consumption of a weaning food supplemented with oligofructose, a prebiotic, on general infant health status." J Pediatr Gastroenterol Nutr, 1999; 29(4): 58A
19. Tsuru S, "Depression of early protection against influenza virus infection by cyclophosphamide and its restoration by protein-bound polysaccharide." Kitasato Arch Exp Med, 1992; 65(2-3): 97-110
20. Suzuki F, et al., "Antiviral and interferon-inducing activities of a new peptidomanna, KS-2, extracted from culture mycelia of Lentinus edodes," J Antibiot (Tokyo), 1979; 32(12): 1336-1345
21. McAnalley B, et al., "Compositions of plant carbohydrates as dietary supplements, Australian Patent No. 734183, 11/22/2001
22. Watson M, Rudd PM, Bland M, Dwek RA, Axford JS, "Sugar printing rheumatic diseases: a potential method for disease differentiation using immunoglobulin G oligosaccharides." Arthritis Rheum. 1999 Aug; 42(8): 1682-90
23. Elkins R, *Miracle Sugars*, Woodland, 2003; p 16
24. Bond A, Kerr M, Hay F, Distinct oligosaccharide content of rheumatoid arthritis-derived immune complexes, Arthritis and Rheumatism, 1995; 38(6): 744-749
25. Kidd P, The use of Mushroom glucans and proteoglycans in cancer treatment, Alternative Med. Review, Thorne Research, Inc, 2000; 5(1): 4-27

Chapter 5, Glyconutrients and Infectious Diseases

1. Rudd PM, et al., Science 2001 Mar 23;291(5512):2370-6
2. Sharon N, Ofek I. Glycoconj J 2000 Jul-Sep;17(7-9):659-64
3. Sharon N, Acta Anat. 1998;161:7-17
4. Zopf D, Roth S, Lancet 1996; 347: 1017-21
5. Feizi T Glycoconj J 2000 Jul-Sep;17(7-9):553-65
6. Vierbuchen M, et al., Verh Dtsch Ges Pathol 1989;73:264-7
7. Beuth J, et. al., Eur J Clin Microbiol 1987 Oct;6(5):591-3
8. Luther P, etal., Zentralb Bakteriol Mikrobio Hyg [A] 1988 Nov; 2701(16-21)
9. Adam EC Am J Respir Crit Care Med 1997Jun;155(6):2102-4
10. Adam EC, et al., J Laryngol Otol 1997 Aug;111(8):760-2
11. Chatterjee S, Glycobiology 1995 May;5(3):327-33
12. Rudiger H, Curr Med Chem 2000 Apr; 7(4):389-416
13. von Bismarck P , et.al., Klin Padiatr 2001 Sep-Oct;213(5):285-7
14. Mysore JV, Gastroenterology 1999;117:1316-25
15. McVeigh P, J Paediatr Child Health 1997 Aug;33(4):281-6
16. Sharon N, Sc Amer 1993, Jan;82-89

Chapter 6, Improving Outcomes in Pregnancy

1. Rommer JJ; "Sterility, Its Causes and Its Treatment," Springfield, Illinois; Charles C. Thomas Publisher, 1952; 54-55.
2. Guyton AG; *Textbook of Medical Physiology*, Philadelphia, PA; WB Saunders Company, 1976; 1106
3. Gardiner T; "Importance of Glyconconjugates in Breastfeeding and Early Nutrition"; Glycoscience & Nutrition July 2000; Vol.1, No 23; 1-10.
4. Larson LA; "Breastfeeding Stimulates the Infant Immune System"; Science & Medicine. Nov/Dec 1997; Vol 4, No 6.
5. McDaniel C; Baumgartner S; "Case Report: early intervention in insulin diabetes with dietary supplementation." Proc Fish Inst Med Res 2002;Apr 2; 2: 9-11.
6. Genius SJ; Genius SK; "Use of Nutraceuticals in Menopause: Case Report." Proc Fish Inst Med Res 1997; 1: 32-34.
7. McDaniel C; Stevens EW; "Nutraceuticals decrease blood glucose and pain in an individual with non-insulin dependent diabetes and myofascial pain syndrome: a case report." Proc Fish Inst Med Res 1997: 1: 30-31.
8. R. K. Murray, "Glycoproteins," Harper's Biochemistry,24th edit.,R. K. Murray, D. K. Granner, P. A. Mayes and V.W. Rodwell (Appleton and Lange,1996), pp. 648-666.

9. Arcadi VC; "Lower Back Pain During Pregnancy" Dynamic Chiropractic; 1994, July 15.
10. Arcadi VC; "Lower Back Pain in Pregnancy, Chiropractic Treatment and Results of 50 Cases" International College of Applied Kinesiology Proceedings; 1995-96; 45-47.
11. Gardiner T; "Biological Activity of Eight Known Dietary Monosaccharides Required for Glycoprotein Synthesis and Cellular Recognition Processes" Glycoscience & Nutr; March 2000: Vol 1, No 13.
12. Campbell BD; Busbee DL; McDaniel HR; "Enhancement of immune function in rodents using a proprietary complex mixture of glyconutritionals." Proc Fisher Inst Med Res; 1997 Nov; 1: 34-37.
13. Ganapini K; "Dietary supplements improve many symptoms of asthma and decrease the need for other medications: a retrospective study." J Am Nutraceutical Assoc. 1997, August: 32-35.
14. Axford JS; "Glycobiology and Medicine: an introduction" JR Soc Med. 1997 May: 90 260-264.
15. Kanmatsuse K; et al.: "Studies on Ganoderma lucidum, I. Efficacy against hypertension and side effects." Yakugaku Zasshi 105 (10); : 942-947, 198
16. Arcadi VC; "How do you treat Hyperemesis Gravidarum(Morning Sickness)?" Dynamic Chiropractic; 1991 March 29.
17. Arcadi VC; "The Fear of Adjusting a Pregnant Woman" Dynamic Chiropractic; 1995 January 1.
18. Arcadi VC; "What is PPPP during Pregnancy? Worldwide Meeting Describes Condition" Dynamic Chiropractic; 1996 February 26.
19. Arcadi VC; "Thoracolumbar Fixations During Pregnancy" ICAK Publication; 1996 August.
20. Mondoa EI; Kitei M; Sugars That Heal, The New Healing Science of Glyconutrients; NY, NY; The Ballantine Publishing Group; 2001 Aug.

Chapter 7, Glyconutrients for Babies and Children

1. Gardiner T., "Importance of Glyconjugates in Breastfeeding and Early Nutrition," Glycoscience & Nutrition, Vol 1, No 23, 1 July 2000.
2. Bezkorovainly A., Nichols .JH., "Glycoproteins from mature human whey," Pediatr. Res., 1976, 10(1): 1-5.
3. Shimizu M., Yamauchi K., Miyauchi Y., et. al., "High-Mr glycoprotein profiles in human milk serum and fat-globule membrane," Biochem. J. 1986, 233(3): 725-730.
4. Hanson L.A., "Breastfeeding Stimulates the Infant Immune System," Science & Medicine, Vol 4 No 6, 1997 Nov/Dec.
5. McDaniel C; Dykman KD; McDaniel HR; Ford CR; Tone CM; "Effects of

Nutraceutical Dietary Intervention in Diabetes Mellitus: A Retrospective Survey." Proc Fisher Inst. Med. Res. 1997 November 1; 1: 19-23.

6. McDaniel C; Baumgartner S; "Case report: early intervention in insulin diabetes with dietary supplementation." Proc Fish Inst. Med. Res. 2002, Apr 2; 2: 9-11.
7. Ganapini K; Dietary supplements improve many symptoms of asthma and decrease the need for other medication: a retrospective study. J Am Nutraceutical Assoc.,1997 August: 32-25.
8. Riesen S; Fals AM; Lee R; "A random open-label controlled study of the effects of asthma treatment combined with glyconutrients and phytonutrients in asthma." Proc Fisher Inst Med Res. 2002 Apr 1; 2: 5-7.
9. R. K. Murray, "Glycoproteins," Harper's Biochemistry,24th edit.,R. K. Murray, D. K. Granner, P. A. Mayes and V.W. Rodwell (Appleton and Lange,1996), pp. 648-666.
10. Arcadi VC; Dykman KD; "Case study: Tay-Sachs Disease Improvement During Nutritional Supplementation." J Am Nutraceutical Assoc. 1997 August: 26-27.
11. Arcadi VC; "Case Report: Prader-Willi Syndrome Improvement with Nutritional Therapy and Chiropractic Care." Proc Fisher Inst Med Res. 2002 April; 2 (3):11-13.
12. Vanderwall M; Pippenger CE; "A retrospective post-marketing survey of clinical symptom changes in cystic fibrosis patients voluntarily supplementing their diets with glyconutrients: preliminary results." Proc Fisher Inst Med Res. 2004; 3: 9-11.
13. Lefkowitz DL; Lefkowitz SS; "Use of a calcium blocker and glyconutrients to treat FSH muscular dystrophy." Glycoscience & Nutrition 2000 July 15; 1: 1-3.
14. Berdow R; Fletcher AJ; Beers MH; The Merck Manual of Diagnosis and Therapy, Sixteenth Edition; Rathway, NJ, Merck Research Publications, 1992: 2267.
15. Dykman KD; McKinley RN; "The effects of glyconutritional supplementation on autistic children." Proceedings of the Annual Meeting of the Pavlovian Society in Dusseldorf, Germany. October 31-November 1. 1998
16. Nisinzweig S; "Phytochemicals and glyconutritionals in autistic children." Proc Fisher Inst Med Res. 1999 Sep; 1: 12-14.
17. Arcadi VC; Padgette-Baird JD; "The Spectrum of Autism: Giving Hope through education and experience." J. Am Nutraceutical, in press
18. Arcadi VC; Case Report: "Ataxic Cerebral Palsy Multidisciplinary Treatment Effects Including Dietary Supplementation" Proc Fisher Inst Med Res. 2002 April; 2(3):7-9.
19. Jaeken J; "Congenital defects of glycosylation (CDG): Pandora's box."

Proceedings of the Royal Society of Medicine;s 5th Jenner Symprosium (Glycobiology and Medicine Conference), July 10-11, 2000.
20. "Axford J; Glycobiology & Medicine: A Millenial Review": Glycoscience & Nutrition: 2001 March 30; 1 (2): 1-7.

Chapter 8, A Living Reality

1. McAnalley BH, Vennum E. "Glycoscience: state of the science review." Glycoscience and Nutrition 2001; 2(14).
2. See,D. "An in vitro screening study of 196 natural products for toxicity and efficacy." JANA 1999;2(1).
3. Maeder T, "Sweet medicines." Scientific American 2002;40-47.
4. R. K. Murray, "Glycoproteins," Harper's Biochemistry,24th edit.,R. K. Murray, D. K. Granner, P. A. Mayes and V.W. Rodwell (Appleton and Lange,1996), pp. 648-666.
5. Ramberg J, McAnalley BH. "Is saccharide supplementation necessary?" Glycoscience and Nutrition 2002; 3(3):1-9.
6. McDaniel HR. "How dietary supplements work?" Proc Fis Inst Med Res. 2002;2(3).
7. Article by Ristine J. $34 million sweetens area's research coffers.2001.
8. Sharon N. "Glycoproteins Now and Then: a personal account." Acta Anatomica 1998,7-15.
9. Sinowatz F, Plendl J, Kolle S. "Protein-carbohydrate interactions during fertilization." Acta Anatomica 1998,196-205.
10. Hodgson J. "Capitalizing on carbohydrates. Bio/Technology." 1990; 8(2):180-111.
11. Mann PL and Waterman RE. "Glycocoding as an information management system in embryonic development." Acta Anatomica 1998,153-161.
12. Villalobo A,Gabius HJ. "Signaling pathways for transduction of the initial message of the glycocode into cellular responses." Acta Anatomica 1998,161:1-4:110-129.
13. Boyd S. "History of Nutrition and Health." Glycoscience and Nutrition 2000;1(2).
14. Kaats G,Pullin D,Squines Jr.W,Keith SC,Parker LK,McDaniel HR. "Phase I of the nutraceutical-intervention longitudinal trials:a meta-analysis of short-term changes in body composition." Proc Fish Inst Med. 2000;2(1).
15. Carbohydrates and Biology. *Science* Magazine 2001.
16. Dykman KD and Dykman RA. "Effect of nutritional supplement on attention deficit hyperactivity disorder." Integ.Phy.Behav.Sci.,Jan-March,33(1):49-60,Jan-March 1998.

17. Omelchuk A, Wells D. "Preliminary investigation into the benefits of glyconutrient supplementation in learning disabled children." Proceedings 2004;3(2).
18. Nugent S. How to Survive on a Toxic Planet. Chapter 9. 2nd edition. Alethia corp.,2004.
19. Kaats G, Keith SC, Wise JA, Pullin MS, Squires Jr, WG. "Effects of baseline total cholesterol levels on diet and exercise interventions." JANA 1999;2(1).
20. Article: "Beating the odds with glyconutritionals." Las Vegas Magazine. July/August 2001.

Chapter 9, Glyconutrients and Cardiovascular Disease
(*For further reading*)

1. Lennarz W.J., ed. 1980. The biochemistry of glycoproteins and proteoglycans . Plenum Press, New York.
2. Ginsburg V. and Robbins P., eds. 1981-1991. Biology of carbohydrates , vol. 1-3. Wiley, New York.
3. Horowitz M. and Pigman W., eds. 1982. The glycoconjugates . Academic Press, New York.
4. Schauer R., ed. 1982. Sialic acids, chemistry, metabolism, and function . Springer-Verlag, New York.
5. Ivatt R.J., ed. 1984. The biology of glycoproteins . Plenum Press, New York.
6. Feizi T. 1989. Carbohydrate recognition in cellular function . Ciba Foundation Symposium, vol. 145. Wiley, New York.
7. Fukuda M., ed. 1992. Cell surface carbohydrates and cell development . CRC Press, Boca Raton, Florida.
8. Allen H.J. and Kisailus E.C., eds. 1992. Glycoconjugates: Composition, structure, and function . Dekker, New York.
9. Fukuda M., ed. 1992. Glycobiology: A practical approach . IRL Press, Oxford, United Kingdom.
10. Roberts D.D. and Mecham R.P., eds. 1993. Cell surface and extracellular glycoconjugates: Structure and function . Academic Press, San Diego.
11. Montreuil J., Vliegenthart J.F.G., and Schachter H., eds. 1995. Glycoproteins, Elsevier
12. Montreuil J., Vliegenthart J.F.G., and Schachter H., eds. 1996. Glycoproteins and disease . Elsevier, New York.
13. Gabius H.J. and Gabius S., eds. 1997. Glycosciences: Status and perspectives. Chapman and Hall, New York.
14. Brockhausen I. and Kuhns W. 1997. Glycoproteins and human disease . R.G. Landes, Austin.

15. Harper's Biochemistry, 26th Edition, Robert Murray, Peter A. Mayes, Victor W. Rodwell, Daryl K. Granner, McGraw-Hill Companies, February 2003.

Chapter 10, Glyconutrients and Cancer

1. Kidd P: The use of mushroom glucans and proteoglycans in cancer treatment. Altern Med Rev 5(1):16, 2000.
2. Kidd, p.8
3. Nanba H; Kubo K: Effect of maitake D-fraction on cancer prevention. Ann N Y Acad Sci 833:204-207, 1997.
4. Nanba H: Activity of maitake D-fraction to inhibit carcinogenesis and metastasis. Ann N Y Acad Sci 768: 243-245, 1995.
5. Matsuo T; Kurahashi Y; Nishida S; et al.: Granulopoietic effects of lentinan in mice: Effects on GM-CFC and 5-FU-induced leucopenia. Gan To Kagaku Ryoho 14(5, pt.1):1310-1314, 1987.
6. Hsu HY: Lian SL: Lin CC: Radioprotective effect of Ganoderma lucidum (Leyss. Ex. Fr.) Karst after X-ray irradiation in mice. Am J Chin Med 18(1-2): 61-69, 1990.
7. Pande S; Kumar M; A: Radioprotective efficacy of Aloe vera leaf extract. Pharmaceut Biol 36(3):227-232, 1998.
8. Egger SF; Brown GS; Kelsey LS; etal.: Hematopoietic augmentation by a beta-(1,4)-linked mannan. Cancer Immunol Immunother 43(4):195-205,1996.
9. Roberts DB; Travis EL: Acemannan-containing wound dressing gel reduces radiation-induced skin reactions in C3H mice. Int J Radiat Oncol Biol Phys 32(4):1047-1052, 1995.
10. Kurashige S; Akuzama Y; Endo F: Effects of Lentinus edodes; Grifola frondosa and Pleurotus ostreatus administration on cancer outbreak, and activities of macrophages and lymphocytes in mice treated with a carcinogen, N-butyl-N-butanolnitrosamine. Immunopharmacol Immunotoxicol 19(2): 175-183, 1997.
11. Mizutani Y; Yoshida O: Activation by the protein-bound polysaccharide PSK (krestin) of cytotoxic lymphocytes that act on fresh autologous tumor cells and T24 human urinary bladder transitional carcinoma cell line in patients with urinary bladder cancer. J Urol 145(5):1082-1087, 1991.
12. Mickey DD: Combined therapeutic effects of an immunomodulator, PSK, and chemotherapy with carboquone on rat bladder carcinoma. Cancer Chemother Pharmacol 15(1):54-58, 1985.
13. Yokoe T; Iino Y; Takei H: HLA antigen as predictive index for the outcome of breast cancer patients with adjuvant immunochemotherapy with PSK.

Anticancer Res 17(4A):2815-2818, 1997.
14. Fujii T; Saito K; Oguchi Y; et al.: Effects of the protein-bound polysaccharide preparation PSK on spontaneous breast cancer in mice. J Int Med Res 16(4):286-293, 1988.
15. Iino Y; Takai Y; Sugamata N; Morishita Y: PSK (krestin) potentiates chemotherapeutic effects of tamoxifen on rat mammary carcinomas. Anticancer Res 12(6B):2101-2103, 1992.
16. Nanba, Kubo, pp.204-207.
17. Torisu M; Hayashi Y; Ishimitsu T; et al.: Significant prolongation of disease-free period gained by oral polysaccharide K (PSK) administration after curative surgical operation of colorectal cancer. Cancer Immunol Immunother 31(5):261-268, 1990.
18. Torisu, Hayashi, Ishimitsu.
19. Kidd, pp. 4-27.
20. Borchers AT; Stern JS; Hackman RM; et al.: Mushrooms, tumors and immunity. Proc Soc Exp Biol Med 221:287, 1999.
21. Taguchi T: Clinical efficacy of lentinan on patients with stomach cancer: End point results of a four-year follow-up survey. Cancer Detect Prev Suppl 1:333-349, 1987.
22. Taguchi T: Effects of lentinan in advanced or recurrent cases of gastric, colorectal, and breast cancer. Gan To Kagaku Ryoho 10(2, pt.2):387-393, 1983.
23. Ogoshi K: Satou H; Isono K; et al.: Possible predictive markers of immunotherapy in esophageal cancer: Retrospective analysis of a randomized study. Cancer Invest 13:363-369, 1995.
24. Nago T; Komatsuda M; Yamauchi K; et al.: Chemoimmunotherapy with krestin in acute leukemia. Tokai J Exp Clin Med 6(2):141-146, 1981.
25. Kidd, pp. 6-7
26. Suto T; Fukuda S; Moriya N; et al.: Clinical study of biological response modifiers as maintenance therapy for hepatocellular carcinoma. Cancer Chemother Pharmacol 33 (suppl):S145-148, 1994.
27. Nanba, pp. 243-245
28. Nanba
29. Nanba, Kubo, pp. 204-207.
30. Shiga J; Maruyama T; Takahashi H; et al.: Effect of PSK, a protein-bound polysaccharide preparation, on liver tumors of Syrian hamsters induced by Thorotrast injection. Acta Pathol Jpn 43(9):475-480, 1993.
31. Hayakawa K; Mitsuhashi N; Saito Y; et al.: Effect of krestin as adjuvant treatment following radical radiotherapy in non-small cell lung cancer patients. Cancer Detect Prev 21(1):71-77, 1997.
32. Yefenof E: Gafanovitch I; Oron E; et al.: Prophylactic intervention in radiation-leukemia-virus induced murine lymphoma by the biological response

modifier polysaccharide K. Cancer Immunol Immunother 41(6):389-396, 1995.

33. Yefenof E; Einat E; Klein E: Potentiation of T cell immunity against radiation-leukemia-virus-induced lymphoma by polysaccharide K. Cancer Immunol Immunother 34(2):133-137, 1991.
34. Go P; Chung CH: Adjuvant PSK immunotherapy in patients with carcinoma of the nasopharynx. J Int Med Res 17(2):141-149, 1989.
35. Chung CH; Go P; Chang KH: PSK Immunotherapy in cancer patients - a preliminary report. Chun Hua Min Kuo Wei Sheng Wu Chi Mien I Hsueh Tsa Chih 20(3):210-216, 1987.
36. Ghoneum M; Jewett A: Production of tumor necrosis factor-alpha and interferon-gamma from human peripheral blood lymphocytes by MGN-3, a modified arabinoxylan from rice bran, and its synergy with interleukin-2 in viro. Cancer Detect Prev 24(4):314-324, 2000.
37. Mickey DD; Bencuya PS; Foulkes K: Effects of the immunomodulator PSK on growth of human prostate adenocarcinoma in immunodeficient mice. Int J Immunopharmacol 11(7):829-838, 1989.
38. Xu R; Peng X; Chen GZ; Chen GL: Effects of Cordycepts sinensis on natural killer activity and colony formation of B16 melanoma. Chin Med J 104(1):97-101, 1992
39. Adachi K; Nanba H; Kuroda H: Potentiation of host-mediated anti-tumor activity in mice by ß-glucan16 melanoma. Chin Med J104(1):97-101, 1992.
40. Hauer J; Anderer FA: Mechanism of stimulation of human natural killer cytotoxicity by arabinogalactan from Larix occidentalis. Cancer Immunol Immunother 36(4):237-244, 1993.
41. Liu C; Ji MR: Effects of Cordyceps sinensis (CS) on in vitro natural killer cells. Chung Kuo Chung His I Chieh Ho Tsa Chih 12(5): 267-269, 259, 1992.
42. Mickey DD; Carvalho L; Foulkes K: Combined therapeutic effects of conventional agents and an immunomodulator, polysaccharide K, on rat prostatic adenocarcinoma. J Urol 142(6):1594-1598, 1989.
43. Pienta KJ; Naik H; Akhtar A; et al.: Inhibition of spontaneous metastasis in a rat prostate cancer model by oral administration of modified citrus pectin. J Natl Cancer Inst 87(5):348-353, 1995.
44. Fullerton SA; Samadi AA; Tortorelis DG; et al.: Induction of apoptosis in human prostatic cancer cells with beta-glucan. Mol Urol 4(1): 7-14, 2000.
45. Harris C; Pierce K; King G; et al.: Efficacy of acemannan in treatment of canine and feline spontaneous neoplasms. Mol Biother 3(4): 207-213, 1991.
46. Maruyama H; Yamazaki K; Murofushi S; et al.: Antitumor activity of Sarcodon aspratus (Berk.) S. ito and Ganoderma lucidum (Fr.) Karst. J Pharmacobiodyn 12(2):118-123, 1989.
47. Wang G; Zhang J; Mizuno T; et al.: Antitumor active polysaccharides from

the Chinese mushroom Songshan lingzhi, the fruiting body of Ganoderma tsugae. Biosci Biotechnol Biochem 57(6):894-900, 1993.
48. Zhang J; Wang G; Li H; et al.: Antitumor active protein-containing glycans from the Chinese mushroom Songshan lingzhi; Ganoderma tsugae mycelium. Biosci Biotechnol Biochem 58(7): 1202-1205, 1994.
49. Ebina T; Fujimiya Y: Antitumor effect of a peptide-glucan preparationextracted from Agaricus blazei in a double-grafted tumor system in mice. Biotherapy 11(4):259-265, 1998.
50. Ralamboranto L; Rakotovao LH; Le Deaut JY; et al.: Immunomodulating properties of an extract isolated and partially purified from Aloe vahombe. 3. Study of antitumoral properties and contribution to the chemical nature and active principle. Arch Inst Pasteur Madagascar 50(1):227-256, 1982.
51. Matsunaga K; Ohhara M; Oguchi Y; et al.: Antimetastatic effect of PSK, a protein-bound polysaccharide, against the B16-BL6 mouse melanoma. Invasion Metastasis 16(1):27-38, 1996.
52. Matsunaga K; Aota M; Nyunoya Y; et al.: Antimour effect of biological response modifier, PSK, on C57BL/6 mice with syngeneic melanoma B16 and its mode of action. Oncology 51(4):303-308, 1994.
53. Ishihara Y; Fujii T; Iijima H; et al.: The role of neutrophils as cyto-toxic cells in lung metastasis: Suppression of tumor cell metastasis by a biological response modifier (PSK). In vitro 12(2): 175-182, 1998.
54. Matsunaga, Ohhara, Oguchi, et al.
55. Li Y; Chen G; Jiang D: Effect of Cordyceps sinesis on erythropoiesis in mouse bone marrow. Chin Med J 106(4):313-316, 1993.
56. Nakazato H; Koike A; Saji S; et al.: Efficacy of immunochemotherapy as adjuvant treatment after curative resection of gastric cancer. Lancet 343:1126, 1994.
57. Takeshita M: Nonspecific cell-mediated immunity in gastric cancer patients - with special reference to immuno-reactivity of the regional lymph node and preoperative immunotherapy. Nippon Geka Gakkai Zasshi 84(8):679-691, 1983.
58. Takeshita M; Kobori T; Sudo E; et al.: Preoperative immunotherapy for gastric cancer patients - immunomodulating effect of levamisole and lentinan on cell-mediated immunity and regional lymph node. Gan To Kagaku Ryoho 9(6):1052-1060, 1982.
59. Kondo M; Torisu M: Evaluation of an anticancer activity of a protein-bound polysaccharide PSK (krestin). In Torisu M, Yoshida T, eds. Basic Mechanisms and Clinical Treatment of Tumor Metastasis. New York: Academic Press, 1985, pp. 623-636.
60. Kidd, pp. 16-18.
61. Romano CF; Lipton A; Harvey HA; et al.: A phase II study of Catrix-S in

solid rumors. J Biol Response Mod 4(6):585-589, 1985.
62. Pucci C; Mittelman A; Chun H; et al.: Treatment of metastatic renal cell carcinoma with Catrix. Proc Annu Meet Am Soc Clin Oncol 13:A769, 1994.
63. Lissoni P; Giani L; Zerbini S; et al.: Biotheraphy with the pineal immunomodulating hormone melatonin versus melatonin plus Aloe vera in untreatable advanced solid neoplasms. Nat Immun 16(1): 27-33, 1998.

Chapter 11, Glyconutrients in Chronic Disease

1. Somersall AC, Bounous, G. Breakthrough in Cell Defense, GoldenEight Publishers, 1999
2. D. Lefkowitz, "Glyconutritionals: Implications in Inflammation," www.glycoscience.org. Copyright 2000. All rights reserved.
3. Presentation - 3rd Annual Conference, New Initiatives in the Prevention and Intervention of FAS/FAE for Aboriginal People of Canada, May 2003, Vanc, BC, Available as a technical syllabus from the Fish. Instit.
4. Sun Ha Jee et al. JAMA, Jan 12, 2005
5. McDaniel C; Dykman K; McDaniel R; Ford C; Tone C: "Effects of Nutraceutical Dietary Intervention in Diabetes Mellitus: A Retrospective Survey." Proc Fish Inst for Med Res 1(1):19-23,1997.

Chapter 12, Glyconutrients and Inflammation

1. Lefkowitz DL, "Glyconutritionals: Implications in Inflammation." GlycoScience & Nutrition. 2000;1(17):1-4
2. Murray RK. "Glycoproteins." In Murray RK, Granner DK, Mayes PA, Rodwell VW (eds): Harper's Biochemistry. Stamford, Appleton and Lange; 2000:677.
3. "Structure and Catalysis." In Lehninger AL, Nelson DL, Cox MM (eds): Principles of Biochemistry. New York, Worth Publishers; 1993: 252-252
4. Gay S, Gay RE, Koopman WJ. "Molecular and cellular mechanisms of joint destruction in rheumatoid arthritis: two cellular mechanisms explain joint destruction?" Ann Rheum Dis 1993;52 Suppl 1:S39-S47
5. DiCorleto PE, de la Motte CA. "Role of cell surface carbohydrate moieties in monocytic cell adhesion to endothelium *in vitro*." J Immunol 1989;143:3666-3672.
6. Kuby J. Immunology. 3rd ed. New York: W.H. Freeman and Company; 1997.
7. Cohen NH, Eigen H, Shaughnessy TE. "Status asthmaticus." Crit Care Clin 1997;13:459-476
8. Lefkowitz DL, Mills KC, Moguilevsky N, Bollen A, Vaz A, Lefkowitz SS.

"Regulation of macrophage function by human recombinant myeloperoxidase." Immunol Lett 1993;36:43-49.

9. Lefkowitz DL, Mills KC, Moguilevsky N. "Enhancement of macrophage-mediated bactericidal activity by macrophage-mannose receptor-ligand interaction." Immunol Cell Biol 1997;75:136-141.
10. Janeway CA, Travers P, Walport M, Capra JD. Immuno Biology: The Immune System in Health and Disease. 4th ed. New York: Garland Publishing; 1999.
11. Stahl PD. "The macrophage mannose receptor: current status." Am J Respir Cell Mol Biol 1997;75:136-141.
12. Stahl PD. "The mannose receptor and other macrophage lectins." Curr Opin Immunol 1992;4:49-52.
13. Lincoln JA, Lefkowitz DL, Grattendick KJ, Lefkowitz SS, Allen RC. "Enzymatically inactive eosinophil peroxidase inhibits proinflammatory cytokine transcription and secretion by macrophages." Cell Immunol 1999;@196:23-33.
14. Lefkowitz SS, Lefkowitz DL. "Macrophage candidicidal activity of a complete glyconutritional formulation versus aloe polymannose." Proc Fisher Inst Med Res 1999;1:5-7.
15. Savill J. "Apoptosis in resolution of inflammation." J Leukoc Biol 1997;61:375-380
16. Hall SE, Savill JS, Henson PM, Haslett C. "Apoptotic neutrophils are phagocytosed by fibroblasts with participation of the fibroblast vitronectin receptor and involvement of a mannose/fucose-specific lectin." J Immunol 1994;153:3218-3227.
17. Murray RK, "Glycoproteins: Crucial Molecules in Many Diseases." Glycoscience & Nutrition (official publication of GlycoScience.com: The Nutrition Science Site). 2003;4(8):1-10
18. Brant WE, Helms CA. Fundamentals of Diagnostic Radiology. 2nd ed. Maryland: Williams & Wilkins; 1999.
19. Lefkowitz DL, Glyconutritionals: "Implications in Rheumatoid Arthritis." GlycoScience & Nutrition. 2000;1(16):1-4
20. Axford JS, "Glycosylation and rheumatic disease." Biochimica et Biophysica Acta. 1999;1455:221-229
21. McAnalley BH, Vennum E, "Introduction to Glyconutritionals." GlycoScience & Nutrition. 2000;1(1):1-5
22. Gardiner T, "Importance of Glycoconjugates in Breastfeeding and Early Nutrition." GlycoScience & Nutrition. 2000;1(23):1-10
23. Boyd, S. The U.S. Centers from Disease Control and Prevention releases Toxin Report.
24. Hipskind T. "Effect of Glyconutritionals on C-reactive protein ANA." Proc

Fisher Inst Med Res;2003.3(1):11-13

25. Proceedings of the Royal Society of Medicine's 5th Jenner Symposium (Glycobiology and Medicine Conference), July 10-11, 2000.
26. Axford JS; "Glycobiology and medicine: an introduction." J R Soc Med. 1997 May; 90:260-264
27. Adams JL, Czuprynski CJ; "Mycobacterial cell wall components induce the production of TNF-alpha, IL-1 and IL-6 by bovine monocytes and the murine macrophage cell line RAW 264.7." Microb Pathog. 1994 Jun;16(6):401-11
28. Barringer TA, Kirk JK, Santaniello AC, Foley KL, Michielutte R; "Effect of a multivitamin and mineral supplement on infection and quality of life a randomized, double-bline, placebo-controlled trail." Ann Intern Med. 2003 Mar 4;138(5):365-71
29. Bochner BS, Undem BJ, Lichtenstein LM; "Immunological aspects of allergic asthma." Annu Rev Immunol. 1994;12:295-335
30. 3Brandi ML; "Natural and synthetic isoflavones in the prevention and treatment of chronic diseases." Calcif Tissue Int. 1997;61 Suppl 1:S5-8.
31. Axford JS; "Glycobiology & Medicine: A Millenial Review." GlycoScience & Nutrition. 2001 Mar 30;2(7):1-5

Chapter 13, Glycoproteins for Fitness & Sports Injury

1. David M. Eisenberg, Roger B. Davis, Susan L. Ettner, Scott Appel, Sonja Wilkey; Maria Van Rompay; Ronald C. Kessler, Trends in Alternative Medicine Use in the United States, 1990-1997: Results of a Follow-up National Survey, JAMA. 1998;280:1569-1575.
2. Diet for a Poisoned Planet, "How to choose safe foods for you and your family" Harmony Books, New York 1990 David Steinman
3. Enzyme Nutrition, The Food Enzyme Concept, Dr. Edward Howell
4. Braving the Elements, Harry B. Gray, John D. Simon, William C. Trogler, University Science Books, Sausalito, California 1995
5. Concepts in Biology, 9th Edition, Eldon D. Enger and Frederick C. Ross, McGraw-Hill Companies, Inc.
6. Keeping Fit, Dr. Patrick J. Bird, PhD. University of Florida, College of Health and Human Performances
Column 507b - 1996

Chapter 14, Glyconutrients and Dental Health

1. Loesche WJ, Abrams J, Terpenning MS et al: "Dental findings in geriatric populations with diverse medical backgrounds." Oral Surg, Oral Med, Oral Path, Pral Rad & Endo 1995; 80(1): 43-54

2. Nutrition Screening Initiative: Nutrition Interventions Manual for Professionals Caring for Older Americans. Washington, DC: Nutrition Screening Initiative, 1992
3. Sullivan DH, Martin W, Flasman N et al: "Oral health problems and involuntary weight loss in a population of frail elderly." J Am Geriatr Soc 1993; 41: 725-731
4. Article:" Australian Aborigines - Living Off the Fat of the Land" at www.westonaprice.org
5. Clark, J.W., Cheraskin, E. and Ringsdorf, W.M., Jr. "An Ecologic Study of Oral Hygiene." Journal of Periodontology/Periodontics 40: #8, 476-480, August 1969
6. Cohen, M.M. "The Effect of Large Doses of Ascorbic Acid on Gingival Tissues at Puberty." Journal of Dental Research 34: #5, 750-751, October 1955.
7. Lane, W.B., Nutrition and Oral Response to Orthodontic Banding. University of Alabama School of Dentistry Thesis, August 1968.
8. Dusterwinkle, S., Cheraskin, E. and Ringsdorf, W.M., Jr. Tissue "Tolerance to Orthodontic Banding: A Study in Multivitamin-Trace Mineral Supplementation." Journal of Periodontology 37: #2, 132-145, March-April 1966.
9. Position of the American Dietetic Association: Oral Health and Nutrition. J Am Diet Assoc.2003; 103:615-625.
10. McDaniel C; Dykman K; McDaniel R; Ford C; Tone C: "Effects of Nutraceutical Dietary Intervention in Diabetes Mellitus: A Retrospective Survey." Proceedings of the Fish Inst for Med Res 1(1):19-23,1997.
11. McKinley R: "The Effect of Dietary Supplements on Periodontal Disease." J Am Nutr Assoc. 1997;Supp.1:20-23.
12 McKinley R: ibid, 1997; Suppl 1:16-19.
13. McKinley R: ibid, 1997; Suppl 1:11-13.

Chapter 15, Glyconutrients and Aging

1. Barhoumi R: Burghardt RG; Busbee DL; McDaniel R: Enhancement of glutathione levels and protection from chemically initiated glutathione depletion in rat liver cells by glyconutritionals. Proc Fisher Inst Med Res 1997; 1:12-16.
2. Packer L, Colman C, The Antioxidant Miracle, NYC: John Wiley, 1999
3. Albert Einstein, Atomic Physics- Film soundtrack, Copyright J. Arthur Rank Organization, Ltd., 1948
4. De los Reyes GC, Koda RT, Lien EJ, Glucosamine and chondroitin sulfates in the treatment of osteoarthritis:a survey, Prog. Drug Res. 2000;55:81-103.

5. Axford JS, Glycosylation and Rheumatic disease, Biochim Biophys Acta, 1999; Oct1455:219-229
6. Medical News and Perspectives, Journal of the American Medical Association, February 23, 2003.
7. McCarty MF, Glucosamine may retard atherogenesis by promoting endothelial production of heparan sulfate proteoglycans. Med Hypothesis 1997Mar;48(3):245-51
8. Darlington LG, Stone TW, Antioxidants and fatty acids in the amelioration of rheumatoid arthritis and related disorders, Br J Nutr 2001 Mar;85(3):251-69
9. Ames BN, Micronutrient deficiencies. A major cause of DNA damage, Ann NY Acad Sci 1999; 889:87-106.
10. Swaim R, Kaplan B, Vitamins as therapy in the 1990s, J Am Bd Fam Pract 1995 May-Jun;8(3):206-16.
11. Lachance PA, Overview of key nutrients: micronutrient aspects, Nutr Rev 1998 Apr; 56(4 Pt 2):S34-9.
12. Mertz.W, Trace minerals and atherosclerosis, Fed Proc. 1982 Sept 41(11): 2807-12
13. Dreizen S, Nutrition and the immune response - a review, Int. J Nutr.Res. 1979; 49(2):220-8.
14. Youngkin EQ, Thomas DJ, Vitamins: common supplements and therapy, Nurse Pract. 1999 Nov;24 (11):50,53,57-60
15. Naurath HJ, Joosten E, Riezler R, Stabler SP, Allen RH, Lindenbaum J, Effects of vitamin B12, folate, and vitamin B6 supplements in elderly people with normal serum vitamin concentrations, Lancet 1995 Jul 8;346(8967):85-9.
16. Williams, Roger J, The Wonderful World Within You, Copyright 1977, reprinted Bio-Communications Press, Wichita, Kansas, 1998
R. K. Murray, "Glycoproteins," Harper's Biochemistry, eds. R. K. Murray, D.
17. K. Granner, P. A. Mayes and V.W. Rodwell (Appleton and Lange, 1996), pp. 648-666.

Chapter 17, Natural Healing and Glyconutrients

1. *Philadelphia Inquirer*, Nov 30, 2000
2. Making Sense of Illness, Robert Aronowitz MD, Cambridge University Press, 1998.
3. *Genome*, Jerry E. Bishop and Michael Waldotz, iUniverse, 1999
4. Fogg-Johnson N, Kaput J., Nutrigenomics: an emerging scientific discipline, *Food Technol* 2003:57(4), 60-67.

Chapter 19, Clinical Trials, Stem Cells and the Future of Glyconutrients

1. Increased Demand for Glycoconjugates During Stress, Gardiner, T., August 25, 2000, Glycoscience and Nutrition, www.glycoscience.org
2. Design and Analysis of Clinical Trials: Concepts and Methodologies, Second Edition, Shein-Chung Chow, Jen-Pei Liu, 2004, John Wiley & Sons US, ISBN: 0471249858
3. Incidence of adverse drug reactions in hospitalized patients: a meta-analysis of prospective studies, Lazarou J, Pomeranz BH, Corey PN, J. Amer Med Assoc. 1998 Apr 15;279(15):1200-5
4. The Centers for Medicaid and Medicaid Services, March 12, 2002. www.cms.hhs.gov/media/press/release.asp?counter=429
5. National Health Expenditure Trends 1975-2004, Canadian Institute of Health Information, 2004, ISBN 1-55392-537-8.
6. NIH budget approved at $28 billion: Concerns over FY 2005 fund, www.natap.org
7. CIHR Annual Report 2003-2004
8. Dr. CE Pippinger, Personal correspondence,
9. Health and Med Res Fdn, 4900 Broadway, San Antonio, TX 78209,
10. Effects of Baseline Total Cholesterol Levels on Diet and Exercise Interventions, JANA, Winter 1999 edition, Vol 2, No 1, PP 42-49
11. Mazess RB, Barden HS, Bisek JP, Hanson J., Dual-energy x-ray absorptiometry for total-body and regional bone-mineral and soft-tissue composition. Am J Clin Nutr 1990;51:1106-12
12. Stem Cell Information, The official National Institutes of Health resource for stem cell research, (www.stemcells.nih.gov/),Accessed Jan 15, '05
13. Pluripotency of mesenchymal stem cells derived from adult marrow, Yuehua Jiang, Balkrishna N. Jahagirdar, R. Lee Reinhardt, Robert E. Schwartz, C. Dirk Keene, Xilma R. Ortiz-Gonzalez, Morayma Reyes, Todd Lenvik, Troy Lund, Mark Blackstad, Jingbo Du, Sara Aldrich, Aaron Lisberg, Walter C. Low, David A. Largaespada, Catherine M. Verfaillie, Nature 418, 41 - 49 (04 Jul 2002),
14. Do No Harm, The Coalition of Americans for Research Ethics, www.stemcellresearch.org) Accessed January 15, '05
15. Adult Stem Cells, David A. Prentice, Ph.D., Accessed Jan 15, '05
16. IPS - Inter Press Service News Agency, "Breakthrough in Treating Diabetes with Adult Stem Cells", Mercela Valente, Buenos Aires, Jan 11, '05, www.ipsnews.net, Accessed Jan 15, '05
17. Presentation - 3rd Annual Conference, New Initiatives in the Prevention and Intervention of FAS/FAE for Aboriginal People of Canada, May 2003, Vanc, BC, Available as a technical syllabus from the Fish Inst Med Res.

APPENDIX 'A'

Eight (8) Vital Sugars

The glyconutrients referred to throughout this book include principally, the eight monosaccharides (vital sugars) commonly found in the oligosaccharide chains of glycoproteins. This is a select subset of the 200 monosacchardies found in nature.

Glucose	Xylose
Galactose	N-Acetylglucosamine
Fucose	N-Acetylgalactosamine
Mannose	N-Acetylneuraminic acid

With growing interest in the science of Glycobiology, these various sugars and their complex carbohydrates are gaining increased recognition for their crucial physiological importance. They are certainly much more than mere energy sources. They derive from a variety of natural sources and end up strategically as glycoproteins and glycolipids in animals and humans.

Although much research remains to be done, there have been many scientific publications regarding the absorption, distribution, metabolism and excretion of these glyconutrients. More interestingly, their biological activities in different glycoconjugate forms are being vigorously characterized.

Galactose

Galactose is one of the two glyconutrients (vital sugars) that are found in relative abundance in the normal diet, especially in dairy products. There it is combined with glucose to form the dissachardie lactose. For the many people who are lactose-intolerant and tend to avoid dairy products, there is always the possibility of inadequate dietary galactose. This sugar may also be obtained in the pectins of some fruits.

Galactose is absorbed in the mouth and the small intestine by active transport. When absorbed, approximately 30% is incorporated into glycogen, 27-47% is oxidized to carbon dioxide and the remainder is used for the synthesis of glycoproteins and glycolipids. It is widely distributed throughout body tissues, particularly in the brain, testes, skin, kidneys and intestinal mucosa. More significantly, galactose is found in different components of the immune system such as immunoglobulins and macrophages. Galactose levels are altered in different disease states such as rheumatoid arthritis, upper airway infections and alcoholism, to name a few.

Galactose is metabolized mainly in the liver and excreted by the kidney. Neither of these processes are altered in diabetics, especially since insulin is not necessary for galactose utilization. However, galactose clearance is reduced in aging.

Galactose enzyme deficiency disorders are known. These are infrequent inborn errors of metabolism but they can have serious medical consequences such as failure to thrive, bacterial sepsis, cataracts, nerve deafness and more.

Galactose can be readily converted into glucose for use as an energy source and alternately, galactose can be formed from glucose via epimerase enzymes. However, a dietary source of galactose appears crucial to maintain an epimerase enzyme - mediated equilibrium.

In biological terms, galactose and its glycoconjugates have been demonstrated to be important in at least:

- immune system modulation;
- inhibition of tumor growth and tumor cell metastatasis;
- wound healing;
- inhibition of cataract formation;
- maintenance of normal colonic bacteria;
- intestinal mucins;
- normal kidney function;
- altered biochemistry leading to arthritis, lupus,
- … and more

Glucose

Glucose is clearly the most familiar of the vital sugars and is a partner with fructose in the common disaccharide 'table sugar' (sucrose). As such, it is overabundant in soft drinks, desserts, processed foods, ice cream, honey, corn syrup, rice, bread, pasta, etc. It is readily absorbed in the intestines and usually quickly distributed throughout the body via the bloodstream. It is reabsorbed in the kidneys and crosses blood-tissue barriers using membrane proteins as specific transporters.

Glucose is widely used as an energy source and as such, it is typically in critical demand. It also serves as a substrate for the potential synthesis of non-glucose containing glycoconjugates, mainly in the liver. Serum glycoproteins incorporate glucose but not quite to the same extent as mannose or galactose.

Hormones, namely insulin and glucagon, regulate the levels of blood glucose. In liver and muscle, it is stored as glycogen, while it forms fatty acids and triglycerides in fatty tissue. As levels fall, the process is reversed. Diabetics in particular, have difficulty metabolizing glucose as tissue cells 'starve' in the midst of 'plenty' blood glucose.

The kidneys excrete glucose as glycopeptide conjugates which are then acid-hydrolyzed in urine to yield the free sugar. However, in health, normal glucose concentrations in urine are extremely low, but not so for poorly-controlled diabetics.

Biologically, glucose is critical as an energy source but is also known to be vital to brain function and an important substrate for glycoconjugates. It is therefore an important player in cellular communication.

Too much glucose can raise insulin levels and lead to obesity and diabetes. On the other hand, too little could have other consequences. Elderly Alzheimer's patients, for example, tend to have lower glucose levels compared to those with organic brain disease resulting from stroke or other vascular disease. Also, glucose metabolism is altered in some cases of depression and eating disorders.

It is probably safe to say, that very few people would come anywhere close to being glucose-deficient in terms of dietary intake. Most North Americans consume far too much, perhaps as much as four times the daily recommended limit.

Fucose

Fucose is readily found in several medicinal mushrooms, some seaweeds like kelp and wakame, as well as beer yeast. It is 'abundant' in human breast milk (NB Fucose should not be confused with 'fructose' or fruit sugar). It is absorbed from the small intestine (at least in vitro) by a non-active diffusion transport process. Many cells though have a specific facilitative transport for fucose, whereas fucose itself can inhibit active transport of other sugars.

Fucose is widely distributed throughout the body in glycoproteins and glycolipids, consistent with a role for these polyconjugates in cell-to-cell communication. It is more prevalent in nerve functions, kidney tubules, testes and skin. However, its distribution is altered in certain disease states such as diabetes and cancer.

Fucose is produced in the sugar-nucleoticle form from mannose by enzyme actions, while other enzymes incorporate dietary fucose into glycoproteins. Different states of enzyme deficiency can have clinical consequences. For example, in leukocyte adhesion deficiency (LAD II), there is severely reduced fucosylation of glycoconjugates resulting in a markedly compromised immune system.

Fucose is excreted mainly in the urine. During the latter stages of pregnancy and during lactation, there is an apparent increase in the concentrations of fucose-containing glycopeptides in human urine. This is consistent with some role for glycoconjugates in the latter-stages of fetal development and transfer of immunity to the newborn.

In biological terms, fucose and its glycoconjugates have been found to have a number of important influences such as:

- neurotransmission
- immune modulation (cf. inflammatory diseases)
- inhibition of cancer growth and metastasis
- prevention and treatment of respiratory infections
- possible regulation of collagen production.

N-Acetylgalactosamine (NAGal)

N-Acetylgalactosamine is probably the least studied and the least known among the eight vital glyconutrients. It is quite abundant in bovine and shark cartilage and in Japan, it is also available from a red algae. It is also a constituent of chondroitin sulfate which is often combined with glucosamine for the treatment of osteoarthritis.

NAGal appears to be absorbed from the intestine by a specific transporter. It is localized within cells in the Golgi apparatus and endoplastic reticulum where active glycoconjugate synthesis occurs. It is particularly concentrated in the brain and nerve tissue, as well as kidney, testes and skin. Its metabolism has not been well studied but we know of its importance in synthesis of glycoconjugates important in cell-to-cell communication.

NAGal may play a role in tumor cell metastasis via its distribution in mucin. Colon cancer cells that metastasize make more mucin, those that make more mucin are more likely to metastasize, and inhibition of mucin synthesis in cancer cells is associated with reduction of that potential.

Lower than normal levels of NAGal have been found in patients with heart disease and its concentration is known to decrease with age.

Xylose

Xylose is unique among the eight vitally necessary sugars in that it is a pentose sugar - it has a ring structure of only five atoms, whereas the others are hexoses (6-atom rings).

Xylose is found in guava, pears, berries, Aloe vera, kelp, echinecea, psyllium, broccoli, spinach, egg plant, peas, green beans, oleva, cabbage and corn. The common sugar substitute Xylitol, is the alcohol formed from fermenting xylose with yeasts. Xylitol is sometimes used in chewing gum and toothpaste. However, it cannot replace the necessary xylose.

Xylose is absorbed from the intestine by passive diffusion and quickly distributed to the liver where it is metabolized. It is also found in kidney, fat and muscle. It is incorporated into glycoproteins after oral administration but not much research has been done on their biological function to date, although we do know some areas of activity:

- xylose glycoconjugates serve a variety of receptor and cell membrane functions including cell-to-cell communication;
- xylose has antibacterial and antifungal properties, particularly with gram-negative organisms and candida;
- xylose promotes the growth of 'friendly flora' in the intestines.

Xylose is easily eliminated from the bloodstream and excreted in urine.

Mannose

Mannose was the first 'active ingredient' among the glyconutrients to be so identified. The Aloe vera leaf gel contins acemannan which is the polysaccharide form of mannose. A polysaccharide of mannose and galactose (galactomannan) is found in fenugreek, carob gum and guar gum. Other sources include black or red currants, goose berries, green beans, cayenne pepper, shiitake mushrooms, kelp, cabbage, egg plant, tomatoes and turnip. In its alcohol form, it is known as mannitol.

Mannose is the foundation of all the vital sugars since it is involved in so many fundamental cell activities. Its deficiency can lead to several physical problems. It is readily absorbed (within 1-hour) from the intestine, by a glucose-tolerant transporter. Its level of concentration in amniotic fluid is comparable to that of blood and it crosses the placenta to nourish the fetus.

Mannose is widely distributed in body fluids and tissues, especially in the liver and intestine. It is directly utilized for glycoprotein synthesis, especially in components of the immune system where it has important modulatory activities. It is also more prevalent in nerves, skin, testes and the retina. There are known metabolic diseases resulting from a loss of activity of certain enzymes involved in mannose glycosylation. Mannose is actively reabsorbed by the kidney.

Many of the biological activities of mannose derive from its function in cell-surface glycoprotein receptors which modulate various aspects of the immune system. Scavenger macrophages, for example, have at least four different receptors that bind mannose which is present on the surface of various pathogens. In wound-healing studies, mannose has been shown to have clear anti-inflammatory action. It clearly suppresses tumor growth and enhances survivability in cancerous animals. Mannose may also inhibit tumor cell metastases. It also acts to prevent some types of bacterial infections. Interestingly, it has gained a reputation as a remedy for urinary tract infections.

N-Acetylglucosamine (GlcNAc or NAG)

N-Acetylglucosamine is best known today by its derivative, glucosamine, which has become quite a popular remedy for osteoarthritis. It is readily available in bovine and shark cartilage and, unlike NACGal it is a constituent of shiitake mushrooms. It is also found as the polysaccharide in chitin, derived from the shells of crustaceans like shrimps and crabs. Chitosan is the modified form of chitin from acid/alkali treatments.

There are three common commercially available forms of glucosamine: N-Acetylglucosamine, glucosamine hydrochloride and sulfate. The first two are seldom used, whereas glucosamine sulfate is fairly widespread. Fortunately, glucosamine appears to be a more efficient precursor than NAG for glycosylation, partly because of much better cellular uptake.

In the synthesis of NAG, dietary glucosamine is first phosphorylated and then acetylated by enzymes. Other enzymes convert NAG into another form that can be metabolized. NAG can also be de-acetylated.

About half of an ingested dose of glucosamine is oxidized and the remainder is distributed into glycoconjugates. These conjugates distribute to cell surface receptors which are important in cell-to-cell communication. NAG is found to be concentrated in the liver and small intestine but also in testes, skin, brain and retina. It appears that NAG is released when some glycoproteins breakdown. It can also be recycled. Animal studies suggest that it is eliminated primarily in carbon dioxide and urine.

Most of the biological activities studied with respect to NAG have actually been conducted with glucosamine. As such, we now understand its importance in several areas:

- It helps repair cartilage while reducing the pain and inflammation in osteoarthritis. Glucosamine is the substrate for glucosaminoglycan (a building block for cartilage) and inhibits its metabolic breakdown.
- It apparently modulates the progression of experimental cancers.
- It decreases insulin secretion without suppressing liver glucose production.
- It is an immune modulator with anti-tumor and antiviral properties.
- It is believed to play a role in the transport of thyroglobulin (an iodine-containing glycoprotein) in the thyroid gland.

N-Acetylneuraminic Acid (NANA)

N-Acetylneuraminic Acid has an interesting history. It was first isolated and named sialic acid. Another scientist isolated a similar crystalline form and called it neuraminic acid. Later, a third scientist proposed a common structure for both. All three agreed on sialic acid as a family name which now covers more than 30 derivatives of neuraminic acid, mostly based on NANA and a close cousin, N-glycolylneuraminic acid.

Sialic acid is found in whey protein isolate or concentrate and in hen's eggs. It appears to be readily absorbed and excreted in urine. It is widely distributed as numerous glycoconjugates throughout mammalian tissues, especially in body fluids like serum, CSF, saliva, urine, amniotic fluid and milk. It is also found in the brain, adrenals, heart, liver, kidney, skin and testes as well as glycoconjugates in macrophages. During pregnancy and lactation, levels are increased especially in the late stage. Sialic acid is also increased in saliva from cancer patients and in breast tumors. In contrast, reduced levels are found in the upper airway epithelium of severely ill patients, as well as in alcoholics and the elderly.

Sialic acid metabolism is important in the biosynthesis of glycoconjugates. It can be formed endogenously from glucosamine and n-acetylmannosamine. It appears to be involved in the metabolism of lipoproteins.

Sialic acid and its glycoconjugates are important in a wide variety of biological functions such as:

- the viscosity of mucous secretions which act as lubricants and defensive agents in body cavities or on surfaces;
- the protection against colonization and infection by bacteria in air ways;
- immune modulation;
- the regulation of glycoprotein synthesis and metabolism in red blood cells as well as the protection of serum glycoproteins.

APPENDIX 'B'

Sources of Glyconutrients

Primary
Appendix 'A' described primary dietary sources for each of the glyconutrients - the eight vital monosaccharides (sugars).

Secondary
Acemannan - a polysaccharide composed mainly of mannose units derived from the Aloe vera leaf gel.

Aloe vera - requires careful harvesting and stabilization of the active ingredient.

Arabinogalactans (Gum Sugars) - complex polysaccharides from the larch tree as well as several grains and vegetables.

Beta-glucans - a class of sugar chains found in cell walls of medicinal mushrooms, baker's yeast, astragalus, and in the brans of oat, rice and barley. They include Maitake-D fraction (extract) from maitake mushroom, and Lentinan from Shiitake mushroom.

Polysaccharides K and P - are extracted from the coriolus mushroom which grows wild on tree trunks in North America and Asia.

Chitin - a polysaccharide composed of N-acetylglucosamine, found in crustacean shells. Chitosan is an acid/base derivative.

Third Generation
These polysaccharide dietary complexes (supplements) are carefully designed and formulated to contain most, if not all eight vital monosaccharides (sugars). They are obtained from the best natural sources including rice, barley and oat brans; a variety of dietary mushrooms; yeast cell walls; Aloe vera; gum sugars and most recently, select seaweed. Supplementation with all the glyconutrients simultaneously and in balance, relieves the burden of complex energy-consuming, enzymatic interconversion of monosaccharides.

INDEX

INDEX

VISIT YOUR FAVORITE BOOKSTORE
FOR ADDITIONAL COPIES OF

The Healing **Power** *of* ^{8}**SugarS**®

An Amazing Breakthrough in Nutrition, Science and Medicine

What Doctors want *YOU* to know about
Glyconutrients ...

Compiled and Edited by

Allan C. Somersall, PhD., MD

$19.95US $21.95CDN paperback

or

visit our website at

www.thehealingpowerofsugars.com

To Order By Mail,
(Shipping $9.25 per copy - add $2.78 S/H for each additional copy)
Enclose Check With Your Order Payable To

The Natural Wellness Group
2-3415 Dixie Road, Suite: 538
Mississauga, Ontario CANADA
L4Y 2B1

Quantity Discounts Available
E-mail Us At: glycobooks@aol.com

Feel free to send your comments about this book to the e-mail or postal address listed above.